Symptom Control in Far Advanced Cancer:
Pain Relief

Symptom Control in Far Advanced Cancer:
Pain Relief

Robert G Twycross MA, DM, FRCP

*Consultant Physician, Sir Michael Sobell House, Churchill Hospital, Oxford,
Honorary Clinical Lecturer, Faculty of Clinical Medicine, Oxford University*

Sylvia A Lack MB, BS

*Consultant in Hospice Care, St Mary's Hospital, Waterbury, Connecticut, USA.
Former Medical Director, The Connecticut Hospice, Branford*

Pitman

PITMAN PUBLISHING LIMITED
128 Long Acre, London WC2E 9AN

Associated Companies
Pitman Publishing Pty Ltd, Melbourne
Pitman Publishing New Zealand Ltd, Wellington

First Published 1983
Reprinted 1984

British Library Cataloguing in Publication Data

Twycross, Robert G.
   Symptom control in far advanced cancer.
   1. Cancer patients   2. Terminal care
   3. Cancer—psychological aspects   4. Cancer—social aspects
   I. Title   II. Lack, Sylvia A.
   362.1′96994   RC 262

ISBN 0 272 79717 0

Text set in 10 on 12 pt Melior Roman
Printed in Great Britain at The Pitman Press, Bath

This book is dedicated to

Deirdre, Alison, Judith, Fiona, John and David

and to Lily and Percy Bennett

Contents

Preface   ix
Drug Names   xi
Abbreviations   xii

Part 1 Pain
1 Pain—and Cancer   3
2 Pain—Assessment   15
3 Pain—A Broader Concept   43

Part 2 Pain Control
4 Modification of Pathological Process   59
5 Non-Drug Measures   79
6 Analgesics   100

Part 3 Pharmacology
7 Non-Narcotic Analgesics   117
8 Weak Narcotic Agonists   149
9 Oral Morphine Sulphate   167
10 Diamorphine   190
11 Brompton Cocktail   200
12 Morphine—Alternative Modes of Administration   207
13 Myths about Morphine   223
14 Alternative Strong Narcotic Agonists   237
15 Narcotic Agonist-Antagonists   253
   Narcotic Antagonists
16 Co-Analgesics   270

Part 4 General

17 Home Care 297

18 More Fundamental Considerations 315

Appendix 325

Index 330

Preface

Out of an estimated 50 million deaths annually in the world, more than 5 million are attributed to cancer. In Europe and North America about one-fifth of the population die of cancer. It is estimated that by the year 2000 the number of cancer deaths will have risen to 8 million annually. Most of those dying of cancer will have distressing symptoms of one kind or another. About two-thirds will experience pain. It is apparent that current health care systems do not always cater adequately for the needs of the patient with far-advanced cancer. This means that many patients continue to suffer unnecessarily. Crowded medical school curricula do not allow a ready solution to present deficiencies. The growing number of hospices—more than thirty in Britain and over one thousand in the USA—is a practical response to the unsatisfactory state of affairs. Constantly stimulated by distressed patients, and forced to work from first principles in a seemingly never ending series of unique clinical situations, the hospices have developed considerable expertise in the management of symptoms as an end in itself. It is out of our own experience in this field that we offer this book to our fellow physicians. Although written with the hospice doctor principally in mind, we hope that the book will prove of interest and value to those working in other settings.

We acknowledge with gratitude the helpful advice and encouragement of many colleagues past and present. Also the inspiration derived from the Courses for Physicians on Symptom Control in Far Advanced Cancer which have been held annually since 1979, alternating between Oxford, England and New Haven, Connecticut. Our debt to both St. Christopher's and St. Joseph's Hospice, London, England, is considerable, particularly to the Medical Director of St. Christopher's Hospice, Dame Cicely Saunders. The path that has led to publication began for both of us at these two centres in 1971. Our greatest teachers, inevitably, have been those people—our patients—whom we have been privileged to help.

We are grateful to those authors and their publishers/editors who have graciously allowed us to reproduce tables or figures. The source of such material is given in the text. Dr. Michael Rance, formerly Head of Biomedical Research, Pharmaceutical Division, Reckitt & Colman, Hull, England, provided most of the chemical formulae of the narcotic analgesics that we have included. Most of the other artwork was undertaken by the Department of Medical Illustration, Oxford University Medical School. The task of typing has been shared by many secretaries over a period of two years. The brunt was borne by Mrs. Sybil Knight, Miss Joanne Robbins and Mrs. Ginnie Cates. We are extremely grateful to them for their patience and quiet determination to see it through, particularly during the final stages.

RGT
SAL

Drug Names

Generic drug names are used throughout the text with few exceptions. Commonly used proprietary names are included in the Index for those readers as yet unfamiliar with official nomenclature.

Generic names are generally the same regardless of the country of use. Important exceptions are:

paracetamol (BP) = *acetominophen* (USP)
pethidine (BP) = *meperidine* (USP)

Readers should also note that:

dioctyl sodium sulfosuccinate (DSS) is now officially known as *docusate sodium.*
prednisolone and its inactive pro-drug, *prednisone* are identical in potency and efficacy.

Abbreviations

The following abbreviations are used in the text.

b.i.d.	twice daily/per 24 hours (alternative, b.d.)	NSAID	nonsteroidal anti-inflammatory drug(s)
BP	British Pharmacopoeia	PO	per os, 'by mouth'
BPC	British Pharmaceutical Codex	PG	prostaglandin
BNF	British National Formulary	PGs	prostaglandins
C	capsule	PGS	prostaglandin synthetase
cm	centimetre(s)	PR	per rectum, 'by rectum'
cGy	centiGray, a measure of irradiation, formerly rad (q.v.)	p.r.n.	*pro re nata*, 'as required'
		q.i.d.	four times a day/per 24 hours (alternative, q.d.s.)
DTF	Drug Tariff Formulary		
E	elixir	q.v.	*quod vide*, 'which see'
EC	enteric-coated	rad	a measure of irradiation now designated cGy (q.v.)
ET	effervescent tablet		
fl. oz.	fluid ounce	SC	subcutaneous injection
g	gram(s)	SI	System Internationale (i.e. international units)
I	injection		
iu	international unit(s)	Supp	suppository
IM	intramuscular injection	Susp	suspension
IV	intravenous injection	Sy	syrup
kg	kilogram(s)	T	tablet
l	litre	t.i.d.	three times a day/per 24 hours (alternative t.d.s)
L	linctus		
M	mixture	USA	United States of America
mg	milligram(s)	USP	United States Pharmacopoeia
ml	millilitre(s)	USNF	United States National Formulary
mm	millimetre(s)		
μg	microgram(s)		

Part One

Pain

Pain

An unpleasant sensory and emotional experience associated with actual or potential tissue damage, or described in terms of such damage.

Note: Pain is always subjective. Each individual learns the application of the word through experiences related to injury in early life. Biologists recognize that those stimuli which cause pain are liable to damage tissue. Accordingly, pain is that experience which we associate with actual or potential tissue damage. It is unquestionably a sensation in a part or parts of the body but it is also always unpleasant and therefore also an emotional experience. Experiences which resemble pain, e.g. pricking, but are not unpleasant, should not be called pain. Unpleasant abnormal experiences (dysaesthesiae) may also be pain but are not necessarily so because, subjectively, they may not have the usual sensory qualities of pain.

Many people report pain in the absence of tissue damage or any likely pathophysiological cause; usually this happens for psychological reasons. There is no way to distinguish their experience from that due to tissue damage if we take the subjective report. If they regard their experience as pain and if they report it in the same ways as pain caused by tissue damage it should be accepted as pain. This definition avoids tying pain to the stimulus.

Taken from a report by the IASP Sub-committee on Taxonomy, 1980 [1]

2

Chapter One

Pain — and Cancer

ARISTOTLE, more than 2,000 years ago, described pain, along with pleasure, as a 'passion of the soul'. He emphasized that pain is not just another sensation by specifically omitting pain when enunciating the doctrine of the five senses. It is still not easy to define pain and more recently the definition reproduced on the opposite page has been proposed. It is noteworthy that the explanatory comment is ten times the length of the actual definition. In practice the most useful definition is:

'Pain is what the patient says hurts.' [1]

Other descriptions include:

'Pain is an intense feeling of discomfort or displeasure.' [2]
'Pain is the conscious awareness of a noxious stimulus.' [3]
'Pain is the resultant of the conflict between the stimulus and the individual.' [4]

For our part, we are happy to accept 'pain is what the patient says hurts' provided an Aristotelian emphasis is preserved; namely, that pain is a somatopsychic experience.

Pain threshold varies between ethnic groups even under controlled conditions in the laboratory, emphasizing that sensation threshold and pain threshold are not the same. What some describe merely as warmth is reported as painful by others [5]. Variation within an ethnic group has been reported by Keele [6], who divided normal subjects into hypersensitives (22 per cent), normosensitives (61 per cent), and hyposensitives (17 per cent). Compared with the former, hyposensitive subjects experience much less pain even, for example, after myocardial infarction.

Nociceptor [1]
A receptor preferentially sensitive to a noxious or potentially noxious stimulus.

Noxious [1]
A noxious stimulus is a tissue damaging stimulus.

Sensation Threshold
The least stimulus at which a person perceives a sensation.
Note: This is uniform for all ethnic groups *under laboratory con-ditions.* Elsewhere, attention and suggestion radically modify the sensation threshold.

Pain Threshold [1]
The least stimulus intensity at which a person perceives pain.

Pain Tolerance Level [1]
The greatest stimulus intensity causing pain that a person is pre-pared to tolerate.

Pain Modulation

It is universally agreed that pain is not simply a matter of impulses travelling along a nerve at a predetermined rate. The following equation does not exist: x units of noxious stimulus = y units of pain experienced. The impact of a noxious stimulus may be modulated in a number of ways. This means that for a given sensory input a person may experience anything from an ache to agony (Figure 1.1).

The Gate Control Theory of Pain [7] is one attempt to explain this phenomenon. It states that neural mechanisms in the dorsal horns of the spinal cord act like a gate which can increase or decrease the flow of nerve impulses from peripheral fibres to the central nervous system (Figure 1.2). Peripheral input is therefore subject to the modulating influence of the gate before it evokes pain perception and a central response. Sensory input is further modulated at successive synapses throughout its course from the spinal cord to the areas in the brain responsible for the perception of pain. In addition, the gate is affected considerably by descending influences from the brain. Melzack and Loeser [8], have extended further the concept of pain mechanisms by postulating the ability of the central nervous system to develop 'pattern generating

4

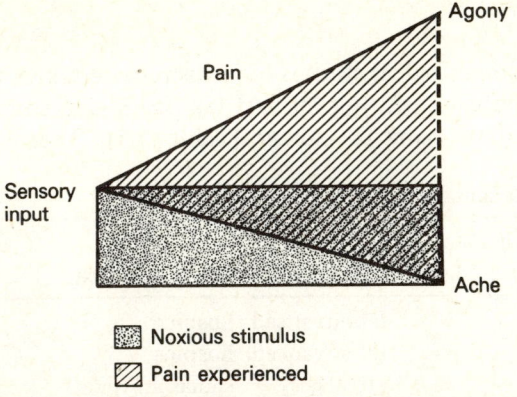

Noxious stimulus

Pain experienced

Figure 1.1 For any given noxious stimulus, the pain experienced varies from ache to agony, and depends on the psychological reaction of the sufferer to his discomfort.

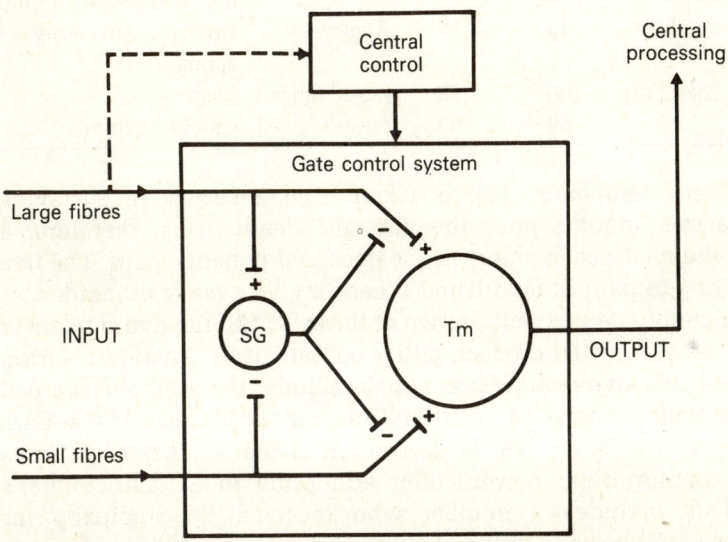

Figure 1.2 Schematic diagram of the gate control theory of pain. SG represents a substantia gelatinosa cell; Tm Cell, a spinal cord transmission cell. Central control refers to cognitive, motivational, and affective processes that modulate descending pain pathways. *Central processing* takes place in the reticular formation, thalamus, and limbic system. Plus (+) denotes an excitatory influence; minus (−) denotes inhibition. Adapted from Melzack, 1973 [7].

mechanisms'. This abnormal activity arises from the transmission pathways from dorsal horn to cortex, proximal to the denervated area, and is capable of producing patterns of impulses which produce pain. This helps to explain the pain of deafferentation seen after trauma to peripheral nerves or spinal cord, which sometimes does not develop for many years after the original injury.

5

Pain in Cancer

Although no large-scale epidemiological studies have been undertaken, a number of small surveys published during the last ten years give some indication of the incidence of pain in cancer (Table 1.1). That of

Table 1.1 Incidence of pain in cancer

Author	Number of patients	% with pain	Stage	Source
Haram [9]	607	66	far-advanced	hospice
Twycross [10]	500	84	far-advanced	hospice
Foley [11]	397	38	all stages	cancer hospital
Wilkes [12]	300	58	far-advanced	hospice
Pannuti et al [13]	291	64	advanced	oncology department
Trotter et al [14]	237	72	advanced	oncology outpatients (not a random sample)
Cartwright et al [15]	215	87	final year	survey of surviving spouses
Norton and Lack [16]	100	75	far-advanced	hospice
Foley [11]	39	60	far-advanced	cancer hospital

Cartwright and associates [15], is taken from a survey of surviving spouses, several months after the patients' death. It is, therefore, a measure of the relatives' memory of the deceased patients' pain. The five reports relating to pain in far-advanced cancer give a range of incidences from 58 per cent to 84 per cent. In two of these [9, 12], the figure refers to pain at the time of initial contact, either outpatient or inpatient. Norton and Lack [16] give an overall figure, which includes those who developed pain during their association with the Connecticut Hospice Home Care Service. Twycross' figure [10] is derived from the number of patients prescribed diamorphine (heroin) after admission to St. Christopher's Hospice. This includes a number who received it principally for dyspnoea or for 'aches and pains of bedfastness'. As a measure of severe pain in cancer it is certainly biased on the high side.

In fact, hospice data is likely to overestimate the incidence of pain in cancer because unrelieved pain is a main reason for referral. It seems reasonable to conclude that perhaps only some two-thirds of patients with advanced cancer experience pain. It is important to appreciate this as, for many people, cancer still means both pain and death. We have seen examples of relatives, and even doctors and nurses, wishing pain onto a patient: 'He says he has no pain; but he *must* have.' Such an attitude leads to the prescription of analgesics where none is necessary. Some patients adopt the attitude, 'I'm waiting for the pain to start.' They unnecessarily jeopardize their present peace of mind and view the future with trepidation; they misinterpret minor aches as the beginning of the inevitable, intractable cancer pain.

Although pain is a common indicator of advancing disease, many patients have pain-free intervals, especially after specific anti-cancer treatment. Some who experience pain in the penultimate stage do not have pain terminally [13]. The incidence of pain varies according to the primary site of the cancer (Table 1.2). Pain is not inevitable even in bone cancer or in cancers affecting the head and neck.

Table 1.2 Primary site and the incidence of pain (%)

Primary site	Incidence of pain (%)
Bone	85
Cervix	85
Oral	80
Stomach	70–75
Lung	50–70
Female GU	70
Pancreas	70
Male GU	60–75
Breast	55–68
Colon-rectum	50–60
Intestine	58
Kidney	55
Lymphoma	20
Leukaemia	5

After Foley, 1979 [11] and Bonica, 1980 [17]

Unrelieved Pain

Data relating to the incidence of unrelieved terminal pain is harder to come by. In one study [18], when first admitted to a hospice, 73 out of 100 patients had had pain for more than 8 weeks, and 57 for more than 16 weeks (Figure 1.3). More than three-quarters of the 73 patients stated that it was severe, very severe or excruciating. Saunders, reviewing 3,362 case notes at St. Christopher's Hospice, states that pain was 'difficult to control' in 34 patients, i.e. 1 per cent [19]. The MacMillan Home Care Service, St. Joseph's Hospice, London, reports that incidence of unrelieved pain in patients cared for at home is higher—about 10 per cent [20]. The higher percentage presumably relates in part to the reluctance of

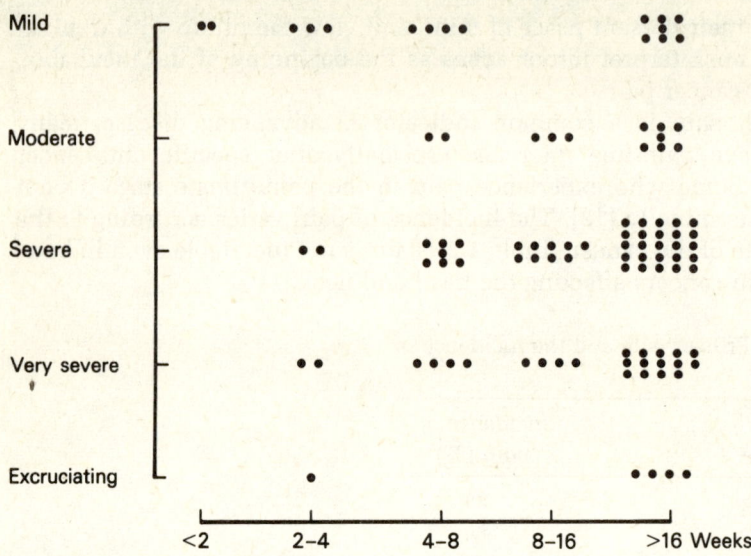

Figure 1.3 Relationship between intensity and duration of pain in 100 consecutively admitted cancer patients with pain. Each ● represents 1 patient.
From Twycross and Fairfield, 1982 [18]

some patients to take tablets or medicine at all. Other patients decline the offer of admission to hospitals for further treatment and prefer to 'soldier on' at home in pain.

Parkes [21] provides data from a study based on visits to the surviving spouses. All patients were under 65 and had died of cancer about a year before. The data relate to the spouses' memory of the patient's pain and, though of value in comparing different modes of care, they are obviously not comparable with records made at the time of the patient's illness. Patients were divided into three groups and the incidence of 'severe and mostly continuous pain' was noted in both preterminal and terminal phases of care (Figure 1.4). In those patients whose care was home-orientated, the incidence of unrelieved pain rose sharply to nearly 30 per cent terminally. In contrast, although a higher percentage experienced pain preterminally (before contact with the hospice), the incidence of pain in patients admitted to St. Christopher's fell to 8 per cent.

Other sources support the contention that cancer pain is often inadequately relieved [22, 23]. Making allowances for the different proportions who die in hospitals or at home, it is reasonable to conclude that about 25 per cent of all cancer patients die without relief from severe pain. This means 30,000 people a year in Britain and 100,000 in the USA.

The Implications of Unrelieved Pain
The implications of unrelieved pain vary according to its cause. In cancer,

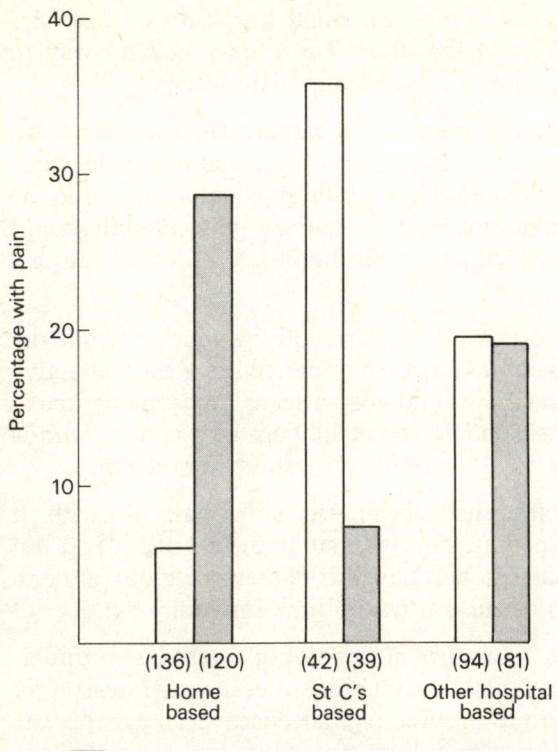

Figure 1.4 Histogram showing percentage with *severe and mostly continuous pain* in groups of terminal cancer patients under 65 who were cared for at home, at St. Christopher's Hospice, or in hospital. Figures in parenthesis refer to the number of spouses interviewed.
From Parkes, 1977 [21]

the pain is usually continuous and tends to get worse. This produces mental and physical exhaustion. The patient becomes demoralized, depressed, and increasingly fearful as yet another day of unrelieved suffering is anticipated. In addition, frequently the patient is incapacitated by pain, and becomes housebound or bedfast.

The National Committee on the Treatment of Intractable Pain was founded in the United States in 1977. It has received thousands of letters from relatives, friends and doctors describing patients who spent their last months in severe pain. Perhaps better than a statistical study, these letters illustrate only too well the meaning of unrelieved pain:

'I have lost my mother with incurable uterine cancer. Her pain was so horrid that she lost her mind and ate her bottom lip completely off from clenching her top teeth so tightly. My 13-year-old sister and I watched

9

this for six weeks. We would enter the small hospital and hear her screams as soon as we closed the door. The nurses had no way to quieten her. She was immune to conventional pain killers.'

'This July we lost our dad with cancer of the kidney. He was a beautiful 65-year-old retired contractor in January. The pain that man went thru' in May and June is undescribable. They would inject morphine into his buttocks and it would run out through his constantly injected flesh and onto the bedsheet. He was stripped of all dignity, food forced into his throat by syringe.'

'I'm sure I am only one of many who saw nothing routine about my husband's suffering an agony of pain when morphine wasn't effective . . . The doctors assured me they could keep him . . . "reasonably free of pain." There is nothing reasonable about the pain of a patient who is terminally ill with cancer . . . Destroying a person before death.'

'My brother just died of terminal cancer. He had a painful death. It deeply hurt us in the immediate family to sit alongside of his bed last week and see him in great pain and have his request for relief, either a shot or pill, turned down because it wasn't time for another shot.'

Parkes [24] also provides a number of horrifying examples of under-treatment. In home-based patients, he concluded that the main reason for poor pain control was failure to provide regular doses of an appropriate analgesic in sufficient quantity to relieve the pain. For example, one 54-year-old man became totally demoralized because of continued pain, and for several months cried almost incessantly. He was so frightened that he clung to his wife and became 'hysterical' whenever she left the room. He received an injection each *week* and was not able to go into a hospital as there was no bed available. Similar accounts given by other respon-dents suggested that neurotic exaggeration was not the explanation.

Reasons for Unrelieved Pain

There are, of course, many reasons for non-relief (Table 1.3). Bonica [17] suggests that the improper application of current knowledge is the most important cause. This is due to a number of interrelated factors. These include:

1 A lack of systematic teaching of medical students, doctors, nurses, and other health professionals;
2 The meagre amount of published information about the treatment of cancer pain.

Bonica has also pointed out that, in 7 of the most important English textbooks and monographs on cancer, less than 20 pages out of a total of nearly 5,500 pages are devoted to the treatment of cancer pain (Table 1.4).

Table 1.3   Common reasons for unrelieved pain

Associated with patient or family
1   Belief by patient that pain in cancer is inevitable and untreatable.
2   Failure by patient to contact physician.
3   Patient misleads doctor by 'putting on a brave face'.
4   Patient fails to take prescribed medication as does not 'believe' in tablets.
5   Belief that one should only take analgesics 'if absolutely necessary'.
6   Non-compliance because patient or family fears 'addiction'.
7   Non-compliance because of a belief that tolerance will rapidly develop, leaving nothing 'for when things get really bad'.
8   Patient stops medication because of side effects and fails to notify doctor.

Associated with doctor or nurse
1   Doctor ignores patient's pain believing that it is inevitable and intractable.
2   Lack of appreciation of the intensity of patient's pain; failure to get behind the 'brave face'.
3   Doctor prescribes an analgesic that is too weak to relieve much or any of the pain.
4   Prescription of an analgesic to be taken 'as required'.
5   Failure to appreciate that standard doses (derived from postoperative studies) have no relevance in the management of cancer pain.
6   Failure to give patient adequate instructions about optimal use of the analgesic prescribed.
7   Due to lack of knowledge about relative analgesic potency, doctor either reduces or fails to increase the absolute analgesic dose when transferring from one preparation to another.
8   Fear that patient will become 'addicted' if a narcotic analgesic is prescribed.
9   Doctor regards morphine/diamorphine as drugs to be reserved until patient is 'really terminal' (moribund), and continues to prescribe inadequate doses of less efficacious drugs.
10 Failure to institute adequate follow-up arrangements in order to monitor patient's progress.
11 Lack of knowledge about 'co-analgesics' and other drugs that are of value in situations where narcotics are only partially effective.
12 Failure to use non-drug measures when appropriate.
13 Failure to give adequate emotional support to the patient and family.

In the 1979, 1980 and 1981 volumes of *The Year Book of Cancer* [25–27], no papers referring to pain control are reviewed in the section Advanced Tumours and Terminal Care. Like Bonica, we conclude that the relief of pain is still not considered important by many oncological scientists and clinicians. This is, to say the least, regrettable, particularly as there are data which suggest that the presence of a hospice leads to improved

Table 1.4   Discussion of pain in oncology textbooks

Title of book	Authors	Year of publication	Total pages	Pages on pain
Cancer Medicine	Holland and Frei	1974	2,018	13
Clinical Oncology	Horton and Hill	1977	819	2½
Cancer Diagnosis, Treatment and Prognosis	Ockerman and Del Regato	1970	783	None
Cancer: Manual for Practitioners	Mass. Division Am. Cancer Soc.	1968	408	None
Clinical Oncology: Manual for Students and Doctors	Comm. Prof. Education U.I.C.C.	1973	322	1¼
Advances in Cancer Surgery	Najerian and Delaney	1976	608	None
Principles of Surgical Oncology	R W Raven (ed)	1976	510	None

From Bonica, 1980 [17]

standards of terminal care and pain relief in surrounding hospitals when measured over a 10 year period [28]. The improvement almost certainly stems from a programme of continuing education and professional interaction.

References

1 IASP Subcommittee on Taxonomy. Pain terms: a list with definitions and notes on usage. *Pain* 1980; **8:** 249–252.

2 Christensen, LV. Cultural, clinical and physiological aspects of pain: a review. *Journal of Oral Rehabilitation* 1980; **7:** 413–421.

3 Gerber J. Personal communication.

4 Leriche R. *The Surgery of Pain*, translated and edited by Young A. Bailliere, Tindall & Cox, London 1939.

5 Hardy JD, Wolff HG and Goodall H. *Pain Sensations and Reactions*. Williams & Wilkins, Baltimore 1952.

6 Keele KD. Pain sensitivity and the pain pattern of cardiac infarction. *Proceedings of Royal Society of Medicine* 1967; **60:** 417–419.

7 Melzack R. *The Puzzle of Pain*. Penguin Books, Harmondsworth, Middlesex 1973.

8 Melzack R and Loeser JD. Phantom body pain in paraplegics: evidence for central 'pattern generating mechanisms' for pain. *Pain* 1978; **4:** 195–210.

9 Haram BJ. Facts and figures in *Management of Terminal Disease*, edited by Saunders CM. Edward Arnold, London 1978, pp 12–18.

10 Twycross RG. Clinical experience with diamorphine in advanced malignant disease. *International Journal of Clinical Pharmacology, Therapy and Toxicology* 1974; **9:** 184–198.

11 Foley KM. Pain syndromes in patients with cancer in *Advances in Pain Research and Therapy, Vol 2* edited by Bonica JJ and Ventafridda V. Raven Press, New York 1979, pp 59–75.

12 Wilkes E. Some problems in cancer management. *Proceedings of the Royal Society of Medicine* 1974; **67:** 23–27.

13 Pannuti E, Rossi AP, Marraro D, Strochi E, Cricca A, Piana E and Pollutri E in *The Continuing Care of Patients with Terminal Cancer*, edited by Twycross RG and Ventafridda V. Pergamon Press, Oxford 1980, pp 75–78.

14 Trotter JM, Scott R, MacBeth FR, McVie JG and Calman KC. Problems of the oncology outpatient: role of the liaison health visitor. *British Medical Journal* 1981; **282:** 122–124.

15 Cartwright A, Hockey L and Anderson ABM. *Life Before Death*. Routledge & Kegan Paul, London 1973.

16 Norton WS and Lack SA. Control of symptoms other than pain in *The Continuing Care of Patients with Terminal Cancer*, edited by Twycross RG and Ventrafridda V. Pergamon Press, Oxford 1980, pp 167–178.

17 Bonica JJ. Cancer pain in *Pain*, edited by Bonica JJ. Raven Press, New York 1980, pp 335–362.

18 Twycross RG and Fairfield S, Pain in far-advanced cancer. *Pain* 1982; **14:** 303–310

19 Saunders CM. Current views of pain relief and terminal care in *The Therapy of Pain*, edited by Swerdlow M. MTP Press Ltd., Lancaster 1981, pp 215–241.

20 Lamerton R. Annual Report of Macmillan Home Care Service St. Joseph's Hospice 1978.

21 Parkes CM. Evaluation of family care in terminal illness in *The Family and Death*, edited by Pritchard ER, Collard J, Orcutt BA, Kutscher AH, Seeland I and Lefkowicz N. Columbia University Press, New York 1977, pp 49–79.

22 Marks RD and Sachar EJ. Undertreatment of medical inpatients with narcotic analgesics. *Annals of Internal Medicine* 1973; **78:** 173–181.

23 Woodbine G. *The Care of Patients Dying from Cancer, a Cross-Sectional Study.* MSc Thesis. University of Southampton 1977.

24 Parkes CM. Home or Hospital? Terminal care as seen by surviving spouses. *Journal of the Royal College of General Practitioners* 1978; **28:** 19–30.

25 Clark RL, Cumley RW and Hickey RC. *The Year Book of Cancer 1979,* Year Book Medical Publisher Inc., Chicago & London 1980, pp 323–331.

26 Clark RL, Cumley RW and Hickey RC. *The Year Book of Cancer 1980,* Year Book Medical Publisher Inc., Chicago & London 1980, pp 327–337.

27 Clark RL, Cumley R W and Hickey RC. *The Year Book of Cancer 1981,* Year Book Medical Publisher Inc., Chicago & London 1981, pp 301–310.

28 Parkes CM and Parkes JLN. 'Hospice' versus 'Hospital' care: re-evaluation after ten years. (In press.)

Chapter Two

Pain — Assessment

Traditionally, we are taught to assess pain by determining its PQRST characteristics (Table 2.1). Unfortunately, a blind belief in the efficacy of so simple an approach may hinder rather than help the doctor in the

Table 2.1   The PQRST characteristics of pain

		'Tell me about your pain' 'Where is it?'
P	Palliative factors	'What makes it less intense?'
	Provocative factors	'What makes it worse?'
Q	Quality	'What is it like?'
R	Radiation	'Does it spread anywhere else?'
S	Severity	'How severe is it?'
T	Temporal factors	'Is it there all the time, or does it come and go?'

After Gray, 1977 [1]

assessment of the patient's pain. Determination of the PQRST characteristics is only the beginning, providing a description of the pain but no more. Complete assessment implies the ability to make a diagnosis and delineate an initial plan of management. This demands:

1   a knowledge of the pathological processes which are potential causes of the pain;
2   a grasp of general and neurological anatomy;
3   an understanding of the phenomenon of referred pain.

From the history and clinical examination, supplemented if necessary

15

by X-ray, scan, or other investigation, it should be possible to develop a clear mental picture of the physical mechanisms underlying the patient's pain. The correct diagnosis can usually be made by asking the patient to point to the site of the pain and describe it fully. Then, assessment completed and diagnosis made, treatment is initiated.

We are familiar with this sequence of events in relation to acute abdominal pain, but often fail to apply the same logical approach when assessing pain in advanced cancer. Yet, assessment in this area needs to be equally thorough. Cancer can cause pain by a variety of mechanisms in any part of the body. A body outline on which to record pain data is a great help in elucidating a complex situation (Figure 2.1).

Direct questions may not produce the required information because patients often put on a brave face for the doctor. This is particularly true if relatives are present during the interview. Unlike patients with acute severe pain, many cancer patients do not groan audibly and appear restless and in distress. When seen by a doctor the patient may simply say, 'I have terrible pain' and not volunteer further information. The pain does, however, disturb sleep, limit activity, and affect mental application. Intensity of pain must be assessed, therefore, not only by the patient's appearance and description, but also by discovering the following details:

1   what drugs have failed to relieve;
2   whether sleep is disturbed;
3   in what way activity is limited.

Helpful questions include:

1   'How long is it since you went out?'
2   'What are you doing around the house?'
3   'Have you given up any hobbies or anything that you usually do?'

As far as possible, note-taking should be avoided when talking with the patients. Receiving the doctor's full attention is therapeutic, and a vital part of pain management. The body chart should, however, be completed in conjunction with the patient who can then verify its accuracy. This makes note-taking a demonstration of the physician's concern, and helps to establish trust.

Assessment of pain in the confused patient is more difficult. An involuntary moan, a wrinkled brow, tense fingers and cautious breathing may betray underlying pain even in a stuporous patient. These signs can sometimes be removed by analgesics.

A detailed history of pain medication is part of assessment, and may be time-consuming to obtain. Whereas, on referral, details of past anti-cancer treatment are usually available, it is still common to receive little or no information about past analgesics and their effects.

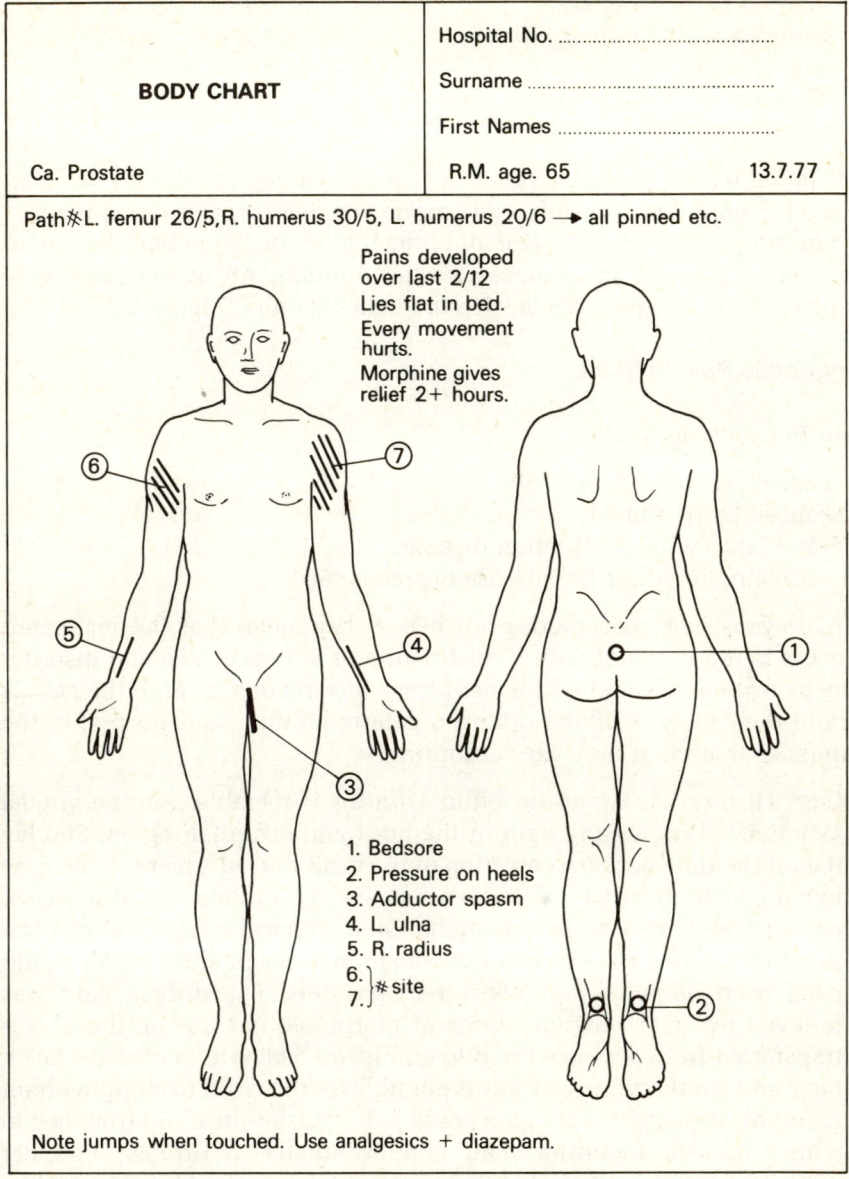

Figure 2.1 Body chart used to record data relating to a 65-year-old man with cancer of the prostate gland.

A pain medication history includes not only a list of drugs but also:

1 dose,
2 route of administration,
3 regular or as required (p.r.n.),

17

4 interval between doses,
5 patient's view on drug efficacy,
6 side effects,
7 duration of use of drug,
8 reason for discontinuation.

If possible, the patient's spouse or closest caregiver† should be interviewed. Sometimes it is only their comments that reveal the true picture. When the pain is relieved, it is not uncommon for the patient to concur spontaneously with the spouse's earlier opinion. An overprinted body chart is useful to help standardize the data obtained (Figure 2.2).

Diagnostic Possibilities

Pain in cancer may be:

1 caused by the cancer itself,
2 caused by treatment,
3 associated with debilitating disease,
4 unrelated to either the disease or treatment.

A diagnosis of cancer does not necessarily mean that the malignant process is the cause of pain. Constipation or a musculoskeletal disorder may be responsible and will benefit from specific treatment. If the pain is due to the cancer, it is important to determine the mechanism(s) of the pain(s) as treatment may vary accordingly.

Case History. A 4-year-old child with an inoperable pontine glioma experienced increasing pain in the head and occipital region. She lay flat all the time because elevation of the head caused a marked increase in pain. With this history, it was necessary to postulate a local source of pain (possibly caused by post-radiation meningeal adhesions) in addition to the diffuse headache of secondary hydrocephalus (which would have been helped by a more erect posture). The diffuse pain was relieved by small, regular doses of morphine, but not until she was transferred from a King's Fund to an Ellison bed (which elevates head, neck and trunk in unison) was it possible for the child to sit up without pain. Subsequently, it became possible to transfer the child from bed to a high-backed, reclining chair and eventually to lift her onto her mother's lap. This suggested that some of the pain had been caused by spasm of the neck muscles, and that the confidence engendered by the ability to sit up in bed allowed additional manoeuvres to be undertaken without pain.

† primary care person (USA)

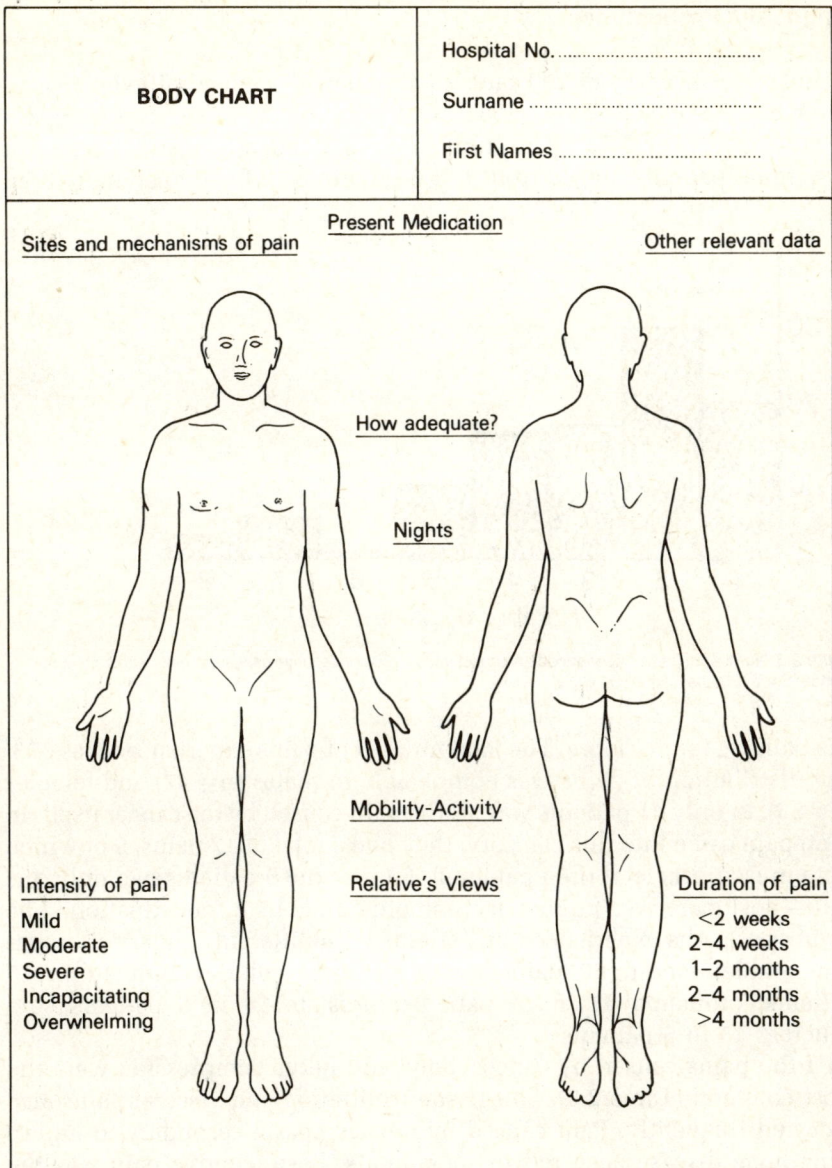

BODY CHART	Hospital No. ....
	Surname ....
	First Names ....

Present Medication

Sites and mechanisms of pain

Other relevant data

How adequate?

Nights

Mobility-Activity

Intensity of pain

Mild
Moderate
Severe
Incapacitating
Overwhelming

Relative's Views

Duration of pain

<2 weeks
2–4 weeks
1–2 months
2–4 months
>4 months

Figure 2.2 Overprinted body chart used at Sir Michael Sobell House, Oxford, for recording pain data.

19

Diagnostic Probabilities

A prospective survey of 100 cancer patients with pain admitted consecutively to Sir Michael Sobell House, Oxford, illustrates the pattern of pain in advanced cancer [2]. The number of anatomically distinct pains in individual patients ranged from 1 to 8 (Figure 2.3). Eighty had more than

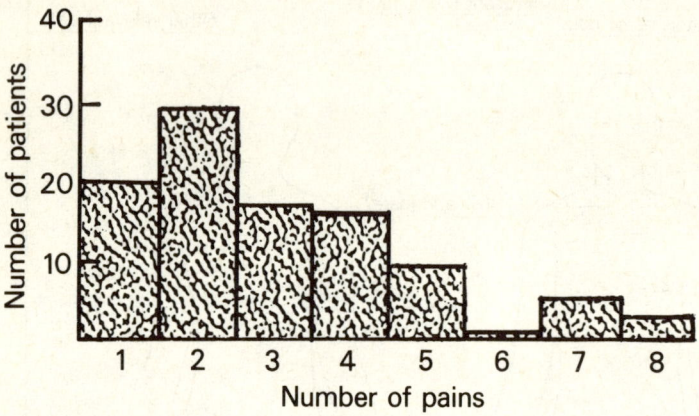

Figure 2.3 Number of pains experienced on admission by 100 consecutive cancer patients with pain at Sir Michael Sobell House, Oxford.

one pain; 34 four or more. The total number of pains experienced was 303. The distribution of pains was comparable in males (n = 47) and females (n = 53). In only 41 patients was all the pain caused by the cancer itself. In 9, no pain came into this category; they had a total of 17 pains, 9 of which were musculoskeletal (in 4 patients). Four of the 9 patients had only one pain—postoperative, pulmonary embolus and, in 2, constipation. The number of pains experienced by patients with different primary sites was comparable: breast, 60 pains in 15 patients; colon-rectum 40 in 15 patients; bronchus 53 in 14 patients; prostate 18 in 6 patients; and pancreas 15 in 5 patients.

Of the pains caused by cancer, bone and nerve compression were the most common (Table 2.2). Soft tissue infiltration and visceral pains also occurred frequently. Pain caused by muscle spasm secondary to underlying bone disease occurred in 11 patients. Postoperative pain was the commonest pain related to treatment and constipation the most common associated pain. Six of the 8 postoperative pains were related to the incisional scar (3 post-mastectomy, 2 post-laparotomy and 1 after a biopsy of a supraclavicular node). In all but one, the pain was chronic, that is, not attributable to recent surgery. Of the other 2, 1 was an upper arm T1 dysaesthetic pain with hyperaesthesia. This was associated with an aching axillary scar pain. This particular pattern of pain, which tends to

Table 2.2 Causes of pain in 100 cancer patients

	Number of pains	Number of patients
Caused by cancer		
Bone	58	31
Nerve compression	56	31
Soft tissue infiltration	35	31
Visceral involvement	33	31
Muscle spasm	14	11
Lymphoedema	4	3
Raised intracranial pressure	2	2
Myopathy	2	2
	204 (67%)	91
Related to treatment		
Postoperative	8	7
Colostomy	2	2
Nerve block	2	1
Postoperative adhesions	1	1
Post-radiation fibrosis	1	1
Oesophageal	1	1
	15 (5%)	12
Associated pains		
Constipation	11	11
Capsulitis of shoulder	4	4
Bedsore	1	1
Post-herpetic neuralgia	1	1
Pulmonary embolus	1	1
Penile spasm (catheter)	1	1
Unrelated pains	19 (6%)	19
Musculoskeletal		
myofascial	24	12
low back	8	8
spinal osteoporosis	4	3
ischial tuberosity	2	1
ankle	2	1
traumatic	2	1
sacroiliac	1	1
	43	27
Other		
osteoarthritis	4	3
migraine	2	2
miscellaneous	16	13
	65 (22%)	39
Total	303 (100%)	100

develop 1 to 2 months after mastectomy, is caused by section of the intercostobrachial nerve (T1–2) close to the lateral chest wall [3]. The other chronic postoperative pain was a deep ache in the right upper thigh. This was caused by a Thompson's hemiarthroplasty inserted 6 months before.

One patient had lower oesophageal pain caused by gastric reflux. This appeared to be associated with delayed gastric emptying, hyperacidity and a reduction in the tone of the gastro-oesophageal junction induced by medication, namely, morphine, dexamethasone and chlorpromazine.

Twenty-seven patients recorded a total of 43 musculoskeletal pains of non-malignant origin. Of those with non-malignant low back pain, in 6 it had been long-standing. Of the other 2, the pain was caused by a large abdominal mass in one case (cp. pregnancy) and in the other by a compensatory lumbar scoliosis associated with a pelvic tilt caused by necrosis of the femoral head. Two other patients had vague but troublesome pain in relation to both ischial tuberosities and around both ankles respectively.

The most common cause of musculoskeletal pain was, however, myofascial. This occurred in 12 patients and accounted for 24 pains. Five of these patients had one myofascial pain and 7 two or more. The maximum number in any one patient was 5. Miscellaneous unrelated pains included tension headache, pain in one or both pinna, several abdominal complaints, urinary retention, coccydynia, restless legs syndrome and artherosclerotic claudication.

The 10 patients who survived for more than a year had a total of 30 pains. Only 2 had just one pain; 4 had 4 or more pains. The pattern in these patients was, therefore, similar to that seen in those who survived for shorter periods.

In retrospect, it is apparent that the concept of four mutually exclusive pain categories is an oversimplification. For example, in the 2 patients with low back pain of recent onset, although classified as unrelated, the pain was clearly caused by the presence of malignant disease, albeit indirectly. Myofascial pains were also classed as unrelated as they are a relatively common form of pain in the general population. The incidence of these pains is almost certainly higher in cancer patients, particularly in those who are cachectic, anxious or exhausted.

Lymphoedema and muscle spasm pains also present a problem of classification. In our patients, neoplastic lymphatic obstruction, either in the axilla, pelvis or groin, is present in almost all those who develop a painful swollen limb. Occasionally, though not in this series, the lymphoedema is secondary to lymphatic fibrosis following successful cancer treatment. Muscle spasm pain was included in the list of cancer induced pains. It represents an indirect form of metastatic bone pain in that the spasm is an involuntary protective response to the underlying discomfort.

The muscle pain sometimes masked the underlying bone pain considerably or completely.

Bone Pain

The majority of osseous metastases are not painful. Those that are cause pain in a variety of ways. These include local bone pain, radiation into surrounding tissues, referred pain, nerve compression, muscle spasm, and associated myofascial pain.

Local bone pain ranges from a dull ache to a deep oppressive intense pain. It is often worse on movement and on weightbearing. Sometimes it is worse at night. With a pathological rib fracture, the pain is most intense when changing from a sitting to a supine posture or vice versa, or when the trunk is rotated laterally. In long bones, weightbearing may cause additional pain as a result of buckling (cp. stress fracture of a metatarsal).

Evaluation of a new bone pain in the patient with known advanced cancer calls for a series of investigative steps and clinical considerations to determine the presence or absence of treatable metastases (Table 2.3). Bone disease is apparent on conventional X-ray films only when there is considerable structural alteration with loss of at least 40 per cent of the mineral content. In hospice practice, where the patient is housebound, or has limited access to investigational equipment, an X-ray will still be the initial step (Table 2.4). If positive, treatment can be initiated straight away.

As patients may have normal skeletal radiographs in the presence of histologically proven metastatic disease, the second step is to arrange for a bone scan. This is more sensitive at detecting metastatic foci. It is also less specific as other bone disorders can produce abnormalities on scanning. Poor specificity is less of a problem in the hospice population with bone pain. Local pain and the known presence of metastases elsewhere increases the likelihood that positive scans reflect neoplastic disease [4]. Bone scan abnormalities must always be correlated with the history and with X-ray studies. Certain cancers are more likely to produce bony metastases (Table 2.5) and 80 per cent are in the axial skeleton [5]. Metastases in the hands and feet are most often from a bronchogenic primary. A normal bone radiograph with abnormal scan is highly suggestive of malignant disease, especially if there is no history to suggest local trauma or osteitis secondary to infection or radiation. In multiple myeloma, the bone scan is less effective than skeletal radiology for detecting bone lesions. A scan may also be difficult to interpret after radiotherapy.

Although plain X-ray and bone scan are the diagnostic procedures of choice there are areas where computed tomography (CT) has been found helpful [6]. CT has been found particularly useful in assessing the cranial vault, orbits, base of the skull, cervicothoracic junction and brachial

Table 2.3 Assessment of bone pain in patients with advanced cancer

Bone pain, → X-ray
known tumour

+ → treat

− → bone scan

    + → correlate with history
        review scan pattern
        check 'negative' X-ray

        − if bone metastases confirmed
                ↳ treat
        − if still doubtful
                ↳ consider bone biopsy

    − → review history, examination, and
        X-ray for possible benign cause

        consider bone biopsy if
        clinical suspicion persists

        consider CT scan if pain is in
        a difficult area

Table 2.4 Diagnostic radiology and cancer pain

1 A 40 to 60% change in bone density is necessary to detect changes on X-ray; pain can occur with less than this.
2 Plain X-rays are inadequate to assess areas where bone shadows overlap:
   1 base of skull,
   2 C7, C8, T1 vertebrae,
   3 sacrum.
3 Tomography of a vertebral body may distinguish between osteoporotic collapse and a metastasis.
4 Plain X-rays detect only 80% of osseous metastases.
5 Bone scans detect 95% of metastases.
6 Bone scans are sometimes negative in myelomatous vertebral collapse.
7 Bone scan may show presence of a metastasis 3 to 6 months before a plain X-ray.
8 Computed tomography not often more helpful than isotope bone scan, but is procedure of choice for evaluation of retroperitoneal, paravertebral, pelvic and skull-base areas.
9 It is sometimes necessary to proceed with treatment on the basis of clinical judgement alone.

Table 2.5 Primary sites commonly associated with osseous metastases

Myeloma	Kidney
Breast	Melanoma
Bronchus	Thyroid
Prostate	

plexus area of the spine, thoracic and lumbar vertebrae and the pelvic bones and sacrum. For the dying patient in poor general condition a halt must be called at some point to invasive and exhausting procedures. A doctor may well elect to proceed with treatment rather than to progress to bone biopsy. However, it is not unusual to have a mobile patient with an obscure pain. With the possibility that carefully planned radiotherapy will relieve the pain, this is one area in advanced cancer care where intensive investigation may be justified.

Referred Pain

Patients with ischaemic heart disease commonly experience referred pain in the upper chest, shoulder, neck and arm. This pain, angina pectoris, is the result of myocardial ischaemia but is manifested at other sites. Similarly, visceral pain may not be experienced immediately over the

Referred Pain

The perception of pain in the skin or other superficial structure caused by a noxious stimulus in a deeper structure at some distance from the site of the pain.

anatomical site. In cancer, referred pain occurs frequently. Perhaps the most common type is that caused by nerve compression, the most important that associated with spinal cord compression, and the least well appreciated that related to myofascial lesions (Table 2.6).

Table 2.6   Origins of referred pain in cancer

Myofascial	Nerve compression
Bone	Spinal cord compression
Visceral	Brain

Why Referred Pain?

Referred pain from compression of peripheral nerves, cauda equina or spinal cord is easily understood, as is referred pain from a lesion in the region of the thalamus. Most referred pain from bone and from myofascial structures is perhaps understandable on the basis of a 'flare' phenomenon—local radiation from the primary source of pain. With visceral pain, an embryological explanation is at least partly necessary. An example is the presence of pain in the ipsilateral shoulder associated with inflammation of the diaphragm in cholecystitis. Both the diaphragm and the shoulder are innervated by fibres derived from the primitive C4 segment. It is then necessary to postulate that the brain 'misinterprets' the afferent impulses that converge on it from both visceral and somatic structures. The pain from the viscus is represented as having come from the embryologically corresponding somatic area. This is known as the Convergence-projection or Convergence-facilitation theory [7].

Myofascial Referred Pain

Musculoskeletal Pain

A term used to describe pain caused by disorders of muscles, ligaments, joints and bones.
Note: It includes myofascial pain.

Myofascial Pain
Pain originating from a muscle and its surrounding fascia.

Myofascial pain commonly accompanies advanced malignant disease. Cachectic patients who need to spend much of the time in bed, are those most likely to develop muscular imbalance and, in consequence, myofascial pain. Diagnosis depends on:

1 awareness of the phenomenon of myofascial pain,
2 a localized trigger point,
3 pain referred in a non-dermatomal manner,
4 a reproducible pattern.

The trigger point (TP) is a small hypersensitive region of a muscle. Pain is triggered whenever the area is stimulated by pressure, extremes of temperature, or movement that stretches the structure containing the TP. Predisposing factors include fatigue, debility and anxiety. Pain is usually local (at the site of the TP) and radiates to other areas in a non-dermatomal manner [8, 9]. In cancer patients, radiation, surgery and weight loss result in a more varied pattern.

A TP may develop in any muscle in the body. There is a tendency for TPs to cluster in certain areas. For example, in the upper trunk, the same person may develop several TPs in the trapezius, levator scapulae, and infraspinatus muscles. The quadratus lumborum is another common area to be affected and may be associated with other TPs in the gluteus medius and tensor fascia lata. A TP in the distal portion of the trapezius may be associated with pain that radiates round the chest to the nipple and down the inner aspect of the ipsilateral arm (see Appendix).

The most reliable method of locating a TP is by gentle palpation of the painful area with the tip of a finger. Pressure to the hypersensitive area in the muscles reproduces or accentuates the pain and causes the patient to wince. The TP may feel indurated. This depends on which muscle is involved and whether the TP is genetic or post-traumatic in origin, or the result of previous treatment.

Referred Bone Pain
Most bone pain is local and not referred. Vertebral and sternal pain, in particular, may include significant lateral radiation. A distinction has to be made between lateral radiation and associated intercostal neuralgia (thoracic vertebrae) or paravertebral muscle spasm (lumbar vertebrae). Pain originating in the upper lumbar vertebrae may present difficulty in diagnosis because of a more marked pattern of reference. For example, L1 pain is usually a local aching mid-back pain with a variable degree of lateral radiation into the paraspinal area. It may be exacerbated by lying or sitting and relieved by standing, though the reverse may also be true. Occasionally, patients will have pain only in the region of the sacroiliac joint(s) or the posterior part of the iliac crest(s) [8]. In patients with such pain, if there is not overlying local tenderness, X-rays should include the whole of the lumbar spine.

27

Referred Visceral Pain

Referred visceral pain is familiar to most physicians. It is initially poorly localized and often referred to the somatic area supplied by the same nerve root. Thus biliary pain may be referred to the area over the right inferior angle of the right scapula (T8). Inflammation of the small intestine or appendix is initially manifested by epigastric and umbilical tenderness (T10). Renal pain may be referred to the ipsilateral testis. Later, with inflammatory involvement of the parietal layer of the peritoneum, accurate localization to the area of stimulation is obtained.

The Brain and Referred Pain

On rare occasions, referred pain relates to a primary or metastatic tumour in the region of the thalamus. Pain will manifest in part or all of the contralateral side of the body. Diagnosis is made with the help of a brain scan, ordered because of the presence of other symptoms and signs suggestive of an intracranial space-occupying lesion. We have not yet seen this syndrome.

Nerve Compression Pain

Trunk and Extremities

The pain relating to each nerve root manifests in an area relating to a fairly constant part of the body surface (Figure 2.4). Access to a dermatomal map is important as few doctors (neurologists apart) can remember the complete pattern. There is inevitably some variation.

Diagnosis of pain secondary to compression of a nerve subserving the trunk or an extremity is easier when there are other signs or symptoms of nerve impairment, such as numbness, weakness and altered tendon reflexes. However, pain usually precedes other sensory and motor changes by weeks or months. Patients often describe less intense nerve compression pain as a constant ache. Some experience intermittent stabbing or shooting pains. When compression results in nerve destruction, the patient may complain of a superficial burning pain, with or without hyperaesthesia.

Metastatic involvement of the spine is the most common cause of nerve root compression pain in patients with far-advanced cancer. Sometimes, a plain X-ray of the appropriate part of the spine is all that is necessary to confirm the presence of a secondary deposit in the relevant vertebra(e). A normal *report* should not be regarded as conclusive. Some X-rays, inevitably, are initially misread, partly because the radiologist is not given sufficient clinical information. 'Normal' X-rays should be reviewed with a radiologist if the history and clinical findings suggest root compression. Sometimes an isotope bone scan is indicated but if after review the X-ray is still considered normal, nerve root compression by an osseous meta-

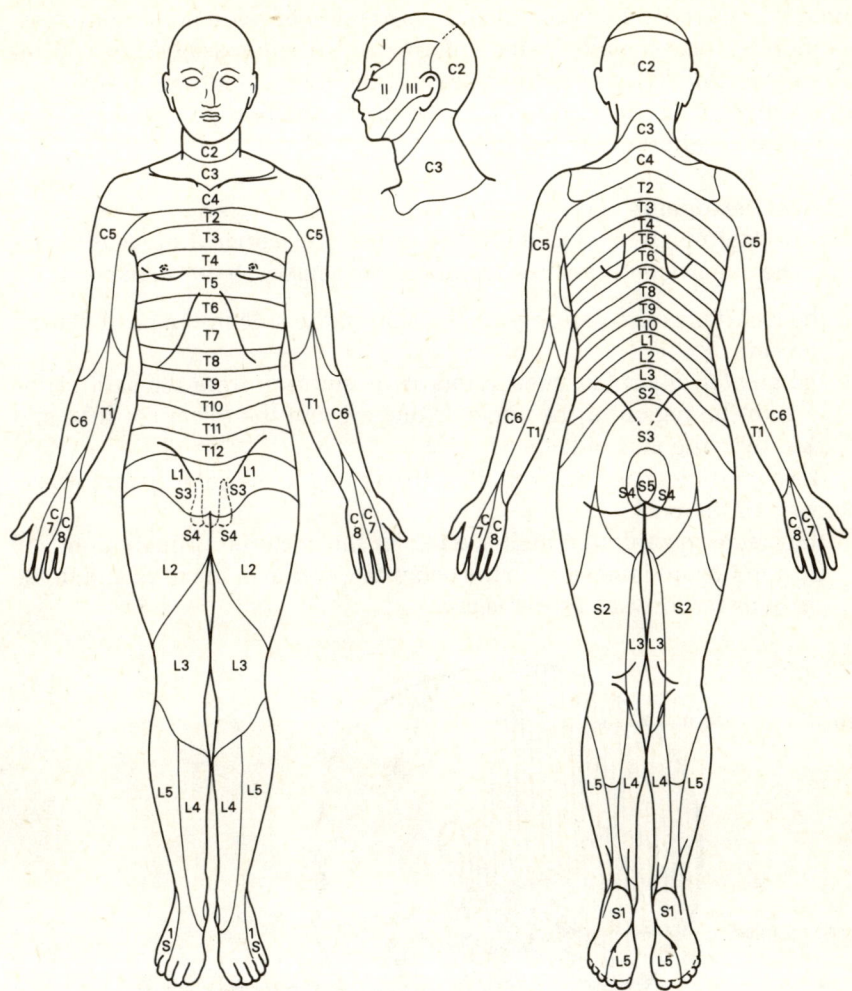

Figure 2.4 Body chart showing dermatomes, i.e., areas in which pain is experienced if corresponding nerve or nerve root is stimulated.
    Note: a variety of 'standard' dermatomal charts exist. We have used this one successfully for several years. It appears to reflect what is seen in cancer pain patients.

stasis is very unlikely. It requires a relatively large lesion with distortion of the bone architecture to produce compression of a neighbouring nerve.

Computed tomography (CT scan) may be necessary in a small number of patients. Though in relation to nerve compression, it is unlikely that a CT scan will detect a relevant bone lesion if a bone scan has not. A CT scan will, however, detect otherwise undetectable soft tissue metastases, such as a neoplastic mass in the neck compressing one or more nerves of the brachial plexus, or a retroperitoneal mass affecting lumbar nerve roots. It is possible for a patient to develop nerve compression months, occasionally years, before a soft tissue mass becomes clinically detectable. CT can help to prevent the long latent period that may exist between the onset of soft tissue nerve compression pain and the institution of appropriate treatment.

Cervical Plexopathy

The cervical plexus is formed of the upper four cervical nerves (Figure 2.5). The superficial branches are primarily sensory. They consist of:

1   the *small occipital*, supplying the skin of the side of the head behind the ear;
2   the *greater auricular*, subserving pain sensation from the skin of the face in the region of the angle of the jaw and the lower ear lobe and skin over the mastoid;
3   the *superficial cervical*, which is distributed to the anterior and lateral parts of the neck;
4   the *greater occipital*, which is a part of the posterior primary ramus of C2 and C3 and is sensory to the occipital portion of the neck and to the scalp as far forward as the vertex.

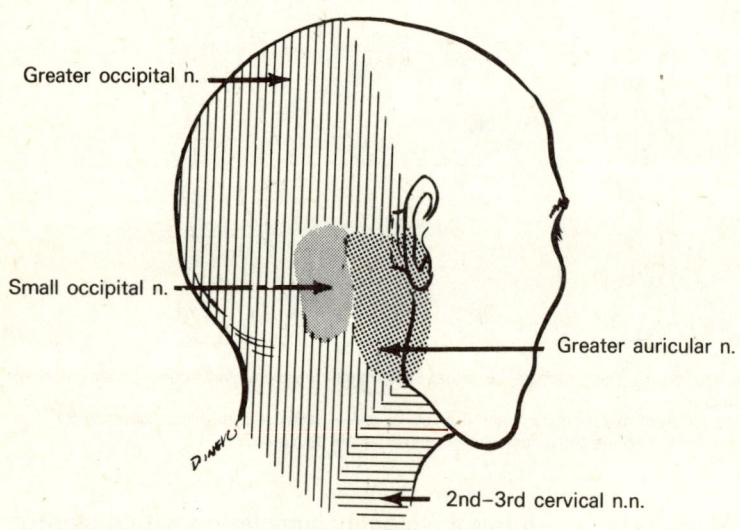

Figure 2.5 Sensory distribution of cervical plexus nerves.
From Boop and Fischer, 1981 [10]

The pain fibres of cranial nerves V, VII, IX and X and of the cervical plexus, enter the CNS in a common tract of descending fibres and grey matter which is continuous down to the C4 level of the spinal cord. This tract is called the spinal tract of the trigeminal. As these fibres descend in the tract they send collaterals to all levels of the nucleus. There is ample opportunity for these sensory nerves to overlap in function centrally. Referred pain patterns may be explicable on this basis. Alteration of the input to this central neural pool may result in changes in other areas. For example, cervical nerve blocks have sometimes reduced the pain of an atypical facial neuralgia.

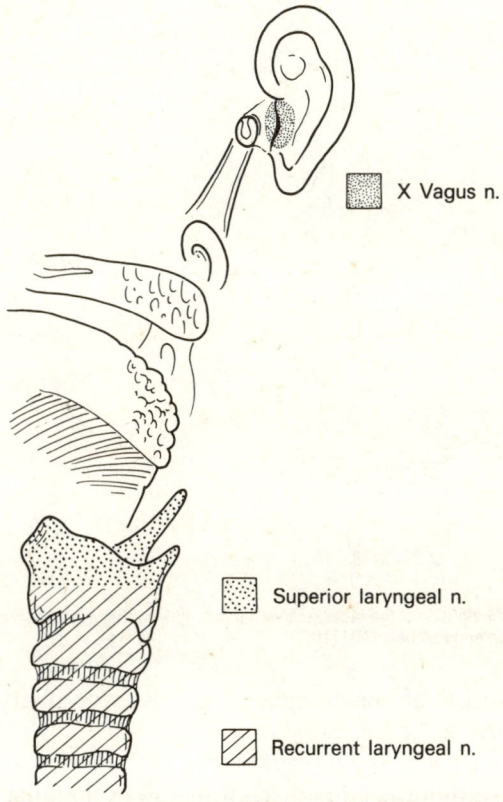

X Vagus n.

Superior laryngeal n.

Recurrent laryngeal n.

Figure 2.6 Sensory distribution of the vagus nerve (cranial X). From Boop and Fischer, 1981 [10]

Pain in the ear may be very difficult to elucidate because there are so many nerves supplying the area. Not only the vagus (Figure 2.6), and glossopharyngeal (Figure 2.7), but the facial (nervus intermedius), the trigeminal (auriculotemporal) and also the greater auricular nerve of the cervical plexus carry pain sensation from this area. From the middle ear and medial aspect of the tympanic membrane, sensory fibres originate in the tympanic branch of the glossopharyngeal nerve (cranial IX). This branch, known as Jacobson's nerve, also subserves sensation from the mastoid cells and upper Eustachian tube. Other sensory fibres in the glossopharyngeal nerve come from the soft palate, tonsillar region,

31

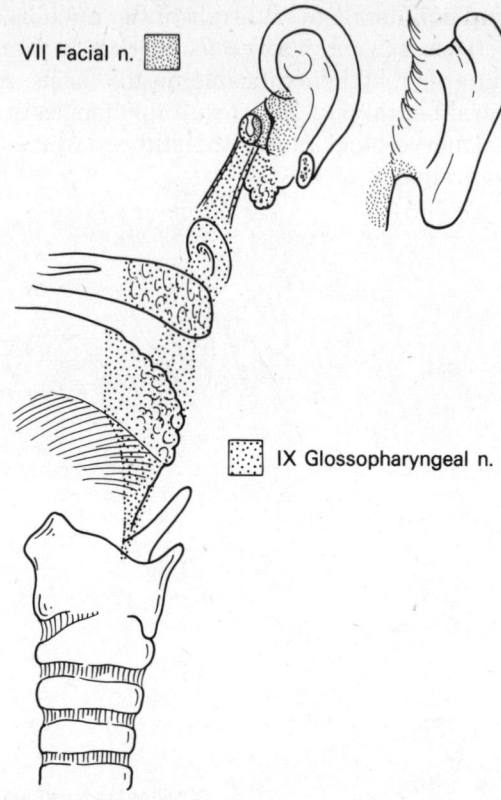

VII Facial n.

IX Glossopharyngeal n.

Figure 2.7 Sensory distribution of the facial (cranial VII) and glossopharyngeal nerves (cranial IX). From Boop and Fischer, 1981 [10]

posterior one-third of the tongue, and posterior pharynx down to the epiglottis (Figure 2.7).

The vagus (cranial X) conveys sensation via the superior laryngeal nerve from the epiglottis and adjacent region of the pharynx and from the vallecula. The recurrent laryngeal nerve supplies the larynx below the vocal folds (Figure 2.6). The vagus also conducts sensation from a small area of the external auditory canal posteriorly and from adjacent skin of the external ear (Figure 2.6).

Brachial Plexopathy

Every so often a patient presents with pain in the arm associated with other symptoms and signs that suggest compression of, or damage to, the brachial plexus. In the majority, there is clear evidence of progressive, metastatic disease from a cancer of the head, neck, breast or bronchus. From time to time, there is no such evidence and, in a patient who has had previous radiotherapy to this area, the question arises, 'could this be caused by post-radiation fibrosis?' Less common causes include acute brachial neuritis, trauma to the plexus during surgery or anaesthesia, and radiation-induced plexus tumours.

The distinction between recurrent disease and post-radiation fibrosis is important because, if metastatic, hormonal treatment or chemotherapy may be appropriate. Difficulty arises when evidence of post-radiation tissue damage is present, but recurrence is also possible. It has been suggested that only surgical exploration and the passage of time will ultimately confirm the aetiology. After five years of progressive plexopathy without evidence of metastasis, the likelihood of a malignant aetiology becomes progressively smaller and the value of the time factor as a criterion becomes greater. The two conditions do, however, differ in a number of respects (Table 2.7), including the presence or absence of severe pain. In short, painless upper trunk lesions with lymphoedema suggest radiation injury, whereas painful lower trunk lesions with Horner's syndrome point to metastatic infiltration [11].

Case History. A 76-year-old woman who had had a mastectomy at the age of 39 for carcinoma, began to experience pain in the left arm. It increased in extent and intensity over a period of 18 months and was associated with loss of function in the hand and forearm. The arm then swelled up and, although no masses were palpable, a presumptive diagnosis of recurrent breast cancer was made. Treatment with tamoxifen was commenced. Within three months the swelling resolved, but the neurological signs and symptoms did not. The pain had changed to a more superficial, burning discomfort with marked hyperaesthesia. She was treated with tricyclic antidepressants and a small regular dose of oral morphine. This achieved a moderate degree of relief. Tamoxifen prevented progression of the neoplastic process and, at the time of writing, the woman is 82 and living reasonably comfortably with her equally elderly husband. Earlier treatment with tamoxifen might well have prevented her continuing pain and functional disability.

Dysaesthetic Pain

Most pain falls within the general definition of 'an unpleasant sensory and emotional experience associated with actual or potential tissue damage, or described in terms of such damage' [13]. This type of pain may be described as nociceptive. Superficial burning pain (with or without hyperaesthesia) falls into a different category and is best referred to as *dysaesthesia* (Table 2.8). The importance of this distinction relates to treatment; most peripheral pain responds to analgesics whereas dysaesthetic pain usually does not. Unless the distinction is clearly made at the time of assessment, a patient may be prescribed strong narcotics

33

Causalgia (13)
A nerve syndrome of sustained burning pain after a traumatic nerve lesion combined with vasomotor and pseudomotor dysfunction and later trophic changes.

Dysaesthesia
An unpleasant tingling, stinging or burning sensation.

Hyperaesthesia (13)
Increased sensitivity to a specified stimulation, excluding special senses.

Hypoaesthesia (13)
Decreased sensitivity to a specified stimulation, excluding special senses.

Hyperalgesia (13)
Increased sensitivity to noxious stimulation.

Hypoalgesia (13)
Diminished sensitivity to noxious stimulation.

Neuralgia (13)
Pain in the distribution of a nerve or nerves.
Note: Common usage often implies a paroxysmal quality. This is especially the case in Europe. More often neuralgia is used for non-paroxysmal pains. The technical usage is as given, and neuralgia should not be reserved for paroxysmal pains.

Neuritis (13)
Inflammation of a nerve or nerves.
Note: Not to be used unless inflammation is thought to be present.

Neuropathy (13)
A disturbance of function or pathological change in a nerve; in one nerve, mononeuropathy; in several nerves, mononeuropathy multiplex; symmetrical and bilateral, polyneuropathy.
Note: Neuritis is a special case of neuropathy and is now reserved for inflammatory processes affecting nerves. Neuropathy is not intended to cover cases like neurapraxia, neuronotmesis, or section of a nerve.

Table 2.7 Metastatic v radiation-induced brachial plexopathy

	Metastatic	Radiation-induced
I Criteria for diagnosis:		
Surgical exploration	Malignancy found in the plexus.	Extensive fibrosis, no neoplasm.
Distant metastases	If multiple, suggests neoplasm, even if tissue diagnosis negative.	If none after 3 years, suggests not neoplastic.
Other	Initial symptoms precede radiation.	Radiation given for non-malignant condition.
II Characteristics†	Pain, paraesthesia and numbness more prominent than weakness in both.	
	Pain usually a steady severe ache, occasionally with burning component.	
	Hyperaesthesia and shooting pains uncommon.	
	Both types tend to follow a progressive downhill course.	
	A few patients experience lessening or disappearance of pain with progression.	
Symptom-free interval	2 months to 16 years‡ (mean 6.5 years)	5 months to 20 years (mean 6.5 years)
If < 1 year after radiation	< 6000 cGy	> 6000 cGy
Severe pain	80% (always an early symptom)	20% (onset sometimes late)
Neurological deficit	C7–8, T1 (72%)	C5–6 (78%)
	+ epidural spread (32%)	
Horner's syndrome	more common	less common
Lymphoedema	less common	more common
Duration of progression	8 months to 6 years (mean 2.5 years)	2 to 30 years (mean 9 years)
Outcome	Death: 8 months to 7 years (mean 4 years)	Survive; 2 to 38 years (mean 11 years)

† After Thomas and Colby, 1972 [11] and Kori et al 1981 [12]
‡ In one patient known to us, the latent period was 37 years

unwittingly, and the dose increased progressively without benefit. The use of a strong narcotic when it is of little or no analgesic value is far more likely to precipitate unwanted side effects.

Table 2.8   Neurological classification of cancer pain

Nociceptive
Nerve compression
Mixed nerve compression and destruction
(partly dysaesthetic)
Nerve destruction (dysaesthetic)
(a) peripheral nerve
(b) cord lesion

Constant superficial burning pain (dysaesthesia) with or without hyperaesthesia, occurs when a tumour infiltrates and causes destruction of a peripheral nerve, nerve plexus, nerve root, or spinal cord. Infiltration is rare in comparison with compression. Investigation is as for nerve and cord compression.

Post-radical Neck Dissection Pain
Some patients experience pain after radical neck dissection as a result of surgical injury or interruption of the cervical nerves. It is dysaesthetic in character. Intermittent stabbing pain may also be present.

Postherpetic Neuralgia
This is included because herpes zoster is not uncommon in patients with cancer, particularly in those with depressed immune responses as a result of chemotherapy or corticosteroids. Pain is not always present, even at the time of the initial eruption. In those who have pain, a proportion will go on to develop postherpetic neuralgia. Commonly, when questioned closely the patient will report several different components to his pain, all in the area of the affected dermatome(s) [14]:

1   a superficial burning pain—most intense at the anterior or posterior limits;
2   hyperaesthesia—which makes all cutaneous stimulation extremely unpleasant;
3   a stabbing pain—this may be precipitated by a relatively minor stimulus, such as extremes of temperature and the wind;
4   a dull ache—especially in the scarred area.

Many patients do not have all four components. The superficial burning pain is the most constant; it is not always accompanied by hyperaesthesia. Some patients are, in fact, hypoaesthetic in the area in which they experience burning sensation. The treatment of dysaesthetic pain is discussed in Chapter 16.

Spinal Cord and Cauda Equina Compression

Spinal cord or cauda equina compression occurs in about 5 per cent of all cancer patients. It is a devastating complication. It usually results from the distortion of a vertebral body or pedicle by a metastasis (Table 2.9).

Table 2.9   Spinal cord compression — classification by mode of spread

	Spread from	Example	% of total
1	Vertebral body or pedicle metastasis	Breast Bronchus Prostate	85%
2	Intevertebral foramina from paravertebral nodes	Lymphoma	10%
3	Intramedullary metastases		4%
4	Haematogenous spread to epidural space		1%

Adapted form Posner, 1977 [15]

Table 2.10   Spinal cord compression — signs and symptoms at presentation†

Pain	80–96%
Weakness	76–97%
Sensory level	51–90%‡
Sphincter dysfunction	40–75%

† Data collated from references [15–21]
‡ Patient may be unaware of sensory loss until examined, especially in the sacral area

Collapse of the vertebral body may or may not be present. About two-thirds of those developing cord compression have carcinoma of the breast, bronchus, or prostate. Of the rest, most will be associated with either renal carcinoma, lymphoma, myeloma, melanoma, sarcoma, or cancer of the head or neck. Eighty per cent occur in the thoracic region, 2 per cent cervical, 2 per cent lumbar (including compression of the cauda equina); the rest occur at the junctions between these regions.

The first symptom is usually pain (Table 2.10) which may have been present from as little as 1 day to as much as 2 years. It is generally exacerbated by coughing, sneezing, and straining. The nature of the pain varies according to the site of compression (Table 2.11). Local pain is not

Table 2.11   Pain associated with spinal cord compression

Site	Local bone pain	Referred pain (cord compression or nerve root pain)
Cervical	May or may not be present	80%
Thoracic	May or may not be present	55%
Lumbar	May or may not be present	90%

Adapted from Posner, 1977 [15]

always present, and may be masked by previously prescribed analgesics. Local tenderness is common. Root pain is often unilateral in cervical or lumbosacral compression, but generally bilateral in patients with a thoracic lesion. True cord compression pain (as distinct from associated root pain) is non-dermatomal in distribution and bilateral. It may be present as a garter or cuff of pain around the thighs, knees or calves. Some patients with cord compression experience more pain when lying flat (therefore worse at night) whereas, with peripheral nerve compression, rest usually reduces pain intensity (therefore nights not disturbed by pain). With thoracic compression, almost all patients have an upgoing plantar response.

Plain X-rays are positive in 80 per cent; an isotope bone scan in 85 per cent. If the plain X-rays are normal, one should proceed directly to a myelogram. As 10 per cent of patients deteriorate after lumbar puncture, the myelogram should be done after consultation with a neurosurgeon with provision to proceed to immediate laminectomy should the patient's condition worsen (see Chapter 4).

Degenerative disc disease, osteoporosis, and epidural spinal cord compression are the most common differential diagnoses to consider in cancer patients complaining of neck or back pain. Degenerative disc disease is rare at C7, T1 or L1. Radiographic differentiation of osteoporosis from osseous metastases may be difficult, especially in the presence of vertebral body collapse. Tomography and CT scan usually allow a distinction to be made. In osteoporotic vertebral body collapse, tomography shows intact vertebral body bony plates and symmetrical collapse. In metastatic disease, the vertebral plates are eroded with associated pedicle destruction and asymmetrical collapse of the body.

Pain in Paraplegia
Three kinds of pain are reported by paraplegia patients [22]:

38

1 *root pain* (or 'girdle pain') localized at or near the level of the cord lesion;
2 *visceral pain* which usually accompanies a distended bladder or bowel;
3 *phantom body pain* which is felt in the areas of complete sensory loss.

More than one-quarter of paraplegics with partial or total spinal cord lesions complain of burning, tingling pain (dysaesthesia) in segments of the body below the level of the lesion. These pains are sometimes replaced by:

'Severe, crushing pressure, by vice-like pinching sensations, by streams of fire running down the leg to the feet and out of the toes, or by a pain produced by the pressure of a knife being buried in the tissue, twisted around rapidly, and finally withdrawn all at the same time.' [23]

These pains may occur after total or partial spinal cord lesions at any level. Some consider that they occur most after lesions of the cauda equina [22, 24]. The onset of pain may be immediate, though commonly the onset is delayed for months or years after injury. In the most severely affected, the pain may recur for years without remitting. Because of the prolonged latent period, few patients with malignant paraplegia experience them. It is necessary, however, to be aware of the phenomenon.

Meningeal Carcinomatosis

Meningeal carcinomatosis is the term used to describe the presence of multiple carcinomatous seedlings on the meninges of the brain and spinal cord. There may also be concomitant invasion of the central nervous system and nerve roots. Pain may be of several types [25]:

1 frontal headache (50 per cent),
2 back pain (46 per cent) (commonly lumbosacral),
3 root pain(s) (32 per cent),
4 neck pain (2 per cent).

Steroid Withdrawal Pain

It has been known for many years that patients receiving corticosteroids for rheumatoid arthritis occasionally develop a syndrome comprising diffuse pains in muscles, tendons, joints and bones, general malaise and pyrexia, asthenia and, sometimes, neuropsychological disturbances. Patients may experience cramps, and the muscular pain may have a burning quality about it, particularly in the intercostals. This condition has been termed *steroid pseudorheumatism* (Table 2.12). An identical

39

Table 2.12   Steroid withdrawal pain or pseudorheumatism [26]

Myalgia and cramps	Malaise
Arthralgia with swelling	Pyrexia
Tendon pains	Tachycardia
Bone pains	Restlessness
Weakness	Emotional lability
Fatigue	Memory deficit

syndrome is sometimes seen in patients receiving large doses of cortico-steroids, or when the dose in such patients is reduced rapidly to a lower maintenance level. The most likely to be affected are:

1 lymphoma and other patients receiving 100 mg of prednisolone daily for several days in association with chemotherapy;
2 patients with spinal cord compression, incipient or actual, receiving 100 mg of dexamethasone for several days;
3 patients on relatively high doses of dexamethasone to reduce intra-cranial pressure caused by brain metastases;
4 on reduction from high dose to low dose;
5 on reduction of average maintenance dose after prolonged course.

Review! Review! Review!

Otherwise known as reassessment, the dictum 'Review! Review! Review!' is basic to cancer pain management. With cancer, one is dealing with a progressive process. This means that new pains may develop or old pains re-emerge. It should not be assumed that a fresh complaint of pain merely calls for an increase in the dose of an analgesic. A new complaint of pain demands reassessment, an explanation to the patient and, only then, modification of drug therapy or other intervention.

The probability that the initial prescription will be inadequate increases with the intensity of pain. Patients should be reassessed within 1 to 2 hours if the pain is overwhelming, or after 1 to 2 days if severe or moderate. If troublesome or unacceptable side effects result, treatment may need to be modified. In addition, the relief of the major pain may allow a second less severe pain to surface.

Case History. An 85-year-old man with carcinoma of the prostate and right femoral metastatic pain was treated with aspirin and morphine. The next day he indicated that, although less severe, pain was still present. Further questioning revealed that the site of pain was now retrosternal and epigastric; he had no femoral pain at all. The dose of morphine was left unaltered, and the prescription of an antacid resulted in complete relief.

In the case of the man with seven pains (Figure 2.1), it was necessary to review progress in relation to each pain. On the second day, he was reluctant to admit that several pains were less intense but, as judged by his reactions to passive movement, they undoubtedly were. Possibly his reluctance was due to a shifting baseline of reference. It was necessary to point out the difference observed by the doctor and to encourage him to recognize that the pains were beginning to ease. It was a case of 'chipping away' at his total pain until, after a week, he was sufficiently more comfortable to be able to sit up in bed.

References

1 Gray J. A pain in the neck—and shoulder. *Pain Topics* 1977: **1**: 6.

2 Twycross RG and Fairfield S. Pain in far-advanced cancer. *Pain* 1982; **14**: 303–310.

3 Granek, I, Ashikari R and Foley KM. Postmastectomy pain syndrome: clinical and anatomical correlates. In press.

4 McKillop JH and McDougall IR. The role of skeletal scanning in clinical oncology. *British Medical Journal* 1980; **281**: 407–409.

5 Schutte HE. The influence of bone pain on the results of bone scans. *Cancer* 1979; **44**: 2039–2043.

6 Kori SH, Krol G and Foley KM. Computed tomographic evaluation of bone and soft tissue metastases in *Bone Metastases* edited by Weiss L and Gilbert HA. GK Hall, Boston 1981, *pp* 245–257.

7 Procacci P and Zoppi M. Pathophysiology and clinical aspects of visceral and referred pain in *Advances in Pain Research and Therapy Volume 5*, edited by Bonica, JJ, Lindblom U and Iggo A. Raven Press, New York 1982, pp 643–658.

8 Travell J and Rinzler SH. The myofascial genesis of pain. *Postgraduate Medicine (Minneapolis)* 1952; **11**: 425–434.

9 Sola AE. Myofascial trigger point therapy. *Resident and Staff Physician* 1981; **27**: 38–45.

10 Boop WC and Fisher JA. Methods of pain control in *Cancer of the Head and Neck* edited by Suen JY and Myers EN. Churchill, New York 1981, pp 821–838.

11 Thomas JE and Colby MY. Radiation-induced or metastatic brachial plexopathy: a diagnostic dilemma. *Journal of the American Medical Association* 1972; **222**: 1392–1395.

12 Kori SH, Foley KM and Posner JB. Brachial plexus lesions in patients with cancer: 100 cases. *Neurobiology* 1981; **31:** 45–50.

13 IASP Subcommittee on Taxonomy. Pain terms: a list with definitions and notes on usage. *Pain* 1980; **8:** 249–252.

14 Raftery H. The management of post herpetic pain using sodium valproate and amitriptyline. *Journal of the Irish Medical Association* 1979; **72:** 399–401.

15 Posner JB. Spinal cord metastases (including cauda equina): diagnosis and treatment in *Neuro-Oncology.* Department of Neurology, MS-K Cancer Center, New York, 1977, pp 19–32.

16 Bright J and McKissock W. Surgical treatment of extradural spinal tumours. *British Medical Journal* 1965; **1:** 1341–4.

17 Gilbert R W, Kim JH and Posner JB. Epidural spinal cord compression from metastatic tumours: diagnosis and treatment. *Annals of Neurology* 1978; **3:** 40–51.

18 Livingstone KE and Perrin RG. The neurosurgical management of spinal metastases causing cord and cauda equina compression. *Journal of Neurosurgery* 1978; **49:** 839–843.

19 Greenberg HS, Kim JH and Posner JB. Epidural spinal cord compression from metastatic tumour: results with a new treatment protocol. *Annals of Neurology* 1979; **8:** 361–366.

20 Young RF, Post EM and King GA. Treatment of spinal epidural metastases. Randomized prospective comparison of laminectomy and radiotherapy. *Journal of Neurosurgery* 1980; **53:** 741–748.

21 Briggs M. Personal Communication (1981).

22 Guttman L. *Spinal Injuries: Comprehensive Management and Research.* Blackwell, Oxford 1973.

23 Davis L and Martin J. Studies upon spinal cord injuries. II. The nature and treatment of pain. *Journal of Neurosurgery* 1947; **4:** 483–491.

24 Botterell EH, Callaghan JC and Jonsse AT. Pain in paraplegia: clinical management and surgical treatment. *Proceedings of the Royal Society of Medicine* 1954; **47:** 281–288.

25 Olson ME, Chernik NL and Posner JB. Infiltration of the leptomeninges by systemic cancer: a clinical and pathologic study. *Archives of Neurology* 1974; **30:** 122–137.

26 Rotstein J and Good RA. Steroid pseudorheumatism. *AMA Archives of Internal Medicine* 1957; **99:** 545–555.

Chapter Three

Pain — A Broader Concept

As stressed in Chapter 1, pain is a dual phenomenon. One part is the perception of a sensation and the other the patient's emotional reaction to it. An individual's sensitivity to pain varies with mood and morale. Attention must be given to factors that modulate pain sensitivity such as anxiety, depression, fatigue, boredom, loneliness and hostility (Table 3.1).

Table 3.1 Factors affecting pain threshold

Threshold lowered	Threshold raised
Discomfort	Relief of symptoms
Insomnia	Sleep
Fatigue	Rest
Anxiety	Sympathy
Fear	Understanding
Anger	Companionship
Sadness	Diversional activity
Depression	Reduction in anxiety
Boredom	Elevation of mood
Introversion	
Mental isolation	Analgesics
Social abandonment	Anxiolytics
	Antidepressants

Death is perhaps the loneliest experience many of us will ever have to face.

Most patients fear the pain of cancer. Cancer and pain are synonymous in the public consciousness. This image is reinforced by graphic television presentations, and by books and magazines. Many patients can relate tales of a hospital room-mate, neighbour or relative who 'died in agony'. Even before the onset of any pain, such memories will haunt the cancer patient and seriously undermine his self-confidence:

'I know I will have a lot of pain.'
'I won't be able to cope with the pain.'
'I'll kill myself if I have a lot of pain.'
'I will die in pain.'
'I will lose control and go crazy with pain.'

These fears often remain unspoken unless the patient is given the opportunity by his doctor to express them and talk about his progress or lack of it (Table 3.2). A patient may need 'permission to talk'. He may feel

Table 3.2   Treating the fear of cancer pain

---

1   Assume the fear exists.
2   Elicit patient's feelings and thoughts regarding their fear of pain in the initial discussion of the treatment plan.
3   Be alert for any unrealistic beliefs/expectations the patient has.
4   *Actively* give realistic information at a level patient can understand.
5   Encourage patient to be an active participant in his pain management.
6   State your own positive belief and expectation that whatever pain the patient experiences can be managed adequately.
7   Follow through consistently with good pain management so trust and security increases and patient's fears decrease.
8   Assume changes in patient's physical/emotional status will affect fear level and continue ongoing process of dealing with fear.

From Hattem, 1981 [1]

inhibited because 'Doctor hasn't got time', or 'Doctor is too busy to be concerned with my problems'. A question such as, 'Are you worried about yourself?' may enable the patient to speak more openly. However, an honest answer is unlikely if the question comes from an unknown doctor standing at the foot of the bed (*see* Chapter 18).

Sir David Smithers, sometime Director of the Department of Radiotherapy, Royal Marsden Hospital, made it a rule that his registrar (resident) should visit terminally ill patients each day [2]. He said that however brilliant a clinical pharmacologist a doctor may be, if he has no time for chat, he knows nothing about terminal care. In this context, chat means 'patient chat' while the doctor listens. Although demanding of both time and emotion, the benefits are considerable. To quote from the experience of one group of general practitioners:

'As the doctor–patient relationship improved, many doctors found they could reduce the drugs. As the true diagnosis of the patient's pain became clear and the patient was helped to deal with the pain of dying, there was less need for sedatives, tranquillizers, and analgesics.' [3]

The control of pain in a patient with advanced cancer requires comprehensive management which considers all sources of distress, whether physical, psychological, spiritual or social. Emotional responses have considerable influence on the experience and perception of pain. Dame Cicely Saunders, Medical Director of St. Christopher's Hospice, England, maintains that a caring person who listens and tries to understand the patient's experience of pain is one of the most important modalities of treatment [4]. The dying have a fundamental need for someone to spend time visiting and listening to them [5, 6].

An example of this appeared in an article describing a vocational training course for general practitioners [7]. At a weekly seminar, patients encountered in routine work were discussed by the trainees in order to demonstrate that psychological factors exist even in apparently straightforward physical illness and vice versa. On one occasion, discussion centred on a patient with bone metastases from disseminated breast cancer whose back pain remained unrelieved by narcotic analgesics. During the seminar, it was suggested that the pain was intractable because the woman was angry as her doctors and relatives would not admit that she was dying or discuss the problems this created. Subsequently, a full and frank discussion confirmed that this was the correct explanation; honest communication resulted in a marked improvement in her mental state and the pain in her back no longer troubled her.

Although the doctor is no longer able to control the disease itself, causing frustration to both physician and patient, it is necessary to establish and maintain a basis of trust. Even mild pain should be taken seriously. This establishes confidence that the doctor does care and has the skills to prevent major discomfort. Such confidence will be a powerful ally if pain becomes a greater problem later on. Confidence is crucial to successful pain management.

The patient may initially resist taking analgesics because of a lifelong habit of never giving in or resorting to drugs. Other reasons for resistance may be fear of constipation, addiction, nightmares experienced with certain drugs in the past, or confusion observed in another patient. These habits and fears need to be identified through sensitive inquiry and adequate history taking. Once the cause for resistance is known, it can be dealt with by discussion and education. It may be necessary to proceed on a step-by-step basis rather than introducing too many new tablets or medicines all at once.

Total Pain

To help emphasize the emotional complexities of pain in advanced cancer, Saunders has coined the phrase 'total pain' [8]. This concept includes aetiological components other than the noxious physical stimulus, namely, psychological, social, spiritual and bureaucratic. Patients with cancer sometimes describe their whole life as painful. Those caring for them must be concerned with all aspects of distress and discomfort [9, 10], if the perception of physical pain is to be alleviated. Although the clinician may be able to discriminate between separate areas of 'life pain', the patient often cannot. To him his pain is total and all enveloping.

Psychological Pain

Persistent cancer pain can be thought of as a vicious circle: physical pain arouses anxiety, anxiety may lead to depression, anxiety or depression causes insomnia, and these in turn exacerbate pain [11, 12]. Control will not be achieved unless pain is viewed and treated with all these components in mind (Figure 3.1).

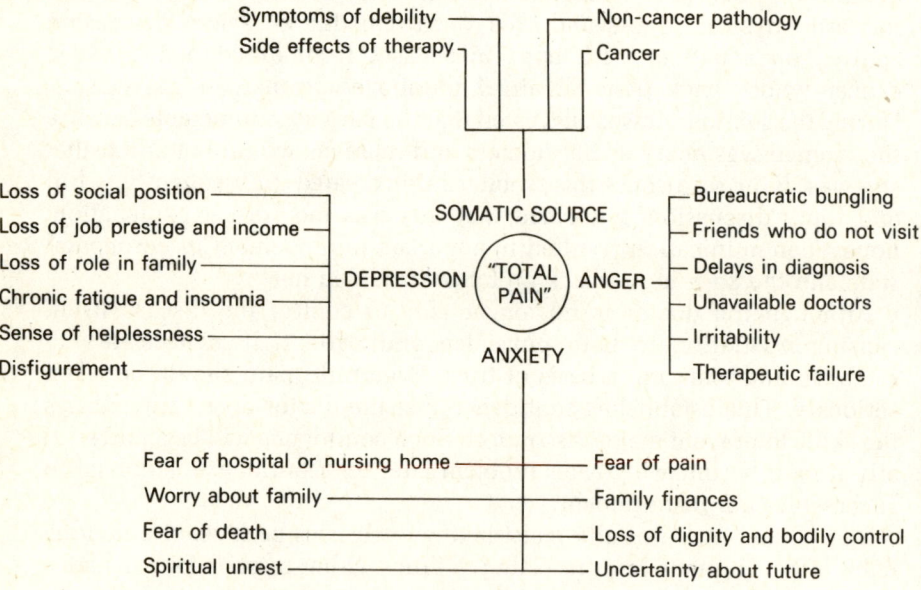

Figure 3.1 Pain is a somatopsychic experience: a diagram indicating some of the many non-physical influences that modify a patient's perception of pain.

Anxiety and depression are part of the long-term nature of advanced cancer pain. Patients whose pain has lasted many months are anxious as they look into the future and anticipate only an increase in pain. Anxiety is also caused by the meaning of the pain. For the cancer patient pain has a sinister meaning and new or worsening pain implies further physical deterioration. Pain takes on an added importance; suffering seems inextricably related to death. The clinical problem of cancer pain includes the problem of attitude toward the pain and towards the illness itself. Hinton states that the incidence of anxiety is greater among those who experience a long terminal illness. He also finds that young people are more anxious during a terminal illness than are older people, with the greatest anxiety and depression occurring in those dying patients under age 50 with young dependent children [13].

Case History. A 56-year-old man had become paraplegic from spinal prostate metastases. He had been in a general hospital for 11 weeks following his paraplegia—which was diagnosed too late for effective treatment—and he was considered terminal. He lay in the hospital with no knowledge of why he had become paraplegic, no knowledge that it had anything to do with his cancer which he thought was cured, with no physiotherapy and few visits from his physician. He received nursing care and was turned every two hours; he had a large sacral bedsore. Thus, he spent two hours out of every four facing the wall instead of the door. This increased his depression and depression increased the pain. Transfer to a hospice, physiotherapy, honesty about his disease and explanation about future expectations, enabled him to be a wheelchair rehabilitated and go home for another three months. Drug doses were unchanged. He required readmission to The Connecticut Hospice for only 24 hours before he died.

Social Pain

Social pain includes the pain of separation. Patients appreciate that they are going to be separated from their family by death. So often the hospital seems to hasten that separation by restrictions on visiting. Nothing that is done in the care of these people should separate them from their family and friends. A patient's pain may be better relieved by allowing grandchildren to visit than by increasing narcotic dosage.

Social isolation contributes to social pain. Friends tend to visit less those who are dying. A bedfast patient on The Connecticut Hospice Home Care programme was distressed when, about a month before her death, church members stopped visiting her. The patient was at a loss to explain this phenomenon, but the feeling of abandonment caused her to focus on her pain. A volunteer began visiting her regularly. Another volunteer, a lay preacher, diplomatically contacted her church and held a series of educational meetings for the members. Gradually they began to trickle back into the home. Arranging for social involvement was important in the management of her pain.

Pain may also relate to interpersonal problems, as shown in the following account.

Case History. A 45-year-old man with advanced pancreatic cancer became so angry and depressed by his deterioration that he disrupted his whole household. He had always been a domineering father, but when suffering from persistent pain, this tendency took on an angry and vicious aspect. Two of his teenage sons ran away from home and his wife tried to commit suicide. At this point he was admitted to The Connecticut Hospice. His pain was greatly exacerbated by the family problems the pain itself had caused. With the help of the social worker, the runaways were found and, in time, brought back into the family. These aspects of care, together with drug therapy, relieved his pain and he, in turn, was then able to establish normal family relationships.

Financial Pain

Case History. A 38-year-old Italian immigrant had come to America with his wife and three small children in the hope of making his fortune. He had set up a small business in horticulture and had minimal medical insurance. He was then found to have advanced carcinoma of the rectum. He was referred to Connecticut Hospice Home Care because of intractable rectal and abdominal pain. When the pain had been reduced by analgesics, he was more able to talk about his problem. It became clear that a main source of his pain was financial. Anxiety over his $12,000 hospital bill exacerbated perception of the organic component of his pain. He knew he was leaving his wife and three young children, a barely-started horticultural business, and a hospital bill which they were trying to pay off at the rate of $50 a week. No increase in morphine dose would render him pain-free while the large bill remained unpaid.

Spiritual Pain

Case History. A Christian woman was in hospital dying of cancer. She was in constant pain. This and the prospect of death created tremendous anxiety. Several relatives spent much of the day with the woman but this appeared not to help. A Church Visitor invited the family members present to pray there and then with her and the patient. Although initially self-conscious, their discomfort gave way to a sense of serenity as they prayed together. The patient's pain completely subsided and, a few days later, she died peacefully in her sleep. Her sister subsequently phoned the Church Visitor to thank her for her help. 'We were all praying for Betty individually, but none of us had realized the importance of praying together *with* her. The experience has deepened our relationship with God and with one another.' [14]

As with much in terminal care and more specifically, in the management of pain, the contribution of any one person or treatment is not generally as dramatic as this. The story is included, in part, to help redress the tendency of the modern doctor to undervalue the role of the clergy and their helpers.

Acute and Chronic Pain

Acute and chronic pain are distinct entities. Severe acute pain is accompanied by a 'fight or flight' response, seen also in acute anxiety. In chronic pain, vegetative features tend to predominate, features which are also commonly seen in organic depression (Table 3.3). This means that a patient may be in severe pain yet not look distressed (*see* Chapter 2). It is all too easy for a doctor, with no experience of chronic pain, to forget this distinction. Doctors' understanding of pain is usually taken from their own experience of acute pain—toothache, headache, bruise or sprain—all of which pass relatively quickly. In contrast, chronic pain is a situation rather than an event and:

1   It is impossible to predict when it will end.
2   It often gets worse rather than better.
3   It lacks positive meaning.
4   It frequently expands to occupy the patient's whole attention and isolates him from the world around him.

Chronic cancer pain is, however, as distinct from chronic pain of non-malignant origin as the latter is from acute pain. Cancer patients in pain exhibit a mixture of both 'fight and flight' and vegetative reactions (Table 3.3). The former is particularly manifest when pain is associated with symptoms of deterioration, such as anorexia, weight loss, decreasing exercise tolerance, and increasing physical dependence. For the patient, this constellation of signs and symptoms has inescapable significance. The message from his body states clearly: 'Unless a miracle happens, I cannot survive for long.' The patient realizes that he is on 'a collision course with death'. Such a realization, even if partly subconscious, evokes an instinctive autonomic response.

'Chronic Pain Syndrome'

In the USA, for up to 10 years, some 30 major units have been treating patients with intractable chronic pain of non-malignant origin. A significant number of such patients have complex social problems and similar patterns of health care utilization. The term 'chronic pain syndrome' (CPS) [15] has been used to describe such cases. A clear distinction must be made between the characteristics and treatment of the CPS patient and

Table 3.3 Acute and chronic pain

	Acute	Chronic
Time course	Transient	Persistent
Meaning to patient	Positive: draws attention to injury or illness	Negative: serves no useful purpose Positive: as patient obtains secondary gain
Accompanying features	Fight or Flight: 1 pupillary dilatation 2 increased sweating 3 increased respiratory rate 4 increased heart rate 5 shunting of blood from viscera to muscles	Vegetative: 1 sleep disturbance 2 anorexia 3 decreased libido 4 constipation 5 somatic preoccupation 6 personality change 7 work inhibition

the cancer pain patient. CPS patients have become dependent on their painful situation as a complex excuse to avoid the challenges of life. They obtain considerable 'secondary gain' from their suffering and have a vested interest in maintaining ill health [16]. They exhibit 'pain behaviour' which has the perpetuation of the sick role as its goal. To achieve this, additional roles may be adopted, such as the 'medication dependent role', the 'rehabilitation role', and the 'diagnosis confounding role' [17]. These patients have been treated by a regimen of 'operant conditioning' (Table 3.4). Operant conditioning focuses on overt pain behaviour and

Table 3.4 Operant conditioning for management of 'chronic pain syndrome'

1 'Contingency contract' between staff and patient specifying goals.
2 Pain behaviour identified and ignored by treatment team.
3 Non-drug treatments, including physical therapy, phased out.
4 Exercise and activities reinforced.
5 Drugs phased out using Fordyce 'Pain Cocktail' method.
6 Assignment to 'work station' in hospital.
7 Family taught to:
   (a) identify pain behaviour
   (b) ignore pain behaviour
   (c) reinforce activity.

After Fordyce, 1981 [18, 19]

seeks to reduce it by modifying the environmental consequences of the patient's actions. This method includes elements very different from the attention needed by the cancer pain patient.

Many CPS patients experience pain in the absence of tissue damage or likely pathological cause. The diagnostic conclusion is that the pain is precipitated and maintained by psychological factors. The patient with advanced cancer almost always has a significant organic cause as the source of pain, though pain perception may be heightened by psychological factors. Secondary gain is not a significant factor and behaviour modification has little or no part to play in treatment. Cancer patients are frequently not properly assessed but, when they are, treatment almost always brings considerable or complete relief. Many CPS patients confound diagnosis and fail to respond to treatment. In order to modify the patients' behaviour, advocates of operant conditioning withhold the attention and benefits that these patients have achieved through their chronic pain role. In contrast, good cancer pain management seeks to support the cancer patient by provision of adequate medication, rest and attention. Non-verbal clues to pain are carefully sought and responded to with appropriate medication and non-drug treatment. Freed from the burden of seeking such help, the patient is enabled to relax and focus on matters of importance to him during the last weeks of his life.

There have been several recent articles on 'chronic pain' [16, 17] in the American medical and nursing press advocating elements of behaviour modification. The irrelevance of such methods for chronic cancer pain must be clearly understood.

Overwhelming Cancer Pain

After several weeks or months of pain, particularly if associated with insomnia, many cancer patients become overwhelmed by pain. Pain envelops their whole mental outlook. Such patients often find it difficult to describe the location or the nature of the pain precisely:

> 'But I'm all pain, doctor.'
> 'The pain is in my chest and in my back and my arm and my head—it's really all over.'
> 'I feel as if my body is enclosed in a pressure balloon and the balloon is slowly collapsing, squeezing every bone and every joint in my body as it closes around me.'

The last statement was made by a woman with a clearly defined site of breast metastasis and source of pain in the lumbar spine. She had earlier described her pain as a knife sticking into her back. By the time she was admitted to St. Christopher's Hospice, she had developed paraparesis and a bedsore, and her entire life had become one pain.

In the majority the response to the pain is vegetative; the patient withdraws mentally and physically, and looks depressed. In some, notably those whose pain is markedly exacerbated, signs of anxiety predominate (Table 3.5). To emphasize this distinction, we have styled overwhelming pain in which withdrawal/depression is prominent as Type 1, and that in which anxiety is prominent as Type 2. A mixture of agitated and depressive features commonly coexist.

In all cases of overwhelming pain, the key to success is breaking the vicious circle of insomnia—fatigue—pain—insomnia. Because the patient is exhausted and demoralized, it may take 3 to 6 weeks to achieve maximum relief. Unless this is understood, staff and patient morale can drop irretrievably after a few days if troublesome pain persists. On the other hand, the doctor can and should promise some early improvement, particularly in relation to rest and comfort at night.

With both types it is advisable, if possible, to review the first day's treatment before deciding on the medication for the first night. Some patients will seem dependent on their former inadequate medication. Presumably this is because it is the best they have had so far. They may be determined that no one, not even the doctor, is going to deprive them of it. In this circumstance, the patient should be allowed to keep his old medication and to use it as necessary *in addition to the new medication*

Table 3.5 Overwhelming pain

Severe pain compounded by:
Insomnia
Fatigue
Mental exhaustion
Loss of morale
Distrust of caregivers

Type 1	*Type 2*
Physical reluctance	Fear of movement or being moved
Depression	Marked anxiety/agitation
Dependence on present	Generally does not have faith
unsatisfactory medication	in any medication

Note: These patients look in pain
May take 3 to 6 weeks to achieve maximum benefit
Initial key to success = obtaining pain-free sleep-full night
Regard Type 2 as a medical emergency: treat with combination of analgesic and anxiolytic

provided it is not an agonist-antagonist (*see* Chapter 15). The patient can be provided with a chart to record when and how much of the old medication is taken.

In Type 2, it is always necessary to begin treatment with both an analgesic *and an anxiolytic*. The choice and dose of each will depend to a large extent on what the patient had previously been taking. If this included narcotic injections, it may be necessary to continue these until the pain is better controlled as the patient cannot accept that an oral preparation will suffice. When more comfortable, the patient will become confident of the doctor's ability to relieve his pain and a progressive changeover to oral medication becomes possible. Type 2 overwhelming pain is best regarded as a medical emergency and a corresponding amount of physician time must be allocated if success is to be achieved. Ideally, one experienced doctor should be responsible for all the medical aspects of care over the first few days in order to establish a satisfactory relationship with both the patient and family.

It is, of course, possible to have marked anxiety and severe pain without the pain being truly overwhelming. Moderate anxiety will usually lessen when pain is relieved and the patient's fears and concerns addressed. Extreme anxiety is not always immediately apparent but may be manifested in one or more of the following ways:

1 attention seeking behaviour,
2 fear of being left alone,
3 hyperkinesis,

4 misperceptions—usually unpleasant,
5 hallucinations—usually unpleasant,
6 nightmares,
7 continued insomnia despite pain relief.

Generally, these patients also need to be prescribed both an analgesic and an anxiolytic.

References

1 Hattem JM. *Treating The Fear of Cancer Pain*. Unpublished paper presented, Third World Congress on Pain, Edinburgh 1981.

2 Smithers D. Where to die? *British Medical Journal* 1973; **1:** 34–35.

3 Harte JD. Personal communication.

4 Saunders CM. Caring for the dying in *The Hour of Our Death*, edited by Lack Sa and Lamerton R. Chapman, London 1975, pp 18–27.

5 Kubler-Ross E. *On Death and Dying*. MacMillan Co, New York 1969.

6 Hinton J. Talking with people about to die. *British Medical Journal* 1974; **3:** 25–27.

7 Special correspondent. Vocational training for general practice. *British Medical Journal* 1971; **2:** 704–705.

8 Saunders CM. *The Management of Terminal Illness*. Hospital Medicine Publications, London 1967.

9 Lack SA. Philosophy and organisation of a hospice program in *Psychosocial Care of the Dying Patient* edited by Garfield C. University of California Press, San Francisco 1976, pp 2–8.

10 Baines MV. Control of other symptoms in *The Management of Terminal Disease*, edited by Saunders CM. Arnold, London 1978, pp 99–118.

11 Lack SA. I want to die while I'm still alive. *Death Education* 1977; **1:** 165–176.

12 Lipman AG. Drug Therapy in Terminally Ill Patients. *American Journal of Hospital Pharmacy* 1975; **32:** 270–276.

13 Hinton J. The physical and mental distress of the dying. *Quarterly Journal of Medicine* 1963; US **32:** 1–21.

14 Shlemon BL, Linn D and Linn M in *To Heal as Jesus Healed* Ave Maria Press, Notre Dame, Indiana 1978, p 49.

15 Black RG. The Chronic Pain Syndrome. *Clinical Medicine* 1975; **82:** 17–20.

16 Aronoff GM and Wilson RR. How to teach your patients to control chronic pain. *Behavioural Medicine* 1978; **5**: 29–35.

17 Bergman JJ and Werblun MN. Chronic pain. A review for the family physician. *Journal of Family Practice* 1978; **7**: 685–693.

18 Fordyce W. An operant conditioning method for managing chronic pain. *Postgraduate Medicine* 1973; **53**: 123–128.

19 Fordyce W. Personal Communication 1981.

Part Two

Pain Control

Chapter Four

Modification
of Pathological Process

Analgesia (GK 'without pain').
1 A state without pain, brought about by the administration of a drug or procedure that relieves pain.
2 Absence of pain on noxious stimulation [1].

Expectations

Is it always possible to relieve cancer pain? The statistics quoted in Chapter 1 suggest that the answer should be: Yes, almost always. In practice, however, it is impossible to give a precise figure for the proportion of patients who obtain *complete* relief. Take, for example, the case of a 66-year-old man with extravesical recurrence of carcinoma of the bladder. He was exhausted and in great distress because of insomnia caused by round-the-clock frequency of micturition and by pain in the pelvic area and the lower limbs. The frequency and insomnia were both corrected by drug therapy. On the other hand, he continued to experience 'a golf ball' sensation in the perineum, 'but it's not really painful', and intermittent pain in the right L5 dermatome. This was usually mild but, on occasion, could be more troublesome. As *lowering* the dose of morphine did not make the pain worse, it was concluded that this particular pain was probably not significantly narcotic responsive. Yet, because of its minor impact on the patient and because nerve blocks are not always without side effects, it was decided not to proceed with intrathecal phenol.

59

The contrast between the man's condition at his initial outpatient attendance and subsequent ones continued to be considerable, despite occasional trouble with constipation or frayed emotions. Was his pain controlled or was it not? In absolute terms, no: but, in his estimation, yes.

In this connection, it should be noted that at St. Christopher's Hospice, when assessing pain control, patients are divided into two broad categories [2]:

1   those in whom there is 'good relief from pain';
2   those in whom 'pain is difficult to control'.

Although apparently vague and lacking in precision, this is in fact a rational and sensible way of summarizing the degree of relief obtained.

In approaching pain control in advanced cancer, it is necessary to bear in mind:

1   Pain relief is not an 'all or none' phenomenon.
2   All pains are not equally narcotic responsive.
3   Some pains continue to be precipitated by activity and/or weightbearing.
4   Relief is not generally a 'once only' exercise; old pains may re-emerge as the disease progresses, or new pains develop.
5   With careful monitoring of drug treatment, it is often possible to control pain without admission to the hospital.
6   Sometimes it takes 3 to 4 weeks of inpatient treatment to achieve satisfactory relief, notably in those who have movement-induced pain and in those whose pain is compounded by severe anxiety or depression.
7   Pain is not usually the only symptom a patient is experiencing; his suffering is linked to the impact of *all* his symptoms.

Fundamentally a doctor is seeking to help a patient move from a position in which he is mastered by the pain to one in which he establishes mastery over the pain. When a patient is mastered by pain, the pain is on the way to becoming overwhelming and all-embracing (*see* Chapter 3).

When sufficiently improved, patients often say:

'I still have the pain, but it doesn't worry me now.'
'It's still there, but it's not what you'd call pain.'
'I can get on with things and forget it now.'

Of course, the doctor's ultimate aim remains complete relief. In practice partial relief is acceptable provided the patient is significantly more comfortable and physically and mentally rested, *and both patient and family are demonstrating their mastery of the situation*. In this situation there is little or no need to pursue the ultimate goal relentlessly with the application of yet more neurolytic or neurosurgical interventions.

Many cancer patients with persistent pain have expectations which are far lower than they need be. All patients must be assured, when first seen, that the situation can be improved and that it is possible to relieve most, if not all, of their pain. Although sometimes it may take 3 to 4 weeks to achieve maximum control, it is always possible to achieve some improvement within 24 to 48 hours.

It is generally wise to aim at 'graded relief'. Moreover, as some pains respond more readily than others, improvement should be assessed in relation to each pain. The initial target must be a pain-free, sleep-full night. Many patients have not had a good night's rest for weeks or months and are exhausted and demoralized. To sleep through the night pain-free and wake refreshed is a boost to both the doctor's and the patient's morale. Next, one aims for relief at rest in bed or chair during the day; finally, for freedom from pain on movement. The former is always eventually possible; the latter is not. Relief at night and when resting during the day gives the patient new hope and incentive, and enables him to begin to live again despite limited mobility. Freed from the day and nightmare of constant pain, his last weeks or months take on a new look.

The doctor must, however, be determined to succeed and be prepared to spend much time assessing and reassessing the patient's pain and other distressing symptoms. In addition, a balance is needed, learned only from experience, between marking time therapeutically so as to capitalize on the beneficial effect of better sleep and improved morale and pressing on decisively to avoid the situation such as that recorded of a 90-year-old man admitted to a London Hospital with bone pain and who died still in pain 3 months later [3].

Treatment Modalities

There is always more to analgesia then analgesics. To obtain the best results a 'broad spectrum' approach is generally necessary, often using

Table 4.1 Pain control

Explanation
Modification of pathological process
Elevation of pain threshold
Interruption of pain pathways
Modification of lifestyle; Immobilization

several different methods at the same time, rather than adopting a sequential pattern (Table 4.1).

61

Explanation

Explanation of the cause(s) of pain is fundamental to success. The patient needs to understand, to make sense of what is happening. Severe pain that does not make sense or, worse, is seen as a threat to one's way of life or existence is always more intense than pain which is understandable. In advanced cancer, several pains may emerge into a diffuse pattern of increasing discomfort. There is need to help the patient discriminate between his various pains, and so make better sense of them. The point has been well illustrated:

'As the Nazis well understood and demonstrated, meaningless and purposeless torture is much harder for the person to accept and resist than is torture which the subject can place in a coherent frame of reference. A perceived senselessness in the universe weakens our belief that our efforts have validity and point. They appear to be essentially futile. This makes it much harder to continue these efforts, including those of coping with pain and stress.'[4]

Although pain may continue to serve as a reminder of the underlying presence and progression of the disease, explanation by the doctor as to the cause of the pain takes much of the mystery and uncertainty from it:

'The pain here is caused by weakness in the bone, and is probably related to the trouble in your breast. This other pain has nothing to do with the breast: it is caused by arthritis in the hip joint—the sort of arthritis many people get as they grow older.'

Whatever negative attributes continue to surround the pain, explanation cuts it down to size psychologically. For the patient whose pain is all non-malignant in origin, the relief will be even greater. It is folly to initiate other pain control measures without preliminary and repeated explanations about the underlying mechanisms, and it reduces the likelihood of a beneficial response to treatment.

Modification of the Pathological Process

Modification of the pathological process should be considered even in far advanced cancer (Table 4.2). It is important though to ensure that the treatment is not worse than the disease. Moreover, because hormone treatment or chemotherapy has been started, this does not mean that analgesics should be withheld. The effect of such treatment on pain may be delayed for several weeks; in the case of chemotherapy in myeloma for 3 to 4 months. A combined approach is therefore necessary. When relief has been obtained and there are no complaints of 'breakthrough' pain, the analgesic regimen can be modified. The dose of morphine can be reduced or a less strong analgesic prescribed.

In this section, we include comments on the correction of hypercalcaemia (modification of a biochemical sequela of disease) and on the pituitary fossa injection of alcohol (modification of the hormonal milieu of the disease). Though, in view of current thinking about the mechanism of action of the latter, it could equally well have been discussed in Chapter 5 under 'Interruption of Pain Pathways'.

Table 4.2 Modification of pathological process

Radiation therapy
Hormone therapy
Chemotherapy
Surgery
Correction of hypercalcaemia
Pituitary fossa injection of alcohol

Radiation

Irradiation should be considered whenever pain is caused directly or indirectly by an osseous metastasis. Although certain tumours metastasize more readily to bone (Table 4.3), all types can and at times do. The

Table 4.3 Primary sites commonly associated with osseous metastasis

Myeloma	Kidney
Breast	Melanoma
Bronchus	Thyroid
Prostate	

sites most frequently affected are mainly in the axial skeleton—vertebral bodies, proximal end of femur, pelvis, ribs, sternum, proximal end of humerus and parts of the skull (Figure 4.1). When deciding on an appropriate schedule for any given patient, it is necessary to consider [5]:

1 the site of the tumour,
2 the area to be irradiated,
3 life expectancy,
4 degree of debility.

In relation to pain relief, as distinct from tumour control, many centres have moved away from 3000 to 4000 cGy (rad) given over 2 to 4 weeks in 10 to 20 treatments to a single dose schedule wherever possible (Table 4.4). Such an approach is particularly useful in the case of metastases of the limb bones. Fractionation is probably necessary only:

1 when there is a high risk of nausea and vomiting despite prophylactic antiemetics, e.g. when irradiating in the region of L1 (behind the stomach) or when treating half or more of the pelvis;

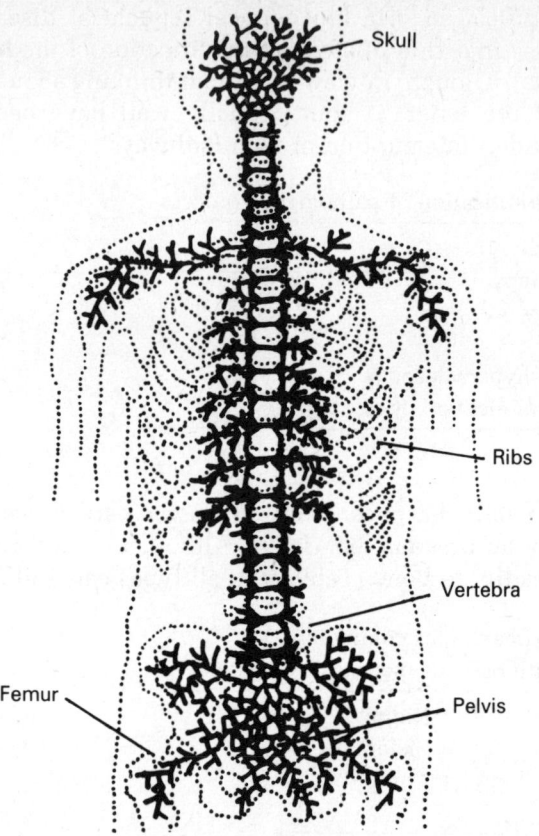

Figure 4.1 Batson's paravertebral venous plexus. Pathway for most osseous metastases.

2   when there is a risk of spinal cord damage (e.g. when irradiating cervical or thoracic vertebrae).

A single dose schedule does, of course, require more time on the one day, and this has to be allowed for. The patient has to be seen and planned, as well as treated. Despite this, there is an overall saving of time both for patient and staff [6].

Radiation therapy gives partial or complete relief in more than 90 per cent of patients experiencing bone pain (Table 4.5), and is associated with recalcification in 80 per cent (Figure 4.2). Radiation is of benefit also in patients experiencing nerve pain caused by compression of one or other of the major plexuses (Table 4.6). Whole-brain irradiation may be indicated; in this circumstance, the patient should be given corticosteroids for several days (prednisolone 30 mg t.i.d.; dexamethasone 4 mg t.i.d.) and

Table 4.4   Short course radiation therapy schedules

cGy (rad)	No. of treatments
2000	4
1800	3
1600	2
1000	1

Table 4.5   Radiation and relief of bone pain in 110 patients (152 treatment fields)

	n	%
Early relief (≤ 2 weeks)	106	70
Early partial relief (≤ 2 weeks) Delayed complete relief (2–12 weeks)	33	22
No relief	13	8
Recurrence of pain	20	14
Permanent relief	119	78

After Allen et al, 1976 [7]
Patients received a range of doses: % relief identical in all treatment groups

Table 4.6   Radiation therapy and pain

Metastatic bone pain
Peripheral nerve compression: brachial plexus
                                              lumbosacral plexus
Cauda equina compression
Spinal cord compression
Raised intracranial pressure†

† Radiotherapy for cerebral secondaries is not generally undertaken in Britain

should be warned that after single dose treatment, he will probably feel 'groggy' for two to three days, and may be drowsy and disorientated. The patient's relatives should also be forewarned.

Spinal cord compression. When pain is thought to be caused by compression of the spinal cord or cauda equina, dexamethasone should be prescribed immediately and radiotherapy commenced as soon as possible. Opinions differ as to the optimum dose of dexamethasone. Most centres prescribe 16 to 20 mg a day in divided dosage. Some start with an IV loading dose of 20 mg. At the Memorial Sloan-Kettering Cancer Center, 100 mg IV is given initially [8]. This dose is repeated by mouth for three days after which it is rapidly tapered to 16 mg (4 mg q.i.d.).

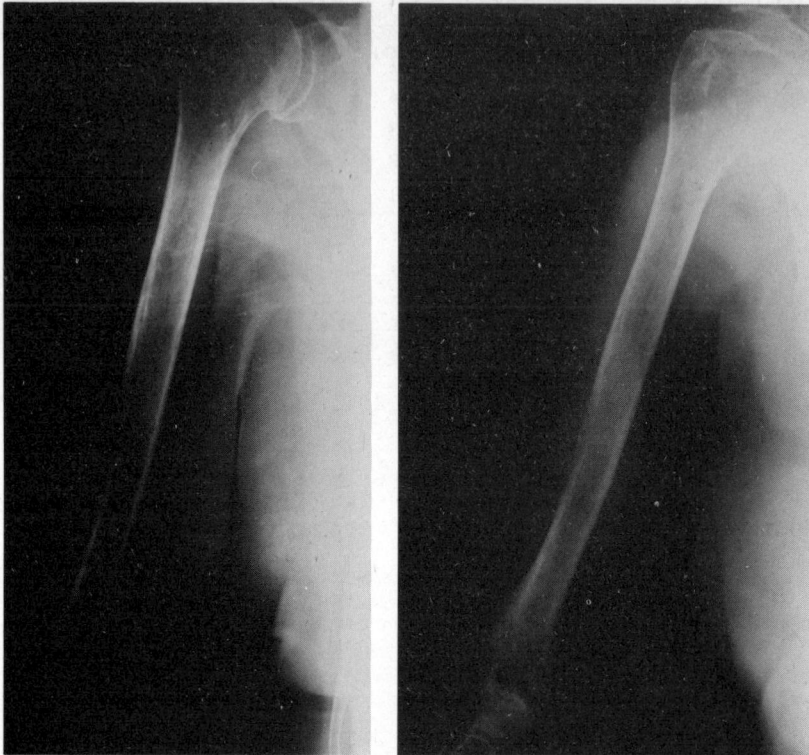

Figure 4.2 Radiographs of the right humerous of an 83-year-old woman with disseminated cancer of the vulva. The one on the left is before irradiation (1000 cGy (rad) in a single dose). The one on the right was taken 9 weeks after treatment, and shows marked recalcification. There was a corresponding improvement in the pain.

Decompression laminectomy is indicated when:

1 symptoms other than pain progress relentlessly even though dexamethasone and radiation have been started;
2 relapse occurs weeks, months, or years after radiation and further radiation cannot be given;
3 the nature of the primary tumour is not known or the diagnosis is in doubt.

Patients with an incomplete block on myelography do better than those with a complete block, as do those with a shorter rather than a longer block. In one series [9], effective pain relief (as judged by patients no longer needing strong narcotic analgesics) was obtained in about half of the patients whether treated by radiation or by laminectomy and radiation.

Hormone Therapy

All breast cancer patients should be reviewed to see if a further hormonal manipulation might be appropriate. Although the sequence of treatments varies from centre to centre, the common manipulations that are employed are shown in Figure 4.3.

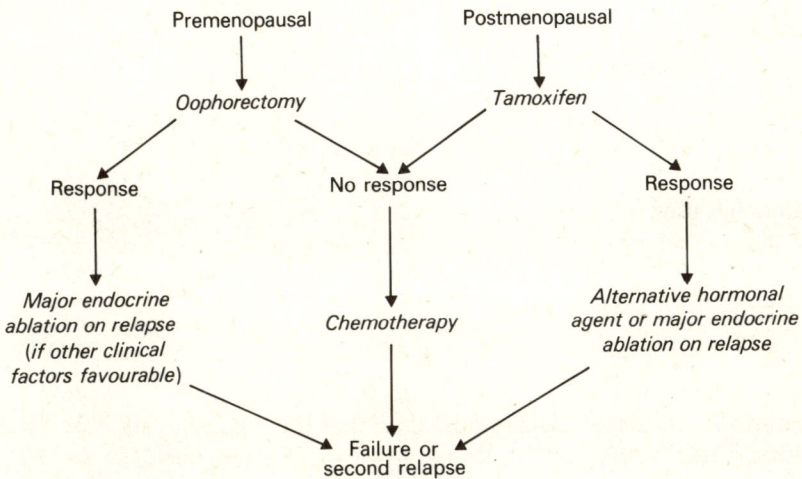

Figure 4.3 Synopsis of hormonal therapy in breast cancer. If oestrogen receptor status known to be negative, *chemotherapy* is generally considered the treatment of choice. Though in postmenopausal women, even if receptor negative, tamoxifen is worth a trial if the disease is slowly progressive. If rapidly progressive in premenopausal women, chemotherapy is the first option.
From Baum, 1980 [10]

In recent years, Pannuti and his associates [11] have explored the use of large doses of medroxyprogesterone acetate (MAP), a semisynthetic pituitary inhibitor. MAP 750 mg IM was given twice daily for 30 days to patients with far-advanced breast cancer, most of whom also had severe pain caused by osseous metastases. Complete or partial relief of pain was noted in over 90 per cent of patients. Improvement is seen within 1 or 2 weeks in almost all of those who are going to respond and is generally maximal in less than a month. Benefit is said to be especially noticeable in patients with multiple osseous metastases 'who were forced to keep completely still' in bed prior to treatment on account of intense movement-precipitated pain. Between 15 per cent and 20 per cent of patients treated with MAP developed abscesses at the site of injection. Other side effects were also noted (Table 4.7). All side effects resolved within 3 weeks of the completion of the course. The average duration of objective remission was 7 months (compared with 1 to 2 years for most other hormone therapies). The duration of pain relief after cessation of treatment is not stated [11].

Table 4.7   Side effects of treatment with IM medroxyprogesterone acetate (MAP) in doses of 500 to 2000 mg/day for 30 days (166 patients)

Side effect	%
Induration ⎫ at site of	7
Abscess ⎭ injections	18
Moonface	16
Tremor	16
Sweating	15
Vaginal bleeding	10
Cramps	9
Thrombophlebitis	1

Modified from Pannuti *et al*, 1979 [11]

Pannuti and his associates postulate that the analgesic effect of MAP is at least partly independent of any anti-cancer effect because:

1 the incidence of pain relief is considerably greater than the incidence of objective remission of the tumour (90 per cent compared with about 45 per cent);
2 some patients obtain significant relief despite obvious clinical progression of the disease.

It is possible that MAP acts by including a selective 'medical hypophysectomy'.

We have not yet used MAP. The fact that many patients were bedfast because of pain suggests that the use of analgesics and radiotherapy may have been more restricted than is generally the case in many centres in Britain and North America.

Hormonal antiandrogen therapy, by oral or intravenous administration of exogenous oestrogens, provides pain relief for the patient with symptomatic metastatic prostate carcinoma. Improvement in pain and sense of wellbeing can be anticipated in 70 per cent within 2 to 3 weeks on oral therapy and 48 hours on intravenous therapy. Many patients entering the terminal phase of their disease will already be on oral diethylstilboestrol 1 mg 8 to 12-hourly. There is little value in increasing the oral dose if bone pain recurs as the relapsed disease tends to be hormone resistant. Intravenous therapy is worthwhile in this circumstance—diethylstilboestrol diphosphonate 500 mg daily as a 4-hour infusion for 5 to 7 days— unless the patient has obvious cardiac insufficiency [12]. The main advantage of intravenous oestrogen therapy is the delivery of a high dose which, if successful, induces rapid remission of symptoms.

Chemotherapy

Patients with tumours that respond well to chemotherapy will not often require pain control in association with far-advanced malignant disease. Apart from those with myeloma or lymphoma, we use chemotherapy only occasionally—generally in patients with breast cancer.

Chemotherapy is also helpful in patients with recurrent painful squamous cell cancers of the head and neck which have already been treated with surgery and/or radiation. About 35 per cent respond to methotrexate or cis-platinum. Marked relief of severe pain is seen in 1 to 2 weeks. Methotrexate 25 to 50 mg/m^2 intravenously once weekly is usually well tolerated even in elderly, debilitated patients. As always, benefits must be weighed carefully against side effects [13].

Surgery

Pathological fracture of a long bone occurs in under 1 per cent of patients with advanced carcinoma but, when it does, it usually inflicts a considerable burden on a patient. All but 1 per cent of such fractures occur proximal to the knee or elbow [14]. Internal fixation or the insertion of a prosthesis should always be considered particularly in the case of a femur, as these measures obviate the need for prolonged bedrest. In addition, pain is either completely relieved or much reduced.

The decision whether to treat surgically depends to a large extent on the patient's general condition. In carcinoma of the bronchus or malignant melanoma, pathological fracture often presages death. This is generally not so in breast cancer, particularly if the tumour is hormone-sensitive. The results of several published series indicate that the median survival after the first or only pathological fracture associated with breast cancer is about 6 months, ranging from 2 months to 4 years [15].

Internal fixation should always be followed by irradiation, otherwise the fracture does not unite. Radiotherapy is commonly delayed until the wound has healed and the stitches removed, but this is not essential. Transcervical and subcapital fractures of the femur, however, do not unite even when treated in this way [14]. With these, the treatment of choice is replacement arthroplasty (Figure 4.4). This controls the pain and the patient can expect to be mobile again within days.

Consideration should sometimes be given to prophylactic nailing. It is easier than the internal fixation of an established, displaced fracture and is less disturbing for the patient. Moreover, when more than half of the cortex has been destroyed, deformity takes place on weight-bearing and this causes pain. Prophylactic nailing also facilitates nursing and should a fracture subsequently occur, it is often symptomless.

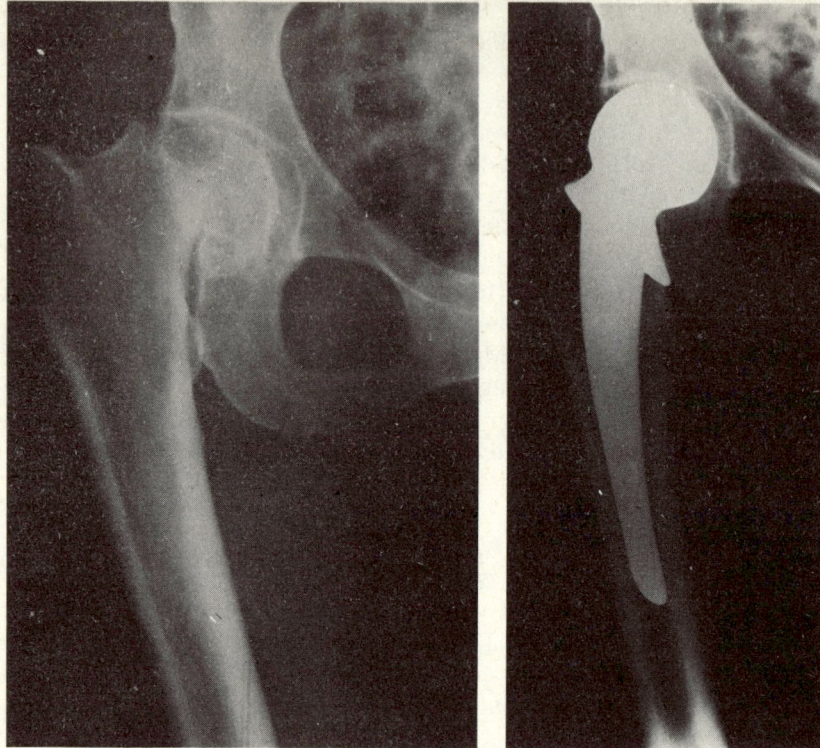

Figure 4.4 Radiographs showing subcapital fracture of right femur in a 58-year-old woman with breast cancer, and after treatment with a Thompson's hip hemiarthroplasty.

Fracture is unlikely when less than 25 per cent of the cortex of a long bone has been eroded, but when erosion is more than 75 per cent, the bone is so weak as often to fracture spontaneously [16]. The indications for prophylactic internal fixation of a long bone are, therefore:

1 increasing pain,
2 destruction of more than half the cortex radiologically.

Local irradiation of a long bone metastasis has been considered a further indication because of an increased risk of fracture [17]. Our experience indicates that irradiation commonly both reduces pain and results in significant recalcification. In other words, irradiation frequently modifies both the above criteria for surgery, and renders such intervention unnecessary.

A more elaborate technique has been described for use when bone destruction is widespread or when the fracture is close to the end of the bone and adequate fixation is not possible by a nail [18]. Lesions are first treated by excision and curettage, and then by appropriate internal fixation with the simultaneous insertion of an acrylic cement into the bone defect. By moulding the cement around the metal device, the shape of the bone can be restored. Although this probably has an adverse effect on fracture healing, fixation is adequate. In patients with advanced disease, any risk of local or general spread of the tumour as a result of curettage is outweighed by the benefits of the procedure. In one series of 73 patients, only 4 failed to regain function in the affected limb [18].

Correction of Hypercalcaemia

Hypercalcaemia occurs in 10 to 20 per cent of all patients with advanced malignant disease. The figure is higher in cancer of the breast and bronchus [19]. In addition to causing nausea, vomiting, constipation, weakness and depression, hypercalcaemia appears to precipitate or exacerbate pain by modifying the patient's pain threshold. Several reports have been published in which hypercalcaemia in malignant disease has been reduced by either SC calcitonin or IV mithramycin. Each report includes examples of patients who have experienced a definite reduction in bone pain, or complete relief, when the plasma calcium concentration returned to normal. Relief was noted in 6 out of 7 [20], 10 out of 15[21] and 5 out of 15 [22] patients, respectively. Lack of response may relate to differences in the mechanisms responsible for the pain. For example, in some the pain may be related to rapid bone resorption (cp. Paget's disease), whereas in others deformity on weight-bearing could be responsible. In the former, benefit from calcitonin or mithramycin might be expected but not in the latter. Whatever the explanation for the inconsistency of benefit, steps should be taken to correct hypercalcaemia if a patient has pain which is not readily relieved by analgesics.

A number of animal studies in which calcitonin was injected into the lateral ventricle of the brain suggest that calcitonin given by this route may have a specific analgesic effect reversible by doses of naloxone 10 to 100 times greater than that required to reverse the effects of morphine [23]. Pain relief in man is, however, always consequent upon a correction of or reduction in hypercalcaemia. This suggests a causal relationship. In the absence of more data, it is not possible to say whether the effect is a peripheral one or one that is centrally mediated.

Urgent management. For a patient who has clear indications for the urgent reversal of malignant hypercalcaemia (Table 4.8), mithramycin is the most effective means of control [24]. This should be given in a dose of $25\,\mu g/kg$ by IV infusion in normal saline, together with calciuretic loop diuretics. In patients with impaired renal function a smaller dose should be used. It is effective within 12 to 36 hours in over 80 per cent of patients. Mithramycin is a cytotoxic antibiotic which is a potent inhibitor of bone

71

resorption, acting directly on the osteoclasts. Impaired renal function is a relative contraindication to its use as the major route of clearance is by the kidneys and side effects are cumulative.

Table 4.8 Indications for urgent reversal of hypercalcaemia in dying patient

1	First episode or long interval since previous one.
2	Prior good quality of life (in patient's opinion).
3	Patient willing to undergo intravenous therapy and requisite blood tests.
4	Severe symptoms attributable to hypercalcaemia.
5	Medical judgement that measures will achieve a durable effect (based on the results of previous treatment).

Intramuscular calcitonin is also effective but very expensive. Effects are transient so it needs to be given every 6 hours until anti-cancer or symptom control measures have had time to exert an effect. As the hospice patient is frequently beyond specific antitumour therapy, the usefulness of calcitonin in this field is limited.

Non-urgent management.   In many hospice patients the urgent need for reversal of hypercalcaemia is less clear-cut. Symptoms are less severe, or less clearly attributable to hypercalcaemia. The patient is reluctant to undergo intravenous therapy or the consequent blood tests; the disease is so advanced and the patient's condition such that aggressive measures are judged inappropriate. In these cases a high daily fluid intake (3 l), gentle diuresis, and prednisolone 40 mg daily will sometimes correct hypercalcaemia. Glucocorticosteroids inhibit bone resorption and inhibit the absorption of calcium by the gut. They are very effective in sarcoidosis and vitamin D intoxication where gut absorption seems to be the major mechanism. However, they are less effective in patients with malignant hypercalcaemia and work in less than 30 per cent of patients with most solid tumours. Moreover their effect takes 7 days to develop. They may be more useful in lowering plasma calcium in haematological and breast cancer [24].

For patients with troublesome hypercalcaemia which fails to respond to other measures, we use mithramycin 25 µg/kg given by slow *IV injection* every 1 to 2 weeks. Although this dose is generally insufficient to suppress marrow function, it is wise to check the patient's blood count before each injection when using mithramycin in this way. A smaller dose should be used in patients with impaired renal function.

Maintenance.   The initial effect may be maintained by using effervescent phosphate tablets and high fluid intake. 500 mg b.i.d. is the best starting dose, increasing by 500 mg a day every 3 to 7 days, if necessary, to a total daily dose of 3 g. Diarrhoea, which may be a limiting factor, and nausea are the main side effects.

Recent work with diphosphonates suggests that they are able to inhibit bone resorption effectively. Although most studies relate to Paget's disease of the bone, several reports deal with their use in hypercalcaemia of malignancy and multiple myeloma [25]. In a group of 10 patients with myeloma, bone pain was reduced, although not abolished, when treated with dichloromethylene diphosphonate [26]. All 10 patients were either hypercalcaemic or had sustained hypercalciuria before treatment.

Diphosphonates do not affect plasma proteins in myeloma. This suggests that the beneficial effects relate to a reduction of osteolysis rather than to improvement in the underlying malignant disease. Diphosphonates should, therefore, generally be used in conjunction with standard anti-cancer chemotherapy in myeloma. In Britain, etidronate disodium is the only readily available diphosphonate. As yet there is only limited data relating to its use in hypercalcaemia and metastatic bone pain.

The symptoms of hypercalcaemia are caused by an elevated *ionized* calcium. The total plasma calcium measures both protein-bound and unbound ionized calcium. Thus, if a patient is significantly hypoalbuminaemic, the plasma calcium concentration may give a false impression of normality. Several centres have recommended ways in which the plasma calcium may be adjusted to take account of a low plasma albumin. Which method one uses is not important, and will depend largely on local custom. A relatively small above-normal calcium concentration sometimes causes definite hypercalcaemic symptoms.

Pituitary Ablation

Hypophysectomy as a means of inducing a remission in potentially hormone-dependent tumours, such as breast and prostate, is not commonly undertaken. The results are not good and the operation is viewed with distaste by most patients and many doctors. On the other hand, there is growing interest in the role of hypophysectomy in the control of pain, particularly in those patients who have multiple bone pains in whom it is difficult to achieve complete relief despite the use of analgesics and radiotherapy. Ablation of the pituitary gland may be achieved in one of several ways:

1 open surgery,
2 yttrium 90 implant,
3 cryosurgery,
4 injection of alcohol.

Although complete destruction of the gland does not always occur with cryosurgery or alcohol injection, the results in terms of pain relief are equally good.

73

Morrica was the first to inject alcohol through needles inserted via the transnasal, trans-sphenoidal route [27]. Up to 2 ml of absolute ethyl alcohol is used. Of some 2,200 patients, 60 per cent experienced complete and immediate relief [28]. Most of the rest became completely pain-free after a second or third injection. In 3.6 per cent (80 patients) pain relief remained incomplete, although even in these it was possible to stop using strong narcotic analgesics. Failure to secure complete relief was commonly attributed to psychological factors. Ninety-two per cent of the patients had hormone-dependent tumours, mostly breast cancer. Results were equally good in patients with hormone-non-dependent tumours, e.g., melanoma and carcinomata of the bronchus, larynx and bladder. Complications included severe bleeding from the internal carotid, hyperthermic crises, hyperphagia and anhydrosis.

Most patients experience frontal headache for 2 to 3 days after the injection. It is thought to be caused by a chemical meningeal reaction and may be associated with a mild pyrexia. The occasional cerebrospinal fluid rhinorrhea may also play a part. Anterolateral spread of the hypobaric alcohol to involve the optic chiasma and nerves to extraocular muscles may result in visual field defects or ocular palsies. If pupillary dilatation is noted during the slow injection of the alcohol, the cannula should be withdrawn and the patient turned on his side. Lipton recommends that, should eye changes occur, 40 to 50 mg of hydrocortisone is injected into the cisterna magna [29]. If this is done, any eye changes disappear within 15 minutes. Since adopting this technique, no patient has sustained a visual field defect.

Other improvements in the technique will also help reduce the overall complication rate of 6 to 10 per cent and, in one series, a mortality rate of 5 per cent [30]. Vasoconstrictors can be applied to the nasal mucosa and the sphenoid sinus irrigated with an antibiotic solution. A fibrosing agent, ethyl cyanoacrylate, may be injected before the removal of the cannula to prevent leakage of the cerebrospinal fluid. After injection, intake of fluids and glucose should be kept high, corticosteroids given, and the polyuria controlled by nasal instillation of the antidiuretic hormone analogue, desmopressin.

Others have not been able to reproduce Morrica's almost total success. Between 70 and 80 per cent of patients gain some benefit, although probably no more than 40 per cent obtain complete relief [31]. Many patients die of the underlying disease within a few months. Relief persists for more than 4 months in only half of those who survive longer.

It is possible that the discrepancies relate to differences in technique. Morrica commonly uses several needles and repeats the procedure until success in achieved. On the other hand, a former colleague disagrees with Morrica's view that pituitary ablation with alcohol is a major step forward in the treatment of diffuse cancer pain. In his opinion, when a patient has diffuse, poorly controlled pain, the use of radio-frequency percutaneous cervical cordotomy is preferable [31].

Life after hypophysectomy is not trouble-free, with the need for hormone replacement. The question arises of which patient with pain should be considered for this procedure. In many studies we suspect that better understanding of narcotic analgesics and adjuvant medication would have eliminated the need for pituitary ablation. In one paper advocating pituitary ablation for metastatic prostate cancer, 12 out of 53 patients referred for pituitary ablation needed only 'frequent non-narcotic analgesics' [32]. Thirty-four had a degree of pain described as 'requiring frequent oral narcotic analgesics'. Analgesic regimens were not discussed and it is not clear whether the narcotics were given on a regular or 'as required' basis. We would advise that pituitary ablation is considered in hormone-dependent patients, only after careful titration of analgesic drugs has failed (see Chapters 6 and 7). In our experience these will be few in number.

How pain relief is produced is not clear. It is known that β-lipotropin, the precursor of β-endorphin, is present in large quantities in the intermediate lobe of the pituitary. A massive release of this substance by autolysis may explain the occasional observation of relief within minutes of the injection. Such a mechanism is unlikely, however, to produce a prolonged effect, and an increased endorphin concentration has not been detected in cerebrospinal fluid after the injection. In most cases relief is obtained after two to three days. A number of other hormonal mechanisms have been postulated [30]. For example, prolactin, one of the pituitary produced hormones, stimulates the production of prostaglandins. These are substances known to play a significant role in the development of metastases in bone, and to have a significant role in the development of metastases in bone, and to have a significant effect on nociception (see Chapter 6). Yet, no correlation between suppression of pituitary function and subsequent relief has been demonstrated [33]. Considerable improvement has been seen after minimal changes in hormone levels, while one patient who had complete hypopituitarism derived no benefit.

Studies with iophendylate (Myodil) have shown that in about 20 per cent of cases, the contrast medium spreads to the region of the infundibular stalk and hypothalamus, and the cavity of the third ventricle is displayed [34]. In postmortem studies, Indian ink has been injected and, in most cases, the dye could be demonstrated histologically in the portal venous system of the pituitary stalk and in the hypothalamus [34]. This indicates injury to the hypothalamus and its thalamic connections.

References

1 IASP Subcommittee on Taxonomy. Pain terms: a list with definitions and notes on usage. *Pain* 1980; **8**: 249–252

2 Haram BJ. Facts and Figures in *The Management of Terminal Disease* edited by Saunders CM. Edward Arnold, London 1978, pp 12–18.

3 Hunt JM, Stollar TD, Littlejohns DW, Twycross RG and Vere DW. Patients with protracted pain: a survey conducted at the London Hospital. *Journal of Medical Ethics* 1977; **3**: 61–73.

4 LeShan L. The world of the patient in severe pain of long duration. *Journal of Chronic Disease* 1964; **17**: 119–126.

5 Gilbert HA, Kagan AR, Nussbaum H, Rao AR, Satzman J, Chan P, Allen B and Forsythe A. Evaluation of radiation therapy for bone metastases: pain relief and quality of life. *American Journal of Roentgenology* 1977; **129**: 1095–1098.

6 Penn CRH. Single dose and fractionated palliative irradiation for osseous metastases. *Clinical Radiology* 1976; **27**: 405–408.

7 Allen KL, Johnson TW and Hibbs GG. Effective bone palliation as related to various treatment regimens. *Cancer* 1976; **37**: 405–408.

8 Posner JB. Spinal cord metastases (including cauda equina): diagnosis and treatment in *Neuro-Oncology* Department of Neurology, MS-K Cancer Centre, New York 1977; pp 19–32.

9 Young RF, Post EM and King GA. Treatment of spinal epidural metastases. *Journal of Neurosurgery* 1980; **53**: 741–748.

10 Baum M. The management of advanced breast cancer. *British Journal of Hospital Medicine* 1980; **23**: 32–39.

11 Pannuti F, Martoni A, Rossi AP and Piana E. The role of endocrine therapy for relief of pain due to advanced cancer in *Advances in Pain Research and Therapy, Vol 2* edited by Bonica JJ and Ventafridda V. Raven Press, New York 1979, pp 145–165.

12 Band PR, Banerjee TK, Patwardhan VC and Eid TC. High dose diethylstilbestrol diphosphonate therapy of prostatic cancer after failure of standard doses of estrogens. *Canadian Medical Association Journal* 1973; **109**: 697–699.

13 Boop WC and Fischer JA. Methods of pain control in *Cancer of the Head and Neck* edited by Suen JY and Myers EN. Churchill-Livingstone, New York, Edinburgh, London and Melbourne 1981, pp 821–838.

14 Galasko CSB. Pathological fracture secondary to metastatic cancer. *Journal of the Royal College of Surgeons of Edinburgh* 1974; **19:** 351–362.

15 Twycross RG. Care of the terminal patient in *Breast Cancer Management— Early and Late* edited by Stoll BA. Heinemann Medical, London 1977, pp 157–163.

16 Fidler M. Prophylactic internal fixation of secondary neoplastic deposits in long bones. *British Medical Journal* 1973; **1:** 341–343.

17 Editorial. Pathological fractures due to bone metastases. *British Medical Journal* 1981; **283:** 748.

18 Yablon IG and Paul GR. The augmentative use of methyl methacrylate in the management of pathological fractures. *Surgery, Gynecology and Obstetrics* 1976; **143:** 177–183.

19 Watson L. Calcium metabolism and cancer. *Australian Annals of Medicine* 1966; **15:** 359–367.

20 Parsons V, Dalley V, Brinkley D, Davies C and Vernon A. The effects of calcitonin on the metabolic disturbances surrounding widespread bony metastases. *Acta Endocrinologica* 1974; **76:** 286–301.

21 Davies J, Trask C and Souhami RL. Effect of mithramycin on widespread painful bone metastases in cancer of the breast. *Cancer Treatment Reports* 1979; **63:** 1835–1838.

22 Coombes RC, Neville AM, Gazet JC, Ford HT, Nash AG, Baker JW and Powles TJ. Agents affecting osteolysis in patients with breast cancer. *Cancer Chemotherapy and Pharmacology* 1979; **3:** 41–44.

23 Bates RFL, Buckley GA, Eglen RM and Strettle RJ. The interaction of naloxone and calcitonin in the production of analgesia in the mouse. *British Journal of Pharmacology* 1981; **74:** 280P.

24 Bockman RS. Hypercalcaemia in malignancy. *Clinics in Endocrinology and Metabolism* 1980; **9:** 317–333.

25 Editorial. Diphosphonates: aimed in a chemical sense. *Lancet* 1981; **2:** 1326–1328.

26 Siris ES, Sherman WH, Baquiran DC, Schlatterer JP, Osserman EF and Canfield RE. Effects of dichloromethylene diphosphonate on skeletal mobilization of calcium in multiple myeloma. *New England Journal of Medicine* 1980; **302:** 310–315.

27 Moricca G. The management of cancer pain in *Progress in Anaesthesiology* (Proceedings of Fourth World Congress on Anaesthesiology). Excerpta Medica, Amsterdam 1968; pp 266–270.

28 Moricca G. Arcuri E and Moricca P. Neuroadenolysis in *Continuing Care of Patients with Terminal Cancer* edited by Twycross RG and Ventafridda V. Pergamon Press, Oxford 1980, pp 155–163.

29 Lipton S. Intractable pain—the present position. *Annals of the Royal College of Surgeons of England* 1981; **63:** 157–163.

30 Editorial. Pituitary ablation for pain relief. *Lancet* 1981; **1:** 1348–1349.

31 Franchi G. Comment of neuroadenolysis in *The Continuing Care of Patients with Terminal Cancer* edited by Twycross RG and Ventafridda V. Pergamon Press, Oxford 1980, p 163.

32 Fitzpatrick JM, Gardiner RA, Williams JP, Riddle PR and O'Donaghue EPN. Pituitary ablation in the relief of pain in advanced prostatic carcinoma. *British Journal of Urology* 1980, **52:** 301–304.

33 Williams NE, Miles JB, Lipton S, Hipkin LJ and Davis JC. Pain relief and pituitary function following injection of alcohol into the pituitary fossa. *Annals of the Royal College of Surgeons of England* 1980; **62:** 202–207.

34 Miles J. Chemical hypophysectomy in *Advances in Pain Research and Therapy Vol. 2* edited by Bonica JJ and Ventafridda V. Raven Press, New York 1979, pp 373–380.

Chapter Five

Non-Drug Measures

Other non-drug treatment modalities are considered in this chapter. It is not possible to discuss the specialist procedures in detail. There are books and papers available which describe these. The most helpful is *Advances in Pain and Therapy, Volume 2* [1]. This is the proceedings of an international symposium on pain in advanced cancer held in 1978. There are four other books in the same series. Three of these relate to successive meetings of the Triennial World Congress on Pain, held under the auspices of the International Association for the Study of Pain (IASP) in 1975 [2], 1978 [3] and 1981 [5]. They cover the whole field of pain and include articles about both drug and non-drug approaches to cancer pain. The fourth is a smaller volume, entirely devoted to Pancoast syndrome [4].

Elevation of Pain Threshold

The somatopsychic nature of pain has already been stressed. A doctor needs to offer 'professional friendship'. He needs to take time not only to listen but also to explain the why and the how of each symptom, and to encourage the patient in *the art of living with cancer*. This is important for both the continuing general care of the patient and the relief of pain. Intensity of pain is modulated by the patient's mood and morale, and also by the significance or meaning of the pain for the patient. There is a continuing need to prevent physical isolation which, on occasion, is tantamount to ostracism. The use of 'TLP'—tender loving physio-therapy—at home or in hospital helps to avoid this [6]. This should be seen as a specific positive contribution and not as a sop for sagging morale, or, worse, as part of a charade to mislead the patient into thinking that he is getting better. For this to be helpful, the therapist must be aware of the real intent behind the request for treatment.

The need for general psychological support for the cancer patient was considered in Chapter 3. Some patients and their families need more intensive help. This can usually be given by a suitably trained doctor or nurse [7] who can spare the time, or by a clinical psychologist, social worker [8], psychiatrist or chaplain. It is necessary, however, to be aware of a number of more specialized forms of treatment (Table 5.1).

Table 5.1   Psychological and related methods of pain control

Distraction [10]	Massage
Imagery [10]	Heat
Relaxation	Pressure
Biofeedback	TENS†
Hypnosis	Acupuncture

† Transcutaneous electrical nerve stimulation

Relaxation Therapy

One of the fundamental messages of relaxation therapy is: 'You can influence your body and your mind and how they react' [9]. For the patient who feels the hopeless and helpless victim of circumstances beyond his control, the use of relaxation techniques can be a step towards the re-establishment of the patient's self-respect: 'At last, there is some-thing I can do!' In relation to pain, the aim is to prevent a vicious spiral of anxiety—muscle tension—muscle pain—more anxiety and so on.

It is important not to give the impression that relaxation will relieve all types of pain. Published reports evaluating relaxation with clinical pain have consisted largely of studies of tension headaches. One of the few well-controlled studies [10] compared relaxation training with frontalis biofeedback and a placebo medication. After 4 weeks both relaxation and biofeedback groups showed a significant decrease in the incidence of headache as compared with the placebo group. There was no significant difference between the relaxation and biofeedback groups. Others have reported similar results [11]. There are no studies reported on relaxation and cancer pain.

Apart from pain associated with or caused by muscle spasm (e.g. myofascial, irritable bowel syndrome), relaxation therapy should be seen as a means of preventing or reducing the secondary muscle spasm that so readily occurs in anxious and frightened patients. In cancer pain manage-ment, relaxation therapy will be an adjunct to other measures.

For maximum benefit, the patient must understand the mechanisms underlying his pain(s) and must comprehend the interaction between anxiety and muscle tone. In fact, the relatively common supraspinatus, levator scapulae and trapezius muscle pains often subside after an explanation as to their cause, without any specific treatment offered or given. Simple guidelines about relaxation are available [12, 13], but it is probably expecting too much of most patients simply to rely on such advice. The use of a trained therapist who is prepared also to listen is helpful for the successful use of this form of treatment in those cancer patients for whom it is appropriate. Advice may be reinforced by the use of tape-recorded instructions. These are of value whether 'pre-packaged' or specifically prepared for the individual.

For relief of persistent pain the patient can be encouraged to practise regularly one of two techniques. These are rhythmic breathing and relaxing with music [13]. For both, the patient should be comfortable with head supported. He should then close his eyes and listen. For rhythmic breathing, the nurse or tape will repeat instructions as in Table 5.2.

Table 5.2   Instructions for patients practising rhythmic breathing

1	Close your eyes.
2	Breathe in and out slowly and deeply.
	In, 2, 3, 4—Out, 2, 3, 4
3	Try to breathe from your abdomen.
4	Every time you breathe out, feel yourself getting more relaxed.
5	Find out how relaxation feels to you, you may feel light and weightless or you may feel very heavy.
6	Every time you breathe out, feel yourself getting more and more relaxed.
7	As you breathe choose a place you remember as peaceful and pleasant. Let your imagination take you there—a beach, a field, a concert. Feel the air, notice the smells. Listen to the sounds.
8	When you are ready to end your relaxation exercise, count slowly from 1 to 3:
	On 1, move your lower body;
	On 2, move your upper body;
	On 3, breathe in deeply, open your eyes and as you breathe out slowly, say to yourself, 'I am relaxed and alert'.

After McCaffrey, 1980 [13]

Relaxing with music (or a favourite poem or Bible passage) may be easier. While listening the patient may imagine himself drifting or floating with the music.

Biofeedback

Many physiological functions are dependent on the autonomic nervous system, e.g. blood pressure and pulse rate. These are traditionally regarded as beyond self-control. Biofeedback is a technique in which a person is made aware of changes in bodily functions, with the aim of eventually controlling the functions to advantage [14]. Biofeedback is the central component of a wide variety of procedures, all of which have the same principal goal of self-control (autoregulation). It has been used in the management of tension headaches, migraine, epilepsy, certain neuromuscular disorders (such as spasmodic torticollis) and anxiety.

The basis for the claims for pain relief frequently made on behalf of the biofeedback are several studies of its use in tension headache [15]. In one study it was shown that, by teaching people to relax the muscles of the forehead, the headaches were significantly reduced in about two-thirds of those studied [16]. A study of the use of biofeedback in chronic non-malignant pain failed to demonstrate any relief [17]. Although, when used in conjunction with hypnosis, over half the patients had decreases in pain of 33 per cent or more. There are no studies on biofeedback with cancer pain. When of benefit, biofeedback probably acts via distraction, suggestion, relaxation, and a sense of control over the pain [18]. Current evidence suggests that biofeedback is no more efficacious, even in headache, than relaxation training. The latter is a simpler and far less costly alternative because it requires no equipment and can be done in groups [15, 19, 20]. Accordingly, biofeedback has no place in the management of cancer pain.

Hypnosis

Hypnosis is an altered state of consciousness characterized by changes in perception and memory. It is a natural ability and has been used for many years as a medical technique for pain relief, muscle relaxation and, sometimes, to facilitate healing. It is also a psychotherapeutic tool to alleviate symptoms, uncover forgotten memories and facilitate behavioural changes.

Hypnotic techniques employed for pain control vary, but generally include some of the following [21, 22]:

1 blocking awareness of the pain;
2 substituting another feeling (such as pressure) for the pain;
3 moving the pain to a smaller or less significant area of the body;
4 changing the meaning of the pain so that it is less important;
5 time distortion;
6 in extreme cases, dissociating the body from the patient's awareness.

Although hypnosis has been in use for longer than any other psychological form of analgesia, clinical research in the area of cancer pain is sparse, methodologically poor and fails to demonstrate convincingly that hypnosis is effective in cancer pain (Table 5.3).

Table 5.3 Hypnosis in cancer pain; experimental designs and treatment outcomes

Authors	N	Design	Control	Dependent measures	Follow-up	Results
Cangello [23]	22	Group outcome	None	Narcotic requests	1–20 weeks	13 patients requested less narcotic medication
Butler [24]	12	Anecdotal case studies	None	Therapist judgement of improvement	None	Some pain alleviation in all patients, unequivocal benefit in 5
Sacerdote [25]	8	Anecdotal case studies	None	Therapist judgement of improvement	No systematic follow-up	All showed pain relief
Sacerdote [26]	4	Anecdotal case studies	None	Self-report	None	Pain reduced or eliminated in all cases
Lea et al [27]	17	Anecdotal case studies	None	Therapist judgement of improvement	None	12 patients judged to have good or excellent improvement

There is no doubt that individual patients have been helped considerably by hypnosis [20]. It has not yet been shown that hypnosis is better than the encouragement and psychological support given by an attentive physician and/or caring team.

Contrary to popular belief, hypnosis is not excessively time-consuming. Group therapy reduces the problem of tiredness in the therapist. As with relaxation, the use of tape-recorded advice helps to maximize the therapeutic effect. It also reduces the possibility of dependence on the physical presence of the therapist. Unless all members of the staff are trained to understand the potential benefits, the efficacy of the treatment is likely to be weakened by scepticism [28]. The main disadvantage of hypnosis is that it is impossible to predict those who will benefit. It also requires a degree of concentration which many oncology patients do not have.

As with relaxation therapy, hypnosis provides the patient with a tool by which he can exert a measure of control over the effects of the cancer. It thereby reduces the sense of helplessness that many patients experience. It heightens a person's ability to concentrate on and to live for the moment. This has the effect of promoting life-enhancing attitudes, and a modification of the way in which the patient views his disease. It does not reduce normal function, nor does it affect the patient's mental capacity in a detrimental way. It has, therefore, a place in the management of cancer pain as an adjunct to more traditional forms of treatment.

Counter-Irritant Cutaneous Stimulation

The relief of chronic pain by counter-irritants is a common practice in primitive cultures and is still a basic principle in the home remedies used by many of our patients in their homes. Menthol ointments, ice packs and hot water bottles are all effective in relieving the aches and pains of bedfast patients. Relief of pain may outlast the duration of the activity of the counter-irritant, but if it does not, even a short period of relief from a niggling ache may serve to improve morale. Although widely used, such methods are little acknowledged in the teaching of pain relief.

Cold can be applied directly to the painful area with an ice pack, cold damp towels or with a re-usable gel pack. Cold packs can provide relief from headache, muscle spasms, joint pains caused by immobility and back pain. Some people prefer hot packs, heating pads or a hot water bottle, especially for back pain and muscle spasm. A hot water bottle may also be helpful for abdominal cramping.

Many analgesic ointments contain menthol, easily detected by its strong odour. An application of menthol ointment to the skin produces a sensation of warmth or cooling that may last several hours. The mechanism by which menthol relieves pain is obscure, but it is frequently effective for joint pain, muscle spasm and tension headache.

Various theories have been invoked to explain counter-irritation, most based on the Gate Control Theory of Pain [29] and/or on the production of endogenous opiates [30]. However, these do not influence the importance of making sure that these modalities are made available to the hospital patient. Massaging an aching back or limb is also an excellent way for a nurse to gain a patient's trust and confidence.

Transcutaneous Electrical Nerve Stimulation

This method of pain modulation was known to the Romans, who used electric eels as current generators. There was a revival of interest in the 19th century when more sophisticated sources of electricity became available. The use of electro-analgesia subsequently waned, because the majority of patients did not benefit from it. In recent years, stimulated by the Gate Control Theory of Pain, there has been renewed interest in transcutaneous electrical nerve stimulation (TENS). It is claimed that TENS works by stimulating the large fibres involved in pain conduction, thereby 'shutting the gate' in the substantia gelatinosa of the dorsal horn of the spinal cord [31]. An important factor in the successful use of TENS is the correct positioning of the electrodes and the optimal adjustment of the electrical output. This is time-consuming and can be done only with the patient's co-operation. Optimum electrical pulse width, intensity, and rate combinations are different for each person.

If an effect is obtained, it is important to continue to use it fairly constantly for at least two days [32]. After that the patient should be allowed to use the stimulator as he likes. This will vary from a few hours to the whole day. Electrodes must not be placed on ulcerated skin or hyperaesthetic areas. It has been suggested that the presence of a trigger point is an indication for TENS [32]. Our impression is, however, that the injection of trigger points with a local anaesthetic is both easier and more efficacious.

Published data shows that TENS may give short-term benefit in many patients treated for various types of chronic pain, but its efficacy usually declines with time. The same is true of cancer patients. In one group of 37 patients, there was a high rate of success in the first few days followed by a rapid decline [32]. Only 4 (11 per cent) experienced reduction of pain after a month. The best results were seen in 3 out of 13 patients with pain associated with head and neck cancer, 3 out of 6 patients with early phantom limb pain and, to a lesser degree, in 6 out of 8 patients with postherpetic neuralgia.

It may be that TENS acts by suggestion, distraction or placebo mechanisms. We have used TENS only on a few occasions, such as in one person who had a distressing thoracic girdle dysaesthesia secondary to compression of the spinal cord at that level.

85

Acupuncture

Acupuncture may be performed in several ways, including the manual rotation of needles and low-frequency or high-frequency stimulation through them. Naloxone, a specific opiate-receptor antagonist, reduces or abolishes low-frequency electro-acupuncture analgesia in animals and man though it has no effect on analgesia induced by high-frequency electro-acupuncture in mice [33]. Naturally occurring opioid peptides are released into the cerebrospinal fluid during acupuncture [33]. The evidence that different forms of acupuncture elicit specific neurohormonal effects gives acupuncture a certain scientific respectability. It has, however, no place in the management of cancer pain.

Interruption of Pain Pathways

Nerve Block

Nociception may be blocked by use of either a local anaesthetic (transient) or one of several destructive (neurolytic) techniques (Table 5.4). Theoretically, local anaesthetic blocks are temporary but, in practice, they may provide partial or complete pain relief for a prolonged period.

Table 5.4 Nerve blocks

Local anaesthesia	(a) lignocaine[1]
	(b) bupivicaine
Neurolysis	(a) chemical: alcohol
	phenol
	chlorocresol
	(b) cold (cryotherapy)
	(c) heat (thermo-coagulation)

[1] lidocaine (USA)

Neurolytic procedures are generally carried out only by suitable trained anaesthetists [34]. If there is a good chance of successful anti-cancer treatment, destructive procedures should be avoided. Moreover, if a patient is expected to survive for several years, neurolytic blocks should be used only with caution. Their complications are real and do not always reverse with time. Urinary and faecal incontinence are particularly distressing.

Neuronal regeneration does take place and, inevitably, the pain will eventually recur. The duration of relief following a successful block varies from several weeks to several months. Understandably, if a patient experienced troublesome, distressing or lasting complications on the first occasion, he is less likely to agree to a repeat block, even though the need may be more pressing.

During the terminal stage, when many patients have a variety of symptoms, often including several pains, drug therapy generally has more to offer than neurolysis. Although, if a patient has a unilateral, relatively localized pain caused principally or entirely by neoplastic nerve compression, a nerve block may be the treatment of choice. This is particularly so if the risk of urinary or anal dysfunction is small, as with blocks in the upper lumbar spine. In general, the place of destructive neurolytic procedures in the management of cancer pain is limited. On the other hand, their use may be crucial in obtaining relief in the minority of patients for whom they are clearly indicated and in whom drug therapy is not proving wholly satisfactory (Table 5.5).

Table 5.5   Sites of pain for which nerve block should be considered

Facial neuralgia
Posterior head and neck pain
Upper limb nerve pressure pain (brachial plexus)
Hemithoracic pain
Epigastric visceral pain (coeliac axis plexus)
Perineal pain
Lower limb nerve pressure pain (lumbosacral plexus)

Pharmacological Considerations

A number of local anaesthetic agents are readily available, more so in the United States than in Britain. In practice, it is necessary to be familiar only with lignocaine[1] and bupivicaine (Table 5.6). The former is short-acting (1 to 2 hours), the latter relatively long-acting (8 to 12 hours). Lignocaine is a substantial vasodilator and is often used with adrenaline by anaesthetists to retard absorption and metabolism. Another advantage of giving lignocaine with adrenaline is that the maximum safe dose is considerably greater, about 1 g as against 500 mg if used alone. Adrenaline should not be used in patients taking monoamine oxidase inhibitors or tricyclic antidepressants, both of which potentiate the pressor effect of sympathomimetic amines.

There is no need to use adrenaline when infiltrating the skin and subcutaneous tissue prior to paracentesis or the injection of depot methylprednisolone. Bupivicaine is not a vasodilator. Unwanted effects are unusual and generally relate to overdosage:

1   CNS excitement—tremor of lips, twitching of corner of mouth;
2   (CNS depression—*rare*);
3   hypotension—faintness, lightheadedness;
4   cardiac arrhythmia—pallor, sweating.

---

[1] lidocaine (USA)

Table 5.6 Local anaesthetic agents

---

1 *Esters*
   (a) *Cocaine hydrochloride* is a naturally occurring plant alkaloid. It is too toxic to be injected. Used only for topical analgesia.
   (b) *Procaine hydrochloride* is the original synthetic local anaesthetic. Unlike cocaine, its surface activity is very poor. Maximum safe dose is about 500 mg. Rapidly absorbed after injection but is effective for up to an hour, *if adrenaline is added* to counter vasodilatation. (Maximum safe dose in this circumstance = 1g.) It is rapidly metabolized by pseudocholinesterase.

2 *Amides*
   (a) *Lignocaine hydrochloride* is slightly more toxic than procaine but, because of its greater potency, a smaller dose is necessary. There is, therefore, little to choose between them in practice. The usual strength used to provide local analgesia is 1%. It is more stable in solution than procaine, much more active topically, and causes less vasodilatation. Action lasts 1–2 hours. Maximum safe dose in the fit adult is about 200 mg (or 500 mg with adrenaline).
   (b) *Bupivicaine hydrochloride* is the longest lasting of the amide local anaesthetics. Its activity can last up to 8–12 hours and even longer in exceptional cases. It has little if any vasodilating effect. It is approximately twice as potent as lignocaine; the standard strength is 0.5%. Maximum safe dose is about 150 mg. Used therapeutically to break 'pain cycles' in chronic conditions.

Occasionally, a hypersensitivity reaction may occur manifesting as profound hypotension and tachycardia after only a small dose.

Local anaesthetics have an antimicrobial property. This helps explain why it is relatively safe to leave, for example, an epidural indwelling catheter *in situ* for several days or even weeks.

Neurolytic agents (e.g. alcohol, phenol and chlorocresol), cause demyelination and degeneration of the dorsal roots. Patchy and cumulative damage to fibres of all sizes extending into the dorsal column of the spinal cord may occur.

Local Anaesthetic Blocks

These fall into three categories:

1 diagnostic,
2 prognostic,
3 therapeutic.

A local anaesthetic nerve block confirms whether a pain is related to compression of a specific nerve and acts as a predictor of the likely outcome of a subsequent neurolytic procedure. Most anaesthetists use local anaesthetics routinely before peripheral (as distinct from intrathecal) blocks. The main use of local anaesthetics, in our experience, is however, therapeutic (Table 5.7).

Table 5.7   Therapeutic local anaesthetic blocks

Sacro-iliac pain
Trigger point related myofascial pain
Solitary rib metastasis
Other bone metastases
Postherpetic neuralgia
(Cervical plexus)

Sacro-Iliac Pain

Patients with advanced cancer sometimes experience pain in the region of one or both sacro-iliac joints. This may relate to an underlying osseous metastasis, notably in breast and prostatic cancer, or to recurrence on the anterior surface of the pelvis from a previously treated intrapelvic cancer, such as rectum, cervix uteri or ovary. In the former it is usually not the only metastasis, and the presence of other osteolytic areas on plain X-ray favour a neoplastic aetiology. In the latter there are often signs of nerve compression of the lower lumbar or higher sacral nerves, or other evidence of recurrence such as an ipsilateral non-functioning kidney. If there are no changes visible on X-ray in relation to the sacro-iliac joint, and no other evidence of recurrence, a bone scan is probably indicated before proceeding with radiation therapy. There may be no strong reason for suspecting a metastasis; the primary site is not one commonly associated with bone involvement, or there may be a preceding history of discomfort and pain in this area. In this situation, the local injection of bupivicaine (Marcaine) and depot methylprednisolone (Depo-Medrone, Depo-Medrol) should be considered, as the discomfort may well be a coincidental non-malignant pain. Non-malignant sacro-iliac pain is more common in patients who have lost weight and, with it, the cushioning effect that adipose tissue normally gives to this region.

The patient should be told:

1 sacro-iliac pain is common in patients with cancer;
2 frequently, it is *not* malignant in origin;
3 an injection of 'local anaesthetic and cortisone' often helps considerably;
4 there will be initial benefit from the local anaesthetic which will tend to wear off 'over the first 6 to 24 hours';
5 the main benefit of the injection will develop over 2 to 3 days as a result of the continuing effect of the 'cortisone'.

Some patients experience more pain after the local anaesthetic has worn off, presumably because of the formation of a haematoma. This can be fairly severe and may take several days to settle. The results after the haematoma pain has resolved are as in other patients: some have marked or complete relief, some moderate relief, and others have none. It is possible that those in whom no relief is obtained have an underlying lesion and the question of irradiation should be reconsidered. Occasionally sacro-iliac pain is referred pain from the upper lumbar vertebrae and, if there is no local tenderness, X-rays should include the lumbar spine.

Injection of the sacro-iliac joint is done with the patient on his side, the painful joint uppermost. Palpation will indicate the site of the sacro-iliac joint: it feels like a ridge of bone in continuity with the posterior part of the iliac crest and is clearly lateral to the midline. Bupivicaine 0.5 per cent (without adrenaline) is used to anaesthetize the skin and subdermal tissue. Usually about 1 to 2 ml is required. With experience it is normally possible to insert the needle into a small, but definite, joint space. With the needle still in the joint space, the syringe is changed and the depot methylprednisolone is injected. This may require a modest amount of pressure. If this is the case, 1 ml (40 mg) only should be injected into the joint space, and then, after withdrawing the needle for a few millimeters, the rest is injected immediately over the joint. The tissues over the joint can then be infiltrated with some 4 to 5 ml of 0.5 per cent bupivicaine.

Trigger Point Related Pain

Although brief stimulation of myofascial trigger points (TP) by dry needling, intense cold, or injection of physiological (normal) saline frequently produces prolonged relief from pain [35], we favour the use of local anaesthetic and depot methylprednisolone. Once the TP has been located by careful palpation, bupivicaine can be injected into it, followed by depot methylprednisolone in a manner comparable to the injection of the sacro-iliac joint or solitary superficial bone metastases (vide infra).

Suggestion and distraction of attention are commonly involved to explain the success of the above methods, but neither is capable of explaining the long duration of relief that is often obtained. When relief is temporary, further blocks may relieve pain for increasingly longer periods of time.

Solitary Rib Metastases

If a patient complains of pain in a rib which is thought to be caused by a metastasis, it is often a good idea to treat locally with bupivicaine and depot methylprednisolone. Having located the tender spot, the intercostal nerve is blocked with 5 ml of 0.5 per cent bupivicaine and then, through a second needle, 2 ml (80 mg) of depot methylprednisolone is injected with the tip of the needle pressing against the now anaesthetized tender spot in the rib. This has resulted in relief in some patients for several months, for example, in breast cancer and myeloma. Sometimes no benefit is obtained or only a transient one related to the immediate effect of the bupivicaine. In these cases, radiation therapy or the use of thoracic intrathecal chlorocresol (vide infra) should be considered. In practice failure with bupivicaine and methylprednisolone usually means that analgesics should be tried or an existing drug regimen modified.

Other Localized Axial Skeletal Secondaries

It is possible to use the same techniques as those employed for non-malignant sacro-iliac or metastatic rib pain in relation to a number of skeletal secondaries, namely, those involving bony prominences. These include parts of the scapula, the iliac crest, and the region of the pubic symphysis.

A recent report highlights the use of 2 per cent lignocaine and penicillin G procaine 'directly into the metastatic bone lesion' [36]. Initially 2 to 3 ml of 2 per cent lignocaine was injected. Those who responded obtained relief for from 24 to 72 hours. A repeat injection was then made using a combination of one part 2 per cent lignocaine and two parts *penicillin G procaine*, 6,000,000 units/ml. The authors thought thus to exploit the local anaesthetic property of the procaine moiety. In addition the lignocaine may be adsorbed onto the surface of the poorly soluble procaine penicillin and be slowly released as the procaine penicillin was solubilized or cleared. Amounts of up to 6 ml were used. Subsequent injections tended to have a longer lasting effect. There is no evidence that this technique is better than the alternative one with bupivicaine and depot methylprednisolone. Both emphasize the value of local injection; one or other should be used when indicated.

Postherpetic Neuralgia

This is included as a proportion of cancer patients develop this type of pain. Unlike acute herpetic pain, postherpetic neuralgia is essentially unresponsive to analgesics. Benefit is obtained in about 70 per cent of cases from antidepressants and/or anticonvulsants (*see* Chapter 16). Residual hyperaesthetic discomfort is usually maximal at the proximal and distal parts of the affected dermatome(s). A subdermal infiltration of 20 ml of 1 per cent lignocaine mixed with 200 mg of hydrocortisone is often helpful. It is wise to use a small-bore spinal needle (22 gauge) as this prevents too rapid and too localized an injection. The needle is inserted in the centre of the area to be treated and moved in a radial fashion subdermally as the lignocaine is injected. Not only is the pain abolished for an hour or so, but when it returns, it is usually not as intense or as widespread. Sometimes relief may last for days or even several weeks. Patients should be told that the injection will take the pain away completely in the treated area for a few hours, after which the discomfort will almost certainly return, but less severely. Repeat injections every 3 weeks for 3 to 4 months can be planned and undertaken as necessary.

Head and Neck Pain

Local anaesthetic nerve blocks of the upper cervical nerves may sometimes be helpful if pain is localized to limited areas supplied by superficial branches of the cervical plexus. The nerves can be injected collectively, as they emerge from under the middle of the posterior border of the sternomastoid muscle.

Neurolytic Blocks

Oro-pharynx

Oro-pharyngeal nerve blocks are hazardous. They are indicated only if narcotic analgesia has utterly failed. Blocks produce difficulty in swallowing, secondary to paralysis of the pharyngeal muscles. Injection of the superior laryngeal branch of the vagus is sometimes carried out for malignant disease of the larynx.

Coeliac Axis Plexus Block

This should be considered in patients with intractable epigastric neoplastic pain, notably pancreatic but also gastric or hepatic. It can be done under local anaesthetic but, in practice, the patient usually has a general anaesthetic. There are no data comparing management of epigastric pain by analgesics and by nerve block. This means that, at present, it is the patients who fail to obtain good relief with narcotics who are considered for a coeliac axis plexus block. The block will not relieve the back pain experienced by some patients. This is indicative of neoplastic extension into the posterior abdominal wall.

Coeliac axis plexus block is generally conducted with the patient lying curled up on the more painful side. A 12 cm needle is inserted below the twelfth rib as far laterally as possible to avoid puncturing the pleura and lung and passed forward to a point just anterior and adjacent to the first lumbar vertebral body. Monitoring with an X-ray image intensifier is essential for the accurate positioning of the tip of the needle. In many cases, 15 to 20 ml of 90 to 95 per cent alcohol on one side is sufficient to relieve pain.

This procedure is almost identical to a lumbar sympathetic block, but one vertebra higher. A coincidental lumbar sympathetic block is, therefore, possible particularly if large amounts of alcohol are used (40 to 50 ml). Transient hypotension, lasting for several days, is common. It is rarely prolonged, let alone incapacitating (Table 5.8). Narcotic analgesics may still be necessary for 1 to 2 days after the block, even when successful.

Lumbar sympathetic blocks using 10 per cent phenol in water are

Table 5.8   Unwanted effects associated with coeliac axis plexus block

Pneumothorax
Puncture of inferior vena cava (right side)†
Puncture of aorta (left side)†
Haemorrhage into adrenal gland (especially on right)—usually associated with the
needle in too lateral a position
Hypotension (usually transient)
Diarrhoea (the result of changes in blood flow to the bowel)
Groin pain (because partial damage to L1 nerve root)

† not necessarily serious

sometimes of benefit in patients with intrapelvic pain, particularly bladder pain or rectal tenesmoid pain [37].

Intrathecal Neurolysis
This may be achieved by use of alcohol (hypobaric), phenol-in-glycerine, or chlorocresol-in-glycerine (both hyperbaric). The most commonly used agent is 5 per cent phenol-in-glycerine. In this concentration there is minimal interference with motor function and with sensations other than pain. Stronger solutions (e.g. 10 per cent) are sometimes used in the treatment of spasticity. Phenol is rapidly fixed to tissues and, in the amount used (0.3 to 0.6 ml), generally effects only one or two nerve routes. If, however, the needle or the patient is badly positioned, the phenol may be injected in such a way that it drips over the cauda equina. This is likely to result in a more diffuse effect.

Chlorocresol 2 per cent is not fixed so readily and is a more attractive agent in the thoracic region where it is necessary to block at least 3 nerve routes to achieve significant relief. Unlike phenol, it has only a slight early local anaesthetic effect prior to neurolysis. It does not, therefore, cause immediate sensory effects like tingling, numbness or warmth. With phenol these are useful guides to the accuracy of the placement of the neurolytic agent.

Phenol 5 per cent damages mainly pain-sensory fibres. Other fibres may be affected in the following order:

1   motor fibres to bladder and rectum,
2   other sensory fibres,
3   somatic motor fibres.

With blocks in the lower lumbar region there is a definite risk of producing bladder and anal dysfunction, particularly in patients with underlying problems such as prostatism (Table 5.9). In one series, the mean duration of benefit was only 3 weeks, ranging from 0 to 3 months

[38]. One-third of patients had a major complication, such as incontinence (urinary, faecal, or both), weakness (occasionally paraplegia) or dysaesthesia. Many patients prefer to have continued pain rather than risk requiring a catheter or anal incontinence. Recovery, which is not always complete, takes place in the reverse order: motor function first, sensation second and, finally, anal and bladder function.

Table 5.9 Complications of intrathecal phenol

Pain at injection site (∵ phenol)
Headache ± vomiting (post-lumbar puncture)
Meningism
Urinary retention
Faecal incontinence
Paraesthesia
Sensory loss
Motor weakness

Other Techniques

These include the replacement of CSF by ice-cold saline and CSF barbotage. The latter refers to the alternate withdrawing and re-injection of 20 ml of CSF through a wide-bore spinal (Twohy) needle with the patient sitting upright [39]. The procedure is repeated up to 20 or 30 times. Neither saline replacement, nor barbotage share the adverse side effects of neurolytic techniques. Both are correspondingly less reliable in terms of relief obtained. Ice-cold saline replacement helps up to 50 per cent of patients, barbotage less. They are of value when cordotomy (vide infra) is not readily available for the patient with bilateral pain below the waist that is not fully controlled by drugs. Ice-cold saline replacement is an extremely painful procedure at the moment of injection. It has, therefore, the added disadvantage of necessitating a general anaesthetic.

Neurosurgery

It is rare to need neurosurgical measures to relieve cancer pain (Table 5.10). Occasionally cordotomy (spinothalamic tractotomy) is necessary. There are two types of cordotomy: surgical and percutaneous. Percutaneous cordotomy means two days in a Pain Relief Unit, whereas open cordotomy generally means two weeks in a neurosurgical ward.

Percutaneous cordotomy is achieved by inserting a needle in the C1/C2 interspace under X-ray image intensification. A thermal lesion is then made in the anterolateral quadrant of the spinal cord using radiofrequency waves. Surgical cordotomy requires a general anaesthetic, is usually done in the upper thoracic region, and the anterolateral quadrant of the cord is cut under direct vision. Cordotomy is used mainly for

Table 5.10 Neurosurgical techniques and cancer pain

Open cordotomy	spinothalamic tractotomy
Percutaneous cordotomy	
Transection of spinal cord	
Thalamotomy†	

† never used so far in our patients

intractable *unilateral* pain located in segments from the mid-thorax downwards. Bilateral percutaneous high cervical cordotomy is hazardous because of the likelihood of sleep apnoea ('Ondine's Curse'), caused by interruption of the motor fibres to the diaphragm. These lie close to the spinothalamic tract and only emerge with the phrenic nerve at the level of C4.

Cordotomy of either variety is not without limitations. The alleviation of the unilateral pain may 'unmask' a severe pain on the contralateral side. Moreover, although seemingly permanent, the versatility of the central nervous system is such that relief does not generally last for more than 6 to 18 months. Although this is sufficient for many patients with terminal cancer, for a substantial minority it is not.

In the last 6 years, we have requested total transection of the spinal cord in 3 patients. All had progressive signs of paraplegia and were catheterized. They experienced severe to excrutiating pain in the spine or adjacent lumbar region on movement as a result of tumour pressing on the spinal cord and nerve roots. Two of the patients experienced complete relief as a result of the procedure. The third no longer had the more local back pain, but, as expected, continued to experience dysaesthetic pain in the legs. One patient was well enough to begin rehabilitation as a paraplegic, though died about 3 weeks later of a pulmonary embolus. The other 2 were too weak to be mobilized, but were free of pain for the first time in many weeks. They died, one 2 months and the other 6 months later.

Immobilization

Some patients continue to experience pain on movement despite analgesics, other drugs, radiotherapy and nerve blocks. In these, the situation may be improved by suggesting commonsense modifications to daily activity (Table 5.11). For example, a man may continue to struggle to stand when shaving unless the doctor suggests that sitting would be a good idea. Such a suggestion is accepted more readily if accompanied by a simple explanation of why weight-bearing precipitates or exacerbates the pain. Individually designed plastic supports for patients with multiple collapsed vertebrae or Thomas splints for femoral pain are occasionally

Table 5.11 Immobilization

Rest
Modification of lifestyle
Cervical collar
Surgical corset
Moulded plastic splints
Slings

necessary to overcome intolerable pain on movement in bedfast patients. The humerus can most satisfactorily be immobilized in the bedfast patient by an arm sling fastened to a torso jacket by means of interlocking Velcro.

Case History. Mrs. NP aged 57 with breast cancer sustained a pathological fracture of the right femoral neck (Figure 5.1). This gave her

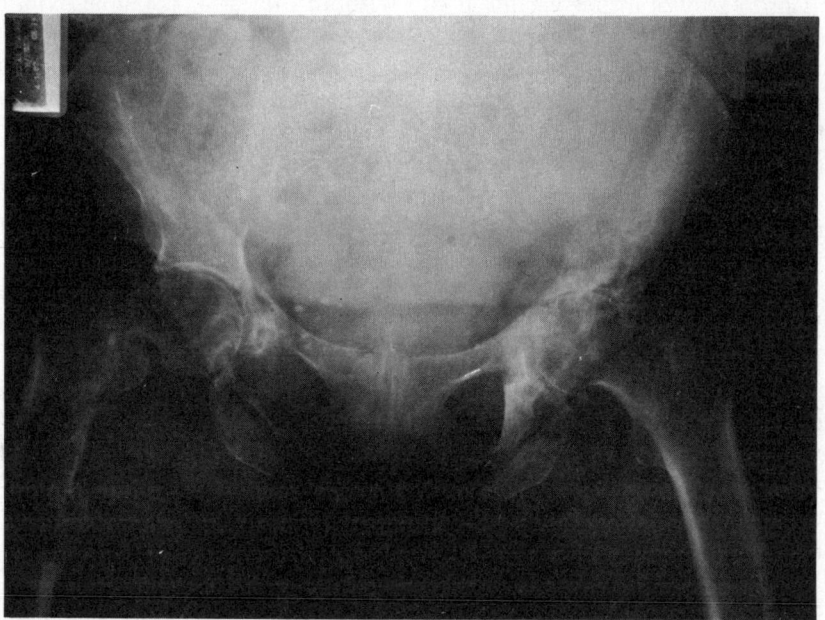

Figure 5.1 Radiograph showing pathological fracture of right neck of femur associated with extensive metastatic disease throughout the length of the bone.

much pain. Because of the extent of the metastatic bone disease, surgical management was not possible. Relief at night and when sitting in a chair was achieved with oral morphine and flurbiprofen. She repeatedly said how wonderful it was to be out of pain (Figure 5.2), yet careless movement of the right thigh was transiently very painful. Before the presence of a fracture was confirmed, she herself limited

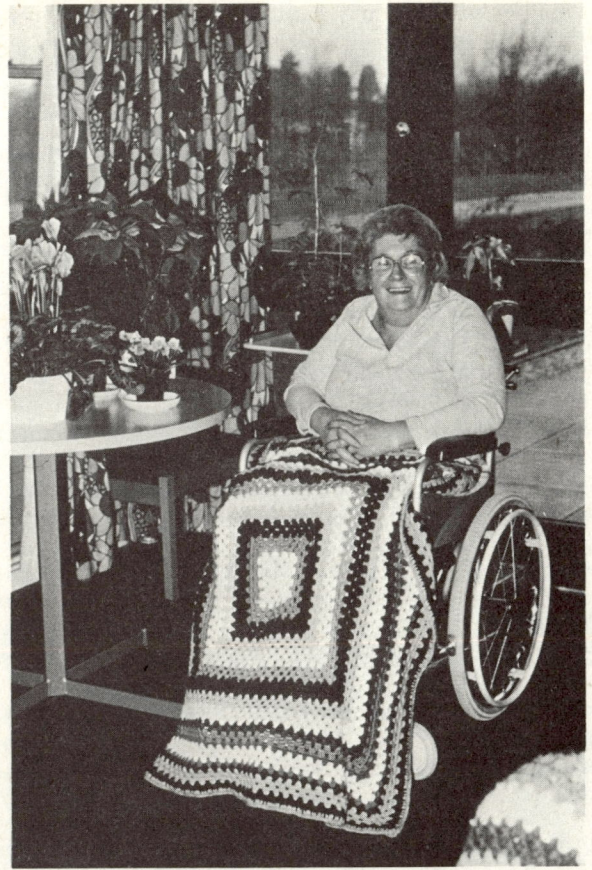

Figure 5.2 Modification of lifestyle. Picture of Mrs. N P dressed and in a wheelchair as she was most days after sustaining a pathological fracture of the right femoral neck.

weight-bearing to a minimum. When transferring from bed to wheelchair, for example, she had learnt to avoid pain by having her daughter hold the legs together and moving them as one.

References

1 *Advances in Pain Research and Therapy, Volume 2* edited by Bonica JJ and Ventafridda A. Raven Press, New York 1979.
2 *Advances in Pain Research and Therapy, Volume 1* edited by Bonica JJ and Albe-Fessard DG. Raven Press, New York 1976.
3 *Advances in Pain Research and Therapy, Volume 3* edited by Bonica JJ, Liebesking JC and Albe-Fessard DG. Raven Press, New York 1979.

4 *Advances in Pain Research and Therapy, Volume 4 Management of Superior Pulmonary Sulcus Syndrome (Pancoast Syndrome)* edited by Bonica JJ, Ventafridda V and Pagni CA. Raven Press, New York 1982.

5 *Advances in Pain Research and Therapy, Volume 5* edited by Bonica JJ, Lindblom U and Iggo A. Raven Press, New York 1983.

6 Lichter I. Communication in *Palliative Care: The Management of Far-Advanced Illness* edited by Doyle D. Croom Helm, Beckenham, Fyshwick and Philadelphia 1984, pp 444–460.

7 Mulhern, RM. A patient with oral cancer. *RN Magazine* 1983. In press.

8 Lynch P. The hospice: changing society's approach to death. *National Association of Social Worker's News* 1978; **23(10):** 5.

9 Jacobson E. *Modern Treatment of Tense Patients.* Charles Thomas, Springfield, Illinois 1970.

10 Cox DJ, Freundlich A and Meyer RG. Differential effectiveness of electromyographic feedback, verbal relaxation, instructions and placebo medication with tension headaches. *Journal of Consultation in Clinical Psychology* 1975; **43:** 892–898.

11 Haynes S, Griffin P, Mooney D and Parise M. Electromyographic feedback and relaxation instructions in the treatment of muscle contraction headaches. *Behavioural Therapy* 1976; **6:** 672–678.

12 McCaffery M, Morra ME, Gross J and Moritz DA. *Dealing with Pain.* American Cancer Society, Connecticut Division, Inc., Yale Comprehensive Cancer Centre 1981, pp 17–22.

13 McCaffery M. Relieving pain with noninvasive techniques. *Nursing* 1980; **10:** 55–57.

14 Kogeorgos J and Scott DF. Biofeedback and its clinical applications. *British Journal of Hospital Medicine* 1981; **25:** 601–605.

15 Turner JA and Chapman RC. Psychological interventions for chronic pain: a critical review. 1. Relaxation training and biofeedback. *Pain* 1982; **12:** 1–21.

16 Budzynski TH, Stoyva JM, Adler CS and Mullaney DJ. EMG biofeedback and tension headaches: a controlled outcome study. *Psychosomatic Medicine* 1973; **35:** 484–496.

17 Melzack R and Perry C. Self-regulation of pain: the use of alpha-biofeedback and hypnotic training for the control of chronic pain. *Experimental Neurology* 1975; **46:** 452–469.

18 Melzack R. Psychologic aspects of pain in *Pain* edited by Bonica JJ. Raven Press, New York 1980, pp 143–154.

19 Turk DC, Meichenbaum DH and Berman WH. Application of biofeedback for the regulation of pain: a critical review. *Psychological Bulletin* 1979; **86:** 1322–1338.

20 Zitman FG. Biofeedback, relaxation training and chronic pain in *Persistent Pain. Modern Methods of Treatment, Volume 3* edited by Lipton S and Miles J. Academic Press, London, Toronto and Sydney; Grune and Stratton, New York and San Francisco 1981, pp 99–117.

21 Barber J and Gitelson J. Cancer pain: psychological management using hypnosis. *CA-A Cancer Journal for Clinicians* 1980; 130–136.

22 Orne MT. Hypnotic control of pain: toward a clarification of the different psychological processes involved in *Pain* edited by Bonica JJ. Raven Press, New York 1980, pp 1550–1572.

23 Cangello VM. The use of hypnotic suggestion for pain relief in malignant disease. *International Journal of Clinical Experimental Hypnosis* 1961; **9:** 17–22.

24 Butler B. The use of hypnosis in the care of the cancer patient. *Cancer* 1954; **7:** 1–14.

25 Sacerdote P. The place of hypnosis in the relief of severe protracted pain. *American Journal of Clinical Hypnosis* 1962; **4:** 150–157.

26 Sacerdote P. Theory and practice of pain control in malignancy and other protracted or recurring painful illnesses. *International Journal of Clinical Experimental Hypnotherapy* 1970; **18:** 160–180.

27 Lea P, Ware P and Monroe R. The hypnotic control of intractable pain. *American Journal of Clinical Hypnosis* 1960; **3:** 3–8.

28 Finer B. Hypnotherapy in pain of advanced cancer in *Advances in Pain Research and Therapy, Volume 2* edited by Bonica JJ and Ventafridda V. Raven Press, New York 1979, pp 223–229.

29 Melzack R. Phantom limb pain: implications for treatment of pathologic pain. *Anesthesiology* 1971; **35:** 409–419.

30 Anonymous. The Pain Paradox. *Lancet* 1976; **i:** 945–946.

31 Melzack R. Prolonged relief of pain by brief intense transcutaneous somatic stimulation. *Pain* 1975; **1:** 357–373.

32 Ventafridda V, Sganzerla EP, Fochi C, Pozzi G and Gordini G. Transcutaneous nerve stimulation in cancer pain in *Advances in Pain Research and Therapy, Volume 2* edited by Bonica JJ and Ventafridda V. Raven Press, New York 1979, pp 509–515.

33 Editorial. How does acupuncture work? *British Medical Journal* 1981; **283:** 746–748.

34 *Relief of Intractable Pain* edited by Swerdlow M. Excerpta Medica, Amsterdam, London and New York (2nd Edition) 1978.

35 Melzack R. Myofascial trigger points: relation to acupuncture and mechanisms of pain. *Archives of Physical Medicine and Rehabilitation* 1981; **62:** 114–117.

36 Zweig JI, Malspies L, Kaus S and Kabakow B. A novel approach to the temporary control of intractable bone pain. *Journal of the American Medical Association* 1980; **244:** 2445.

37 Clarke IMC. Personal communication.

38 Evans R. Personal communication.

39 Lloyd JW, Hughes JT and Davies-Jones GAB. Relief of severe intractable pain by barbotage of cerebro-spinal fluid. *Lancet* 1972; **i:** 354–355.

Chapter Six

Analgesics

> *Analgesic*
> A drug which modifies the perception of pain without loss of consciousness.

Many drugs affect pain (Table 6.1). Some affect it indirectly, such as antibiotics in cystitis or sinusitis and penicillinamine or gold in rheumatoid arthritis. These drugs act by modifying the pathological process and fall outside the definition of analgesic. Spasmolytics are another group of pain modulating drugs (Table 6.2). When used in conjunction with an analgesic in cancer pain patients, it is convenient to describe such agents as 'co-analgesics' (*see* Chapter 16).

Table 6.1   Drugs that relieve pain

Category	Mode of action
Antibiotics	Modification of pathological process
Anti-rheumatoid drugs	Modification of pathological process
Spasmolytic	Reduction of muscle spasm
Anticonvulsant	Control of paroxysmal neuralgia
Anxiolytic	Reduction of anxiety
Antidepressant	Alleviation of depression
Analgesic	Modulation of pain threshold

Table 6.2   Spasmolytic drugs

Muscle type	Drug
Somatic	baclofen
	diazepam
	dantrolene
Smooth	probanthine and related drugs
	flavoxate (bladder only)
Cardiac	verapamil

Classification of Analgesics

There is no universally agreed classification of analgesics. The classification into *non-addictive* and *addictive* is, thankfully, falling into disrepute. The use of the terms *mild* and *strong* is also not to be encouraged. Weak narcotics such as codeine are usually classed in the former. This obscures their pharmacological relationship with morphine and other narcotic drugs. Moreover, there are occasions when morphine (a 'strong analgesic') does not relieve pain which aspirin (a 'weak analgesic') does. *Antipyretic*

Table 6.3   Classification of analgesics

	1 *Non-narcotics*
	aspirin
	paracetamol[1]
	nefopam*
2 *Narcotic agonists*	3 *Narcotic agonist-antagonists*
Weak	*Weak*
codeine	pentazocine
dextropropoxyphene	
ethoheptazine	
oxycodone[2]	
Strong	*Strong*
morphine	butorphanol
diamorphine*	buprenorphine
hydromorphone**	nalbuphine
oxymorphone**	
methadone	

* not available in the USA
** not available in Britain
[1] acetaminophen (USA)
[2] see page 157 for comment

101

and *narcotic* have much in their favour, except that a drug such as nefopam* (*see* Chapter 7) does not fit into either category. The basic division into *non-narcotic* and *narcotic* is, however, important. The advent of drugs that have morphine-like (agonist) properties when used alone but act as antagonists when given after or in association with morphine has complicated the issue. As agonists and agonist-antagonists should not be prescribed concurrently, the classification in Table 6.3 has much to commend it. There is need also for a separate classification of drugs for use in rheumatoid arthritis (Table 6.4). The use of the term *simple* in relation to paracetamol[1] is not a comment on its mode of action. It is a shorthand way of saying that it is simply an analgesic (and antipyretic) and has no anti-inflammatory properties.

Table 6.4   Classification of drugs used in rheumatoid arthritis

Type of drug	Example
Simple analgesics	paracetamol[1]
Analgesics with minor anti-inflammatory properties	propionic acid derivatives
Analgesics with major anti-inflammatory properties	aspirin, indomethacin
Pure anti-inflammatory drugs	corticosteroids
Compounds with more specific action in rheumatoid arthritis	gold, penicillamine
Anti-inflammatory immunosuppressives	azathioprine

After Huskission, 1974 [1]
[1] acetaminophen (USA)

Narcotic (GK. narkotikos, benumbing)
A generic designation for all exogenous substances which bind specifically to the opiate receptors and produce some agonist actions. Drugs that meet this definition may or may not have a pharmacological profile similar to that of morphine.

Note: Some authors regard the term as obsolete and prefer the use of the word 'opioid' [2].

Mode of Analgesic Action

It is generally considered that aspirin and non-steroidal anti-inflammatory drugs (NSAID) act peripherally and narcotics centrally, that is,

* not available in the USA
[1] acetaminophen (USA).

within the central nervous system. Paracetamol and nefopam also act centrally but via different mechanisms. Recently published data [3] indicate, however, that such concepts are almost certainly an oversimplification. Aspirin and related drugs appear to act at several sites in relation to prostaglandin synthesis, some peripheral and some central. The same holds true for morphine.

The central and peripheral effects of morphine are both mediated by specific receptors and are both antagonized by naloxone. It has been suggested that narcotics may produce analgesia by inhibiting the activation of an enzyme, adenylate-cyclase, the production of which is stimulated by prostaglandins [3]. If this is confirmed, it augers far-reaching developments in the field of analgesics. It may well prove possible to develop a new class of analgesics that would act selectively on peripheral opiate receptors, thereby reducing or eliminating unwanted central effects.

Misuse of Analgesics

Poor pain control is often related to a failure to provide an adequate dose of an appropriate analgesic regularly. Colin MacInnes, novelist and social commentator who died of cancer in 1976, asked whether the medical profession stints its use of analgesics by tradition rather than from well reasoned principles [4]. He wondered if this was due partly to a masochistic streak in doctor and patient alike. Whether this is so, other important reasons for under-prescribing and under-administration include:

1   use of analgesics on an 'as required' rather than a regular basis;
2   lack of knowledge about narcotic analgesic pharmacology;
3   use of standard rather than individually determined doses;
4   fear of causing respiratory depression;
5   fear of causing addiction;
6   other fears about narcotic analgesics.

Table 6.5   Administration of analgesics

Method	Synonyms
As required	pro re nata (p.r.n.)
Regular	time-contingent, scheduled

1   *Use of analgesics on an 'as required' rather than a regular basis*
'As required' medication means that the doctor prescribes a drug to be given at the discretion of a nurse or on request by the patient. 'Regular' medication means that the patient receives a drug at specific stated times (Table 6.5). In a study of prescribing for severe pain [5], it was found that

74 per cent of all prescriptions for strong narcotics were 'as required', regardless of the aetiology of the pain, and despite the fact that analgesics were required on average for 11 days. In relation to persistent pain, notably cancer, Hunt and associates [6] found that when analgesics were prescribed 'as required' they were seldom used, sometimes never, despite the fact that patients were known to be in pain. Great reliance was placed by the nurses on patients asking for analgesics, or admitting to needing them when asked at the time of the routine drug rounds.

Even postoperatively with diminishing pain, 'as required' IM medication is commonly unsatisfactory, or at best, less satisfactory than continuous IV administration [7, 8]. The reasons given for an alternative approach in the management of postoperative pain are even more compelling in relation to persistent pain in cancer. As required medication is unsatisfactory because:

1 some patients do not appreciate that the onus is on them to ask for an analgesic if in pain;
2 shortage of nurses causes an inevitable delay between the re-appearance of pain and the request being made;
3 auxiliary nurses are not allowed to administer drugs, particularly those on the Controlled Drug Register;
4 fear of causing respiratory depression or drug dependence makes many nurses frightened to administer strong narcotics 'until absolutely necessary';
5 parallel fears concerning dependence may cause the patient not to ask unless the pain becomes very severe.

2 *Lack of knowledge about narcotic analgesic pharmacology*
It is reasonable to expect all doctors to have sufficient knowledge to make a rational choice of analgesic preparation, dose and frequency of administration. Unfortunately, this is not yet the case. For example, within a few days, a patient received the following drugs in this order [5]:

pethidine[1] (dose not stated)
codeine 15 mg—paracetamol 300 mg
aspirin 325 mg—codeine 30 mg (Empirin with Codeine No 3)
dextropropoxyphene napsylate 100 mg—paracetamol 650 mg (Darvocet-N 100)
chlorzoxazone 250 mg—paracetamol 300 mg (Flexaphen)

Almost certainly, proprietary names were used when prescribing these preparations and, if asked, the doctor(s) concerned would not have been able to identify correctly the content of some, if not all, of the compound tablets.

[1] meperidine (USA)

The tendency to indulge in pharmacological roulette or to 'kangaroo' from analgesic to analgesic is seen commonly with both weak and strong narcotics. A patient is well controlled on, for example, dextromoramide* 5 mg or hydromorphone** 2 mg 4-hourly. The pain recurs, and the medication is changed to morphine instead of adjusting upwards the dose of the previously satisfactory analgesic. This is done, presumably, on the grounds that the dextromoramide or hydromorphone has 'failed'. No thought is given to the fact that when using a strong narcotic agonist, the dose can be adjusted upwards considerably. What makes 'kangaroo jumping' with strong narcotics more hazardous is the widespread belief that morphine and diamorphine (heroin)* are the most potent of strong narcotics. Therefore, regardless of dose, doctors believe these drugs must be more efficacious. It is no wonder that both doctor and patient despair when morphine or diamorphine proves no better than the previously used analgesic, and sometimes worse.

It is still not uncommon to find terminal cancer patients prescribed opium/morphine/diamorphine 4-hourly with a weak narcotic-non-narcotic compound tablet boarded to be given midway between each main 4-hourly administration. As a result, the patient is tied unnecessarily to a 2-hourly regimen. Other patients, who have been adequately controlled on a certain dose of morphine are advised, when pain recurs or a new pain develops, to reduce the interval between administration from 4 hours to 3, or even 2 hours, rather than continue on the more convenient 4-hourly regimen with an increased dose. When pethidine is used, doses that are too small and too infrequent are commonplace[9]. It is perhaps part of the medical profession's general ignorance about narcotics that has resulted in the Brompton Cocktail becoming the panacea for cancer pain in the minds of many doctors (see Chapter 11).

3 *Use of standard rather than individually determined doses*
It is part of clinical folklore that most analgesics should be given in a certain predetermined dose or, perhaps, over a very limited range of doses. The concept of individual dose requirements is still foreign to many doctors and nurses when it comes to analgesics. There is, however, considerable published evidence which shows that individual need varies considerably both postoperatively [10] and in advanced cancer.

Many patients are denied relief because of a failure to 'optimize' the dose of the prescribed analgesic. There is no justification for this, as relief is not an all-or-none phenomenon. Many patients will report some relief for some time—however little and however short—that will guide the

---

* not available in the USA
** not available in Britain

doctor in the upward adjustment of dose until the optimum for the patient is achieved.

4   *Fears about the adverse side effects of narcotic analgesics*
These are a major stumbling block and do much to prevent good pain control. Because of the need to eradicate unfounded fears, a later chapter has been devoted to this aspect of the problem (Chapter 13). Suffice it to say that the danger of *possible* respiratory depression is grossly exaggerated in the minds of many doctors and nurses. Further, when addiction is defined, it is found *not* to be a problem (*see* page 226). Other fears relate to what have become self-perpetuating myths. These probably owe their origin ultimately to the innate fear in all of us of losing control of the situation. Narcotics, with their unsavoury reputation as 'euphoriant' and 'addictive', are seen as likely causes of loss of control. It is then only a matter of time before such drugs become suspect or evil. Once a cultural belief is established, albeit erroneous, it takes much time and effort to correct it.

Principles of Analgesic Use

1   Analgesics should be prescribed within the context of 'total patient care' and 'broad spectrum' pain control.
2   Keep it simple.
3   Use oral medication wherever possible.
4   Do not use mixtures routinely.
5   Persistent pain requires prophylactic therapy.
6   Doses should be determined on an individual basis.
7   Adjuvant medication is generally necessary.
8   It is sometimes necessary to balance the degree of relief against unwanted side effects.
9   Not all pain is relieved by narcotic or other analgesics.
10   Psychotropic drugs should not be given routinely.
11   Insomnia must be treated vigorously.
12   Inpatient admission is sometimes necessary to achieve pain control.

1   *Analgesics should be prescribed within the context of 'total patient care' and 'broad spectrum' pain control*
Analgesics are the backbone of the management of cancer pain. They are taken by the patient initially when pain is first experienced. They are adjuncts to anti-cancer treatment if necessary and remain a key therapeutic modality when other non-drug treatments are spent. The use of analgesics is not, however, synonymous with analgesia. Analgesics can never be more than part of a comprehensive multi-modality approach to pain control (*see* page 61).

2 Keep it simple

The three basic analgesics are aspirin, codeine and morphine. The rest should be considered alternatives of fashion or convenience. Appreciating this helps to prevent the doctor 'kangarooing' from analgesic to analgesic in a desperate search for some drug that will suit the patient better. If a non-narcotic-weak narcotic preparation such as aspirin-codeine, paracetamol-dextropropoxyphene, fails to relieve, it is usually better to move directly to a small dose of oral morphine sulphate than, for example, to prescribe dihydrocodeine.

It is necessary to be familiar with one or two alternatives for use in patients who cannot tolerate the standard preparation. Aspirin has two alternatives. Paracetamol, which has no anti-inflammatory effect, is one; NSAID as a group is the other. Which alternative is appropriate depends on whether there is a need for a peripheral anti-inflammatory effect. The individual doctor's basic analgesic ladder, with alternatives, should comprise no more than 9 or 10 drugs in total (Table 6.6). Other alternatives are available. Some of these are discussed later (see Chapters 8 and 14). It is better to know and understand a few drugs well than to have a passing acquaintance with the whole range.

Table 6.6   A basic analgesic ladder

Category	Parent drug	Alternatives
Non-narcotic	aspirin	paracetamol[1]
		flurbiprofen*
		naproxen
Weak narcotic	codeine	dextropropoxyphene
		oxycodone (USA)
Strong narcotic	morphine	papaveretum (Britain)
		phenazocine* (Britain)
		hydromorphone** (USA)
		oxymorphone** (USA)

* not available in the USA
** not available in Britain
[1] acetaminophen (USA)

(a)   With mild or moderate pain, use a non-narcotic in the first instance.

(b)   It may be appropriate to prescribe aspirin in addition to a narcotic, especially in patients with bone pain (see Chapter 7).

(c)   It is logical to combine analgesics that act via different mechanisms, for example:

   aspirin and paracetamol,
   paracetamol and codeine,
   aspirin and morphine,
   aspirin and oxycodone

However, it is not always wise, from the point of view of patient compliance, nor is it always therapeutically necessary.

(d) It is pharmacological nonsense to prescribe two weak narcotics simultaneously; likewise two strong narcotics.

(e) There is sometimes a place for a patient on a strong narcotic to have another narcotic (weak or strong) as a second 'as required' analgesic for occasional troublesome pain, although, generally, patients should be advised to take an extra dose of their regular medication if 'breakthough' pain occurs.

(f) If one weak narcotic preparation does not control the pain, do not waste time by prescribing an alternative; move to something definitely stronger.

(g) Morphine or an alternative strong narcotic should be used when non-narcotics and weak narcotics fail to control the pain.

(h) The severity of the pain determines the choice of analgesic, not the doctor's estimate of life expectancy—which is often wrong. A patient should not be made to wait in pain until the last days or hours of life.
    'Morphine exists to be given not merely to be withheld'

(i) The top of the analgesic ladder is not reached simply by prescribing morphine. Morphine may be given in a wide range of doses from as little as 2.5 mg to more than 500 mg (Figure 6.1).

(j) Do not prescribe narcotic agonist-antagonists with a narcotic agonist.

3 *Do not use mixtures routinely*

At some centres, morphine is always prescribed with a second drug, either cocaine (a stimulant) or a phenothiazine (a tranquillizer). Sometimes both are added. In these circumstances, increasing the dose of morphine can be hazardous if, by increasing the *volume* of the mixture taken, the dose of the adjunctive medication is also automatically increased regardless of need. Depending on the adjunctive drug, this can lead to agitation and restlessness or to somnolence. It is far better to give adjunctive medication separately, either as a syrup or a tablet/capsule. The dose of each pharmacologically active substance can then be adjusted individually against patient need.

4 *Use oral medication whenever possible*

The route of administration is a significant consideration because it has a substantial impact on the patient's way of life. The patient taking oral medication is free to move around, travel in a car and, most important, be at home. If pain is controlled by intravenous injection the patient usually cannot go home. Injections promote dependence on the person administering the drug. Apart from the last 2 to 3 days of life, only some 15 per cent of patients receiving hospice care require injections to control their pain at any one time (Figure 6.2). Oral administration eliminates muscle

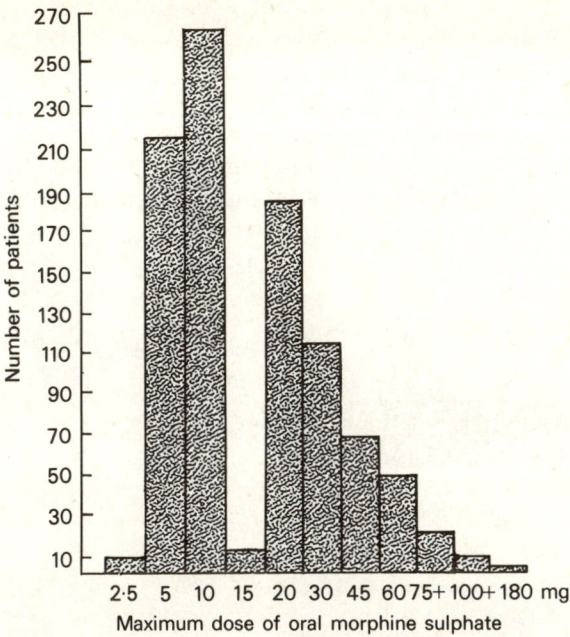

Figure 6.1 Histogram of maximum 4-hourly doses of orally administered morphine sulphate in 955 patients at St. Christopher's Hospice (1978–79). Median dose = 10 mg.
    Note: '75+' means 75, 80 or 90 mg, and '100+' means 100, 110 or 120 mg. Higher doses, up to 1200 mg, have been used occasionally by the authors.

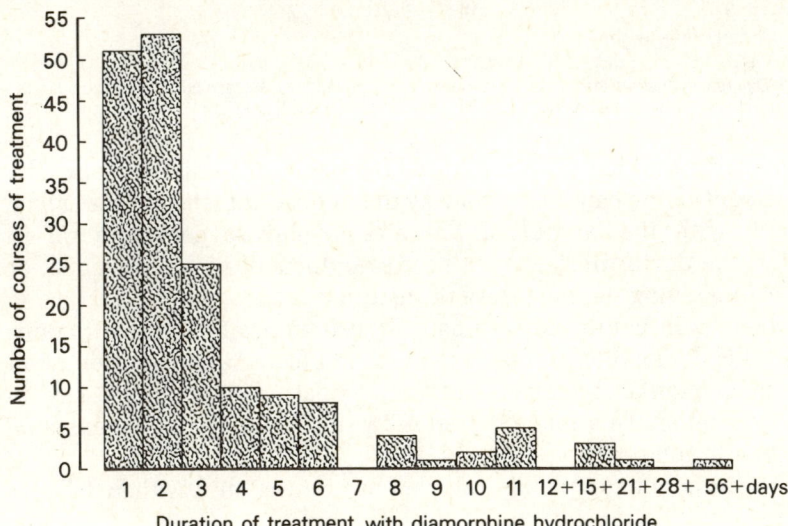

Figure 6.2 Histogram of duration of treatment with regular injections of diamorphine hydrochloride. 145 patients received a total of 173 courses of treatment by injection. Parent patient population = 210, admitted to Sir Michael Sobell House, Oxford, in 1978.

trauma, enables the patient to maintain control over his own drug administration and helps to retain his options over where to spend his last days.

5   Persistent pain requires prophylactic therapy

Continuous pain relief is superior to the sporadic pain relief provided by inadequate dosage or too long an interval between the doses (Figure 6.3).

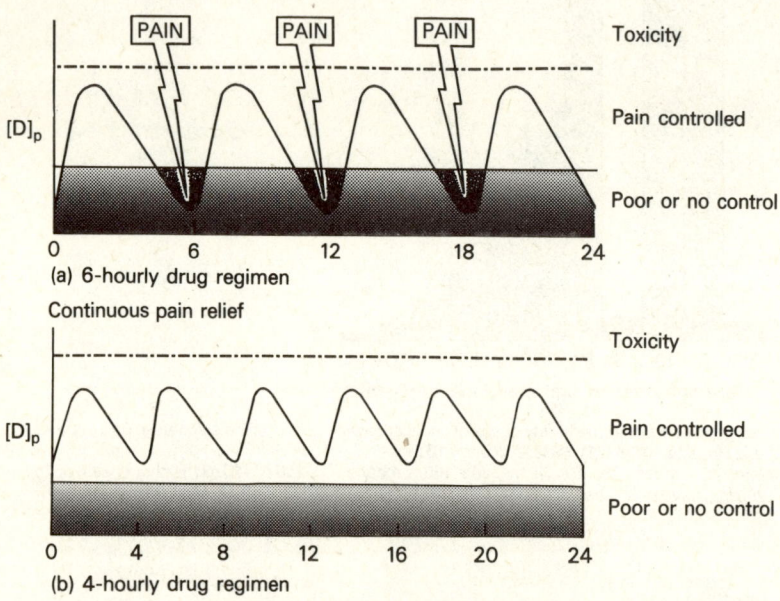

Figure 6.3 Diagram to illustrate the results of 'as required' and overspaced regular medication (a) compared with regular 4-hourly morphine sulphate (b). $[D]_p$ = plasma concentration of drug.

'Four-hourly p.r.n.' has no place in the treatment of persistent pain. The aim is to control the pain in such a way that it does not return. This can be compared with the control of the plasma glucose concentration in diabetics: the doctor does not wait for symptoms of hyperglycaemia, or coma, before giving the next dose of insulin.

Recurring pain is unnecessary pain. It also erodes the patient's confidence in his doctor and generates anxiety and fear. Administration of an analgesic at regular intervals and in adequate dosage is the key to continuous relief. This method results in smaller doses and keeps side effects to a minimum.

If the pain is not completely relieved but returns in less than 4 hours either:

(a)   increase the regular dose;
(b)   decrease the time interval to 3 hours.

The correct course of action can be ascertained by asking the patient the following questions:

'Does the medicine ever take the pain away completely?'
'Does the pain return before it is time for the next dose of medicine?'

If the answer to the first question is no, then the dose should be increased. If the answer to the second question is yes, the dose should also be increased: on most occasions, this will correct the deficit in pain relief. Should it not, the time interval should be decreased. We stress, however, that in practice it is rarely necessary to use a 3-hourly regimen.

If a strong analgesic other than morphine is used, the physician must be familiar with its pharmacology. For example, pethidine is effective for an average of two to three hours. Yet it is commonly boarded to be given every 4 hours or every 6 hours [9]. This is clearly insufficient and forces the patient to be in pain for at least 3 out of every 6 hours.

6   *Doses should be determined on an individual basis*
The effective analgesic dose varies considerably from patient to patient. The right dose of an analgesic is that which gives adequate pain relief for at least 3, and preferably 4 or more hours. 'Maximum' or 'recommended' doses derived mainly from postoperative parenteral single-dose studies, are not applicable in cancer. The dose of morphine and other strong narcotic agonists (except pethidine) can be increased almost indefinitely. On the other hand, the non-narcotics, weak narcotic agonists and narcotic agonist-antagonists tend to reach a plateau of maximum effect after 2 or 3 upward dose adjustments. Indeed the analgesic effect of buprenorphine, an agonist-antagonist may *decrease* above the optimal dose (*see* Chapter 15). Thus, if the upper effective dose has been reached with one of these agents, the dose should not be increased further but a stronger drug should be prescribed.

7   *Adjuvant medication is generally necessary*
Laxatives are almost always necessary, especially with patients receiving a narcotic. Unless fairly experienced, an antiemetic should be prescribed routinely with oral morphine or other strong narcotics. There are many situations where a better result is obtained by adding a second drug that relieves pain in a different way rather than increasing the dose of morphine indefinitely (*see* Chapter 16).

8   *It is sometimes necessary to balance the degree of relief against*
    unwanted side effects
Examples include aspirin and gastric irritation, and morphine and gastric stasis. Generally, there are ways round these problems but occasionally a compromise is necessary (*see* Chapters 7 and 9).

111

9 *Not all pain is responsive to narcotic or other analgesics*
Common pains not relieved by narcotics are listed in Table 6.7. Narcotics
do not usually relieve pain caused by degenerative nerve damage (dysaesthesia and stabbing pains), but the occasional patient does respond. The
site of the neurological lesion and the type of pain determine whether or
not narcotics will be of benefit (Table 6.8).

Table 6.7   Narcotic unresponsive pains

Sedative response only: narcotic should not be used
Tension headache
Postherpetic neuralgia
Dysaesthesia
Stabbing

Variable response: narcotic best avoided
Gastric distention
Muscle spasm

Partial response: but narcotic often necessary
Bone
Nerve compression
Activity precipitated (bone or nerve compression)
'Tenesmoid' (rectum or bladder)
Decubitus (superficial component)

Table 6.8   Neurological classification of pain: implications for therapy

	Type of pain		*Treatment*
1	Nociceptive		analgesics
2	Nerve compression		analgesics
			corticosteroids
			nerve blocks
3	Nerve destruction		psychotropic drugs
	(dysaesthetic)		(especially antidepressants)
		narcotics	*peripheral nerve—*
		corticosteroids	occasionally useful;
		nerve blocks	*cord lesion—*
		cordotomy	of no benefit
4	Mixed nerve		treated as mixed 2 and 3
	compression and destruction		(?) stellate ganglion block
	(partly dysaesthetic)		for upper limb pain

10 *Psychotropic drugs should not be used routinely*
If the patient is very anxious, an anxiolytic should be prescribed. If a
patient remains depressed after several days of much improved pain
relief, an antidepressant may be necessary.

11   Insomnia must be treated vigorously
Discomfort is worse at night when the patient is alone with his pain and his fears. The cumulative effect of many sleepless, pain-filled nights is a substantial lowering of the patient's pain threshold with a concomitant increase in pain intensity.

12   Admission is sometimes necessary to achieve pain control
Particularly in a hospice, a patient is affected by far more than drug changes [11, 12]. He is surrounded by a team of people who are confident that the pain will come under control. Peer support comes from the other patients in the four or five bed unit who relate their own stories of having achieved good pain control [13]. The patient sees the others receive their medicine regularly and observes that they are alert and functioning normally.

Anxieties About Prescribing

'Freedom from any anxiety about prescribing may amount to dangerous ignorance.'[14]

Most doctors have anxieties about prescribing [14], just as most patients have anxieties about the drugs they take. Unless doctors recognize their own anxieties, they are unlikely to be able to understand or to deal sensibly with those of the patient. Some of the more common fears doctors, patients and families have about strong narcotics are discussed in Chapter 13. A recognition that, generally, such fears are ill-founded or exaggerated helps to allay anxiety. Even so, in the individual patient, there remains the possibility that what a doctor prescribes may upset rather than help the patient. It is not possible, for example, to predict who will have anaphylactic shock after receiving penicillin, or a perforated peptic·ulcer from corticosteroid therapy. It is normal and necessary to be anxious about prescribing.

It is important for the doctor not to detail minutely every possible small-print adverse reaction because compliance will be markedly reduced. Common side effects should be mentioned, advice about driving and alcohol given, and a 'hot-line' for advice should be available if something unusual happens [15]. In practice, it is better to make light of this, so as to help neutralize the patient's concern: 'If you find something odd happens—such as your toenails fall out or your hair goes green—let me/us know. You can get hold of me/one of us by phoning . . ., but let me emphasize, I don't expect this to be necessary. In any case, Sister/Nurse will be in touch by phone and plans to visit you after a day or two to see how things are going.'

113

References

1 Huskisson EC. Recent drugs and the rheumatic diseases *Reports on Rheumatic Diseases, No. 54* The Arthritis and Rheumatism Council, London 1974.

2 Jaffe JH and Martin WR. Opioid analgesics and antagonists in *The Pharmacological Basic of Therapeutics* edited by Gilman AG, Goodman LS and Gilman A, McMillan, New York, Toronto and London 1980, pp 494–534.

3 Ferreira S. Peripheral and central analgesia. *Pain* 1981; supplement 1: 54.

4 MacInnes C. Cancer ward. *New Society* 1976; **36:** 232–234.

5 Aguwa CN and Olusanya OA. Analgesic prescribing for severe pain studied. *Drug Intelligence and Clinical Pharmacy* 1978; **12:** 556.

6 Hunt JM, Stollar TD, Littlejohns DW, Twycross RG and Vere DW. Patients with protracted pain: a survey conducted at the London Hospital. *Journal of Medical Ethics* 1977; **3:** 61–73.

7 Nayman J. Measurement and control of postoperative pain. *Annals of the Royal College of Surgeons of England* 1979; **61:** 419–426.

8 Rutter PC, Murphy F and Dudley HAF. Morphine: controlled trial of different methods of administration for postoperative pain relief. *British Medical Journal* 1980; **280:** 12–13.

9 Marks RM and Sachar EJ. Undertreatment of medical inpatients with narcotic analgesics. *Annals of Internal Medicine* 1973; **78:** 173–181.

10 Catling JA, Pinto DM, Jordan C and Jones JG. Respiratory effects of analgesia after cholecystectomy: comparison of continuous and intermittent papaveretum. *British Medical Journal* 1980; **281:** 478–480.

11 Melzack R, Ofiesh JG and Mount BM. The brompton mixture: effects on pain in cancer patients. *Canadian Medical Association Journal* 1976; **115;** 125–129.

12 Lack SA. Institutional Living—Referral: Hospice in *The Later Years, Social Applications of Gerontology* edited by Kalish RA. Brooks/Cole Publishing Company Monterey, California 1977, p 351.

13 Buckingham RW, Lack SA, Mount BM, MacLean LD and Collins JT. Living with the dying. Use of the technique of participant observation. *Canadian Medical Association Journal* 1976; **115:** 1211–1215.

14 Julian P and Herxheimer A. Doctors' anxieties in prescribing. *Journal of the Royal College of General Practitioners* 1977; **27:** 662–665.

15 Lack SA. Hospice. A concept of care in the final stage of life. *Connecticut Medicine* 1979; **43:** 367–372.

Part Three

Pharmacology

Chapter Seven

Non-Narcotic Analgesics

Several review articles on aspirin and paracetamol[1] have appeared in recent years. We have not therefore set out to be comprehensive. Analgesic nephropathy is not discussed [1], nor is the treatment of overdosage [2, 3]. Our aim is simply to highlight those aspects which are relevant and important to the physician when considering the use of non-narcotic analgesics in patients with cancer (Table 7.1).

Table 7.1 Commonly available non-narcotic drugs

aspirin
NSAID[2]
paracetamol[1]
nefopam*

* not available in the USA
[1] acetaminophen (USA)
[2] non-steroidal anti-inflammatory drugs

Aspirin

Aspirin in small doses is *not* anti-inflammatory. 600 mg produces relief which begins within 30 minutes of taking it; this lasts for up to 6 hours. Further doses have the same effect. A daily intake of at least 3.6 g is generally considered to be the minimum significant anti-inflammatory dose. Several days are required to achieve maximum relief. It is not known how much aspirin *per se* reaches sites of inflammation. From animal studies with chemically induced inflammation it is known that aspirin has an effect in certain models where sodium salicylate does not.

[1] acetaminophen (USA)

Drug portrait

Aspirin (acetylsalicylic acid; ASA) is a semisynthetic derivative of salicylic acid, a naturally occurring substance (Figure 7.1). It is the 'parent' non-steroidal anti-inflammatory drug (NSAID). In small doses, aspirin is simply analgesic and antipyretic. In larger doses (more than 3.6 g a day in normoalbuminaemic patients) it also has an anti-inflammatory effect. Aspirin appears to act at more than one site and via more than one mechanism [4, 5]. Its primary action is almost certainly at the site of pain. Aspirin is readily absorbed from the upper gastrointestinal tract. Considerable between-patient variation exists in plasma concentration after identical doses. At low doses increments result in proportional increases in blood level. Doses up to 1200 mg, possibly 1800 mg, provide increasing dose-related relief. Aspirin has a plasma half-life of about 15 minutes. It is rapidly hydrolyzed to salicylate by plasma and hepatic esterases. The salicylate remains detectable in the serum for several hours and almost certainly is responsible for the latter part of the effects of aspirin. Eighty per cent of the salicylate is converted to salicylurate by conjugation with glycine. This is then excreted in the urine. In overdosage, this pathway becomes saturated, and a small increase in dose results in a relatively large increase in plasma concentration. A single dose is effective for some 4 to 6 hours.

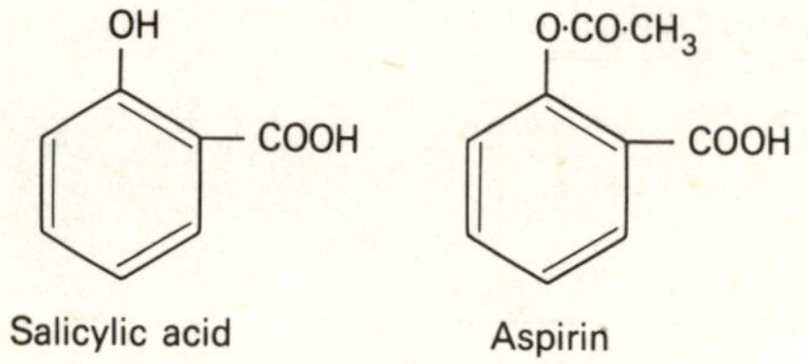

Figure 7.1 Chemical formulae of salicylic acid and aspirin.

This suggests that the initial effect of aspirin is mediated via the intact molecule. Almost certainly, however, the continuing effect is mediated by the salicylate (Figure 7.2). The site of action of aspirin is primarily at the site of pain, in contrast to narcotics which act in the CNS. This was demonstrated in cross-circulatory experiments in which analgesics could be delivered either to the CNS or to the splanchnic circulation in dogs.

Aspirin and salicylate are uricosuric in high doses (>5 g/day). Medium dosage (2 to 3 g/day) usually does not alter urate excretion. Low doses (1 to 2 g/day) may lead to an elevation of plasma urate concentration because of

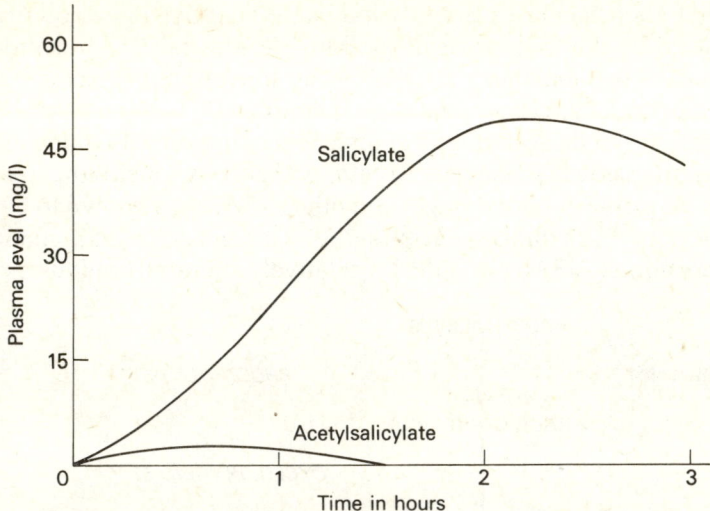

Figure 7.2 Blood levels of acetylsalicylic acid and salicylate after oral ingestion of 650 mg of aspirin. From Leonards, 1976 [6].

a competitive effect on tubular secretion [7]. Both medium and low doses block the uricosuric effect of probenecid. Plasma protein binding can displace oral hypoglycaemia (Table 7.2).

Table 7.2 Main salicylate drug interactions

Drug	Effect
Anticoagulant	potentiate
Uricosuric agent	antagonize
Oral hypoglycaemic	potentiate
Corticosteroid	increase gastric irritation
NSAID	? antagonize

Although most cells can resynthesize cyclo-oxygenase, platelets cannot. Thus, the acetylation of their microsomal enzyme lasts for the life of the platelet. This is why once a day treatment with aspirin is possible in prophylaxis against cerebrovascular and cardiovascular thrombosis, but round the clock administration is necessary to maintain effective control in inflammatory conditions.

Bone Pain
In recent years, the role of aspirin in the management of cancer pain has assumed greater importance because of discoveries about osteolytic factors produced by osseous metastases. The growth of an osseous metastasis appears to be linked with induced bone resorption. Initially

119

this is mediated via osteoclastic activity but, subsequently, an osteolytic agent is produced by the tumour itself [8]. Most studies relating to solid tumours implicate prostaglandin E_2 (PGE$_2$), as the principal factor in volved [8]. Other work has shown that prostaglandins (PGs) of the E series cause pain when injected subdermally at high concentrations [9]. In lower concentrations, the same PGs exacerbate pain, probably by sensitizing free nerve endings. Aspirin (in high dosage) and other NSAID are known to be potent inhibitors of PG synthesis (Figure 7.3). This suggests that, compared with morphine, NSAID should be relatively more efficacious in

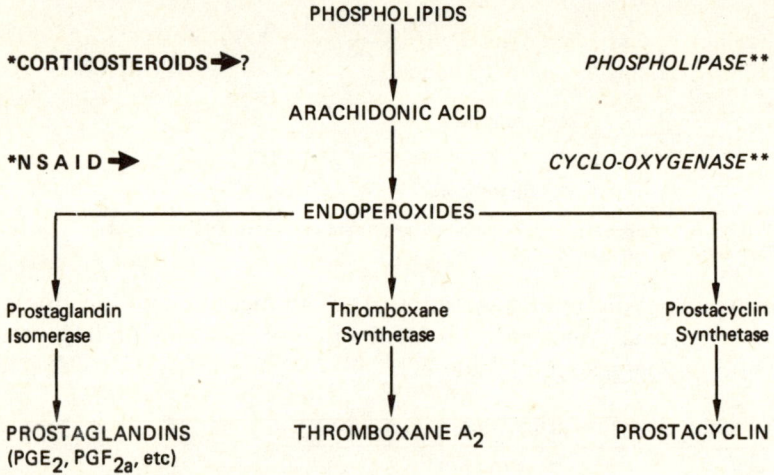

Figure 7.3 Simplified scheme for prostaglandin biosynthesis, showing sites of enzyme action (**) and sites of drug inhibition (*).

bone pain than in pain caused by soft tissue infiltration. Our experience would support such a hypothesis.

Response to PG inhibitors is, however, variable; a fact which can be explained if certain cancer cell types synthesize osteolytic agents other than or in addition to PGE$_2$. In patients with hypercalcaemia in association with multiple myeloma or a reticulosis, the urinary excretion of PG metabolites is normal. Bone resorption appears to be due to secretion of 'osteoclast activating factor' by tumour cells [10]. Other candidates include ectopic parathyroid hormone and active vitamin D metabolites or related sterols. Although complex, as further research elucidates the relative importance of these substances, the ability to relieve bone pain by pharmacological means should improve (Table 7.3).

1 Is there a NSAID of choice?

In the early 1970s, aspirin (3 g or more/day), indomethacin (75 to 150 mg/day) and phenylbutazone (400 to 600 mg/day) were being used by

Table 7.3 Osseous metastases and NSAID

1	Majority are not painful.
2	In carcinoma, bone secondaries produce a prostaglandin (PG).
3	PG induces local osteoclastic activity.
4.	PG also sensitizes the free nerve endings. This makes them more responsive to noxious stimuli.
5	NSAID inhibit production of PG, and so reduce the sensitivity of the free nerve endings.
6	NSAID may sometimes slow down the progression of osseous metastases.
7	Not all osseous metastases produce an osteolytic PG.
8	Some do only at the early stages of 'colonization'. This may account for the variable analgesic effect of NSAID.
9	Myeloma and lymphoma deposits do not produce PG; yet NSAID are often of definite analgesic benefit.
10	Pain relating to soft tissue metastases is sometimes greatly eased by NSAID.
11	Some soft tissue metastases have been shown to produce PG.

See Galasko, 1981 [8]; Mundy and Spiro, 1981 [10]

different centres. Phenylbutazone and indomethacin have little to commend them. Both give rise to troublesome side effects, Because of the risk of a serious blood dyscrasia, it is unjustifiable to use phenylbutazone in patients whose life expectancy is more than a few weeks, particularly now that safer alternatives exist. Indomethacin is not well tolerated by many cancer patients (vide infra). In a number of acute inflammatory conditions other than rheumatoid arthritis and in seronegative spondyloarthropathies, the newer NSAID can be more effective than aspirin. We still, however, consider the humble aspirin as the NSAID of choice for cancer pain. If not well tolerated we prescribe one of the following instead:

aspirin-glycine (Paynocil)	600 mg 4-hourly	⎫
flurbiprofen	100 mg b.i.d.	⎬ in Britain
benorylate suspension	10 ml b.i.d.	⎭
choline salicylate (Arthropan liquid)	870 mg 4-hourly	⎫ in the USA
naproxen (Naprosyn)	250–500 mg b.i.d	⎭

2   *Is prednisolone (or other corticosteroid) as effective as NSAID?*
Corticosteroids prevent the release of PGs by their 'stabilizing' effect on cell membranes; they do not inhibit PG synthesis. They also have an impact on other elements of the inflammatory process that are not connected with PGs and are of considerable symptomatic benefit in certain patients with advanced cancer. Yet, in the absence of evidence from controlled studies, the answer to the question is probably no. Until more data is available, it would seem best on the basis of clinical

experience to use aspirin for bone pain, and prednisolone when there is nerve compression or both (*see* Chapter 16). Sometimes, however, particularly with pelvic malignancy it may be necessary to use both aspirin (or alternative) and prednisolone.

3   *Should NSAID be used alone or in combination with a narcotic?*
The NSAID have been described as '40 to 50 per cent' drugs, a reminder that they relieve only that proportion of the pain related to the production of PGs. It is, however, possible that elevation of the peripheral pain threshold by administration of a NSAID may be enough to raise the patient's total pain threshold to a degree sufficient to relieve the pain completely. When aspirin is used, this is more likely because of its suggested multifocal action; the same will be true of benorylate. A decision to use a NSAID alone or in combination with a narcotic will, in practice, depend on the intensity of pain. If severe, a combination should be used, at least initially.

4   *Can NSAID be used in combination with each other?*
The large number of NSAID of differing chemical structure and varying mechanisms of action may tempt the physician to use two NSAID simultaneously. Although this is common in rheumatological practice our impression is that it is less common in terminal care. Published data indicate that NSAID should not be used in combination for the following reasons [11]:

1   Aspirin reduces the blood levels of many NSAID (Table 7.4), though clinical trials suggest that this may not be of therapeutic importance.
2   Multiple drugs are antagonistic or at least less than additive in animal models of inflammation.

Table 7.4   Interaction between non-steroidal anti-inflammatory drugs

Interacting drugs	Effects
Aspirin – flurbiprofen	Decreased plasma flurbiprofen†
Aspirin – naproxen	Decreased plasma naproxen†
Aspirin – diflunisal	Decreased plasma diflunisal
Indomethacin – diflunisal	Increased plasma indomethacin†
Aspirin – diclofenac	Decreased plasma diclofenac
Aspirin – fenoprofen	Decreased plasma fenoprofen
Aspirin – ibuprofen	Decreased plasma ibuprofen†
Aspirin – tolmetin	Decreased plasma tolmetin†

After Brooks, 1980 [12]
† Does not appear to be of significance in clinical trials

3 There is no good clinical data to suggest that combination use of NSAID is beneficial.
4 There is some evidence that combination of NSAID produce an increase in adverse reactions [13].

Some centres recommend the combined use of a strong NSAID (e.g. indomethacin, naproxen or flurbiprofen) and a fenamate in bone pain. As yet, the efficacy of such combinations has not been assessed objectively by controlled trial. Until new studies become available, NSAID should be used one at a time. This approach will not compromise therapy and will minimize adverse reactions and the cost to the patient or National Health Service.

Aspirin Toxicity

Dyspepsia is said to occur in 25 per cent of patients who take aspirin regularly [14]. This refers to standard 'insoluble' aspirin and probably explains why doctors in the USA are often reluctant to prescribe it. Their concern may also be related to the fact that, even with far-advanced cancer, many patients are still receiving aggressive chemotherapy. This is a situation in which aspirin is generally contraindicated because of its adverse effect on haemostasis. On the other hand, gastric intolerance is much less with all the alternative forms of aspirin, including soluble aspirin [15]. This is the most commonly used aspirin preparation in Britain, though it is not yet available in North America.

PGs inhibit gastric acid secretion and also have a protective effect on the mucosal cells. Inhibition of PG synthesis by aspirin will result in increased gastric acid secretion and, at the same time, the mucosa will become more vulnerable. Blood flow in the mucosa is also reduced and damage may occur in relatively ischaemic areas particularly if the dispersal of aspirin particles is slow.

Animal studies have shown that stress induced by prolonged physical restraint (comparable to anxiety and fear in man?) increases the incidence and number of gastric erosions considerably. Even a small quantity of food, such as a biscuit, counteracts this to a large extent. As a general rule, therefore, patients should not take aspirin on a completely empty stomach. A cup of tea or hot water with the 'on waking' medication may make all the difference between tolerance and intolerance. In patients who continue to have gastric intolerance to aspirin or an alternative NSAID, cimetidine 400 mg b.i.d. should be prescribed. Cimetidine reduces the incidence of gastric erosions but does not affect plasma salicylate levels. Antacids are also effective, but reduce aspirin absorption.

Aspirin may cause or exacerbate constipation. Because of this, it has been suggested that aspirin might be used in radiation-induced diarrhoea.

We do not use it for this, preferring codeine or an alternative anti-diarrhoeal. Other NSAID share this property to a certain extent though some may cause diarrhoea.

Table 7.5   Unwanted effects of aspirin

Gastric irritation:	dyspepsia
	epigastric pain
	haematemesis
	melaena
	anaemia
Salicylism:	tinnitus
	deafness
	vertigo
	depression
Hypersensitivity:	bronchospasm (in atopic patients)
	pruritis
	urticaria
	angioneurotic oedema

Aspirin has other adverse effects (Table 7.5). As with all NSAID, it may induce hypersensitivity reactions. Asthmatic attacks may be precipitated in patients with vasomotor rhinitis, nasal polyposis and bronchial asthma. Urticaria and angioneurotic oedema may occur in non-atopic individuals. On the other hand, sodium salicylate, a weaker inhibitor of PG synthesis, does not precipitate hypersensitivity reactions. This is of particular interest because of the new generation of cation-salicylate derivatives (see page 126).

Tinnitus and deafness are an early warning of toxicity. These clear when the dose is reduced or the aspirin discontinued. Toxic manifestations are related to the concentration of the free drug. As this varies inversely with the plasma albumin concentration, hypoalbuminaemic patients are more susceptible to toxic manifestations. This is important in patients with cancer, many of whom come into this category.

Aspirin, as well as other NSAID, cause a transient decrease in renal function. The postulated mechanism is the inhibition of the renal synthesis of PG, which appears to be important in the autoregulation of renal blood flow. Aspirin can also block the diuretic effect of spironolactone by inhibiting its binding to the tubular-cell receptor.

Preparations of Aspirin
Standard Aspirin (BP, USP) causes more gastric intolerance than other preparations. The rate of absorption varies according to the formulation.

Coarser particles have a slower dissolution rate and correspondingly slower absorption. They also cause more gastric erosions and occult blood loss. Some of the cheaper over-the-counter preparations in the USA are of the coarser particle variety. These are manufactured by a quicker and, therefore, cheaper one stage process called Wet Granulation. More expensive formulations (BP, USP) are made by a two stage process called Slugging or Dry Granulation.

*Soluble Aspirin (BP)** is a combination of aspirin, calcium carbonate and citric acid. When the tablet is dropped into water the calcium carbonate and citric acid react with effervescence and disperse the aspirin into a fine

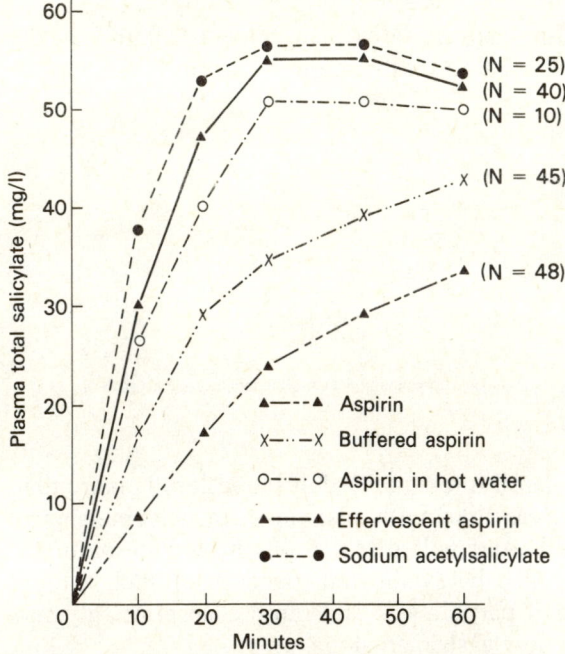

Figure 7.4 Total plasma levels of salicylate after ingestion of various aspirin preparations. Total dose was equivalent to 640 mg of aspirin in all cases. N = no. of patients.
From Leonards, 1963 [16]

suspension. Strictly speaking, this preparation should not be described as soluble but as dispersible. Soluble aspirin is more rapidly absorbed (Figure 7.4) and produces only half as much occult bleeding. There is, however, no close correlation between occult bleeding and gastric symptoms.

* not available in the USA

Buffered aspirin is a mixture of aspirin and antacids. Examples are Bufferin, containing aspirin, magnesium carbonate and aluminium glycinate and Ascriptin, containing aspirin and magnesium-aluminium hydroxide. By decreasing gastric activity, such preparations reduce the likelihood of mucosal damage by hydrogen ions consequent upon initial injury to cells by aspirin. Bufferin produces only about one-third of the occult blood loss of soluble aspirin. Buffered preparations are more slowly absorbed from the stomach than dispersible and effervescent forms (Figure 7.4), but on the other hand, speed up gastric emptying. Effervescent buffered aspirin (e.g. Alka-Seltzer) contains sodium bicarbonate. This make it undesirable for long term use because of the amount of sodium and bicarbonate it contains.

Cation-aspirins. Aluminium-aspirin (aloxiprin, Palaprin forte) is the prototype cation-aspirin (Figure 7.5). Liberation of aspirin is slow in the

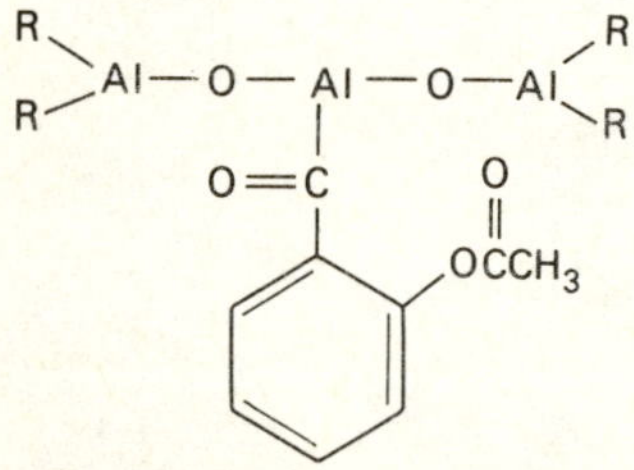

Figure 7.5 Chemical formula of aloxiprin; aluminium polyoxaspirin. R = acetylsalicyl radical (as depicted under the central aluminium atom).

stomach but rapid in the small intestine. Occult blood loss is more than with soluble aspirin but less than with plain aspirin. Glycine-aspirin (Paynocil) is highly soluble and will dissolve on the tongue or in the mouth. It can, of course, also be swallowed. Because of such a rapid dissolution time, very small particle size and rapid absorption, glycine-aspirin causes remarkably few gastric erosions.

Enteric-coated aspirin (Nu-Seals) releases the aspirin only in the relatively alkaline environment of the small intestine. It has been suggested that absorption is not always complete, probably not so much of a problem in costive patients. The *size* of the tablet is, however, a deterrent to many.

Microencapsulated aspirin (Levius, Bayer Timed-Release) consists of small aspirin particles individually encapsulated and bound together as a tablet. The aim is to achieve the slow release of aspirin in both the stomach and the small bowel. There are few trials comparing this preparation with alternative formulations.

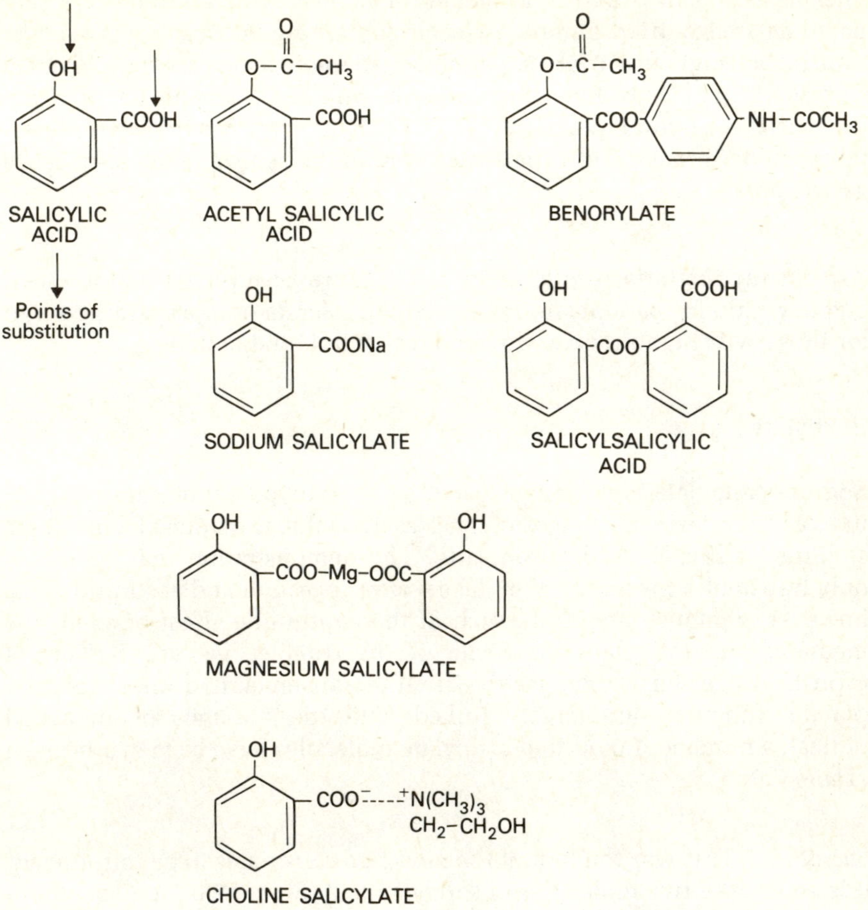

Figure 7.6 Chemical formulae of salicylic acid derivatives.

Esterified aspirin. Benorylate is an ester of aspirin and paracetamol (Figure 7.6). It is absorbed intact and is rapidly hydrolyzed within 15 minutes in the bloodstream to the two constituent substances. It is generally given twice daily as a suspension. Each 10 ml contains 4 g of benorylate yielding approximately 2 g of both aspirin and paracetamol. It causes less faecal blood loss than soluble aspirin. Tablets are also available containing 750 mg. As only half of this is aspirin, 9 to 10 tablets a day are necessary to obtain a definite anti-inflammatory effect.

Injectable aspirin. Although it is generally possible to administer non-narcotic analgesics by mouth, it is important to note that a preparation of injectable aspirin is available in Italy. Lysine-aspirin (Flectadol) is prepared in freeze-dried ampoules, each containing 900 mg (equivalent to aspirin 500 mg) In a trial in patients undergoing major gynaecological surgery, 1.8 g of IM lysine-aspirin was shown to be as effective as 10 mg of IM morphine hydrochloride [17]. No trials appear to have been undertaken in terminal cancer patients. Parenteral aspirin may also cause gastric erosions.

Aspirin suppositories available in the USA are used on 1:1 oral to rectal potency ratio for patients no longer able to tolerate oral preparations and for those wishing to reduce the amount of oral medication.

Salicylates

Sodium salicylate is no longer used. It is not as potent as aspirin when used as an occasional analgesic. It is less irritant to the stomach but causes sodium loading if used chronically. The demonstration that aspirin is only transiently present in the plasma after ingestion and absorption has, however, demonstrated that much of the continuing effect of aspirin is mediated via salicylate. As some of the troublesome side effects of aspirin—hypersensitivity, gastric irritation, anaemia, and impairment of platelet function—are largely linked with the presence of an acetyl radical, a number of modified salicylate molecules have been synthesized (Table 7.6).

*Salsalate.** This was the first of the modified salicylates to be introduced. It is an ester of two molecules of salicylic acid (Figure 7.6). It is insoluble in gastric juice and causes little gastric bleeding. It is relatively slow in onset compared with other NSAID but lasts longer. The manufacturer's recommendation indicates that twice daily administration is generally appropriate.

Choline-salicylate. This is available in the USA but not in Britain. Choline salicylate is a crystalline, odourless powder which is very soluble in water (Figure 7.6). It is marketed in the USA as Arthropan, an aqueous mint-flavoured solution. Each 5 ml contains 870 mg salicylate content equivalent to aspirin 648 mg. It is reported to be less irritant to the gastric mucosa [18]. It is used at The Connecticut Hospice, Branford, for patients who have difficulty swallowing tablets. Its expense precludes use as the first line salicylate.

* not available in the USA

Table 7.6   Salicylic acid derivatives

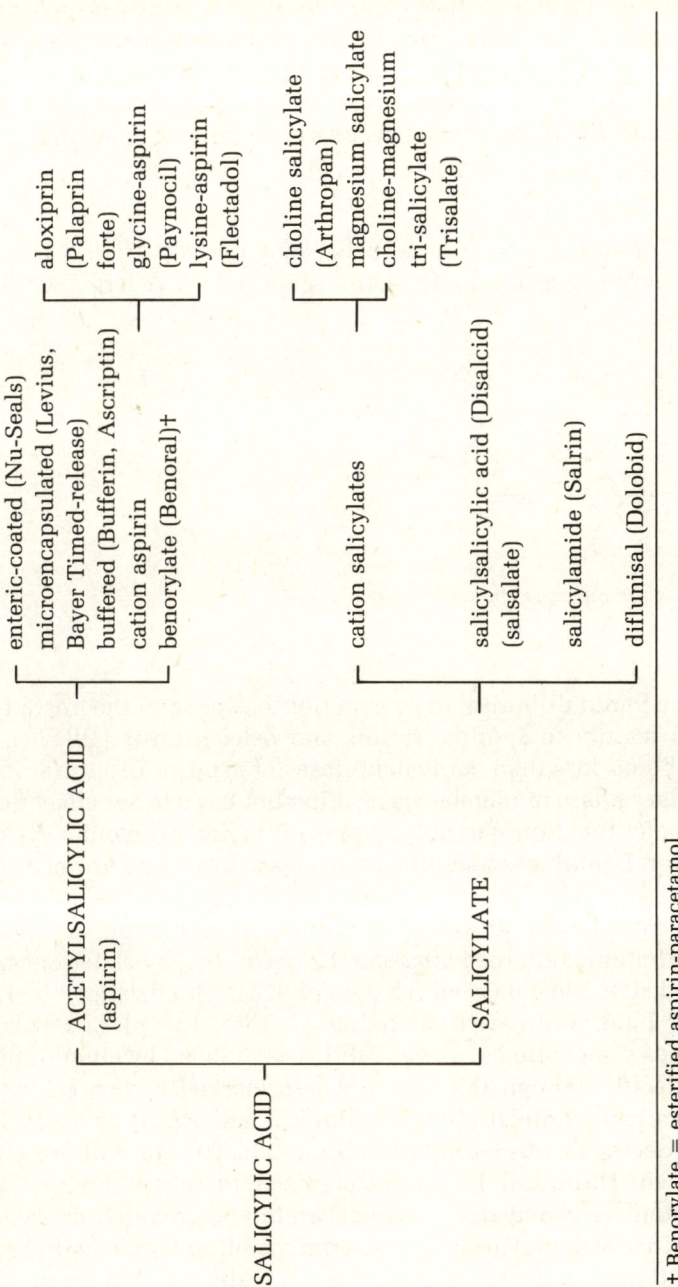

SALICYLIC ACID
ACETYLSALICYLIC ACID (aspirin)
- enteric-coated (Nu-Seals)
- microencapsulated (Levius, Bayer Timed-release)
- buffered (Bufferin, Ascriptin)
- cation aspirin
- benorylate (Benoral)+
  - aloxiprin (Palaprin forte)
  - glycine-aspirin (Paynocil)
  - lysine-aspirin (Flectadol)

SALICYLATE
- cation salicylates
  - choline salicylate (Arthropan)
  - magnesium salicylate
  - choline-magnesium tri-salicylate (Trisalate)
- salicylsalicylic acid (Disalcid) (salsalate)
- salicylamide (Salrin)
- diflunisal (Dolobid)

+ Benorylate = esterified aspirin-paracetamol

Choline magnesium trisalicylate. This is a mixture of choline salicylate and magnesium salicylate (Figure 7.6). It has recently been introduced in Britain as Trisalate. Each tablet contains 500 mg of salicylate and a dose schedule of 2 or 3 tablets *twice* a day is recommended. The plasma half-life varies in a dose-dependent manner. At the lower dose the average plasma half-life of trisalicylate is nearly 8 hours; at the higher dose it is 18 hours.

Diflunisal. Diflunisal is a salicylic acid derivative with a duration of action of between 8 and 12 hours (Figure 7.7). A large trial in general

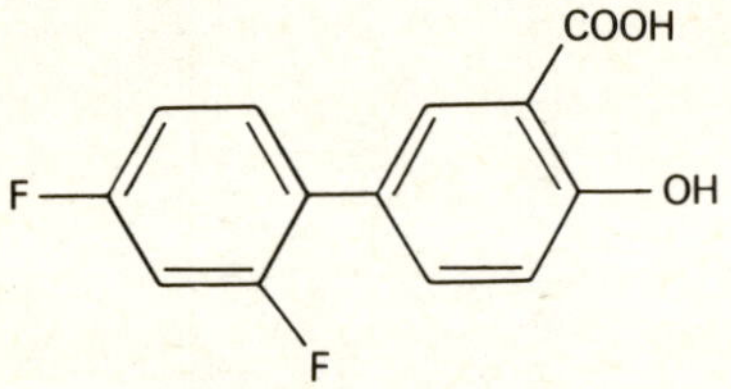

Figure 7.7 Chemical formula of diflunisal.

practice found diflunisal to be superior to aspirin in the treatment of pain related mainly to sprains, strains and osteoarthritis [19]. It causes less faecal blood loss than equivalent doses of aspirin. Diflunisal inhibits the secondary phase of platelet aggregation but has a lesser effect than aspirin on platelet function, possibly because it is not as potent a PG synthetase inhibitor. It produces a significant decrease in plasma uric acid concentration.

Diflunisal is well absorbed after oral administration, and peak plasma concentration is attained after about 2 hours. Steady-state concentration is reached after 3 to 4 days with a dose of 125 mg b.i.d., after 7 to 9 days with 500 mg b.i.d. With each doubling of dose, the plasma concentration increases some 3 times. Bioavailability is reduced by aluminium-containing antacids, though this effect is less marked in non-fasting subjects. Concomitant administration of diflunisal and aspirin (2.4 g a day) significantly decreases plasma concentration [20]. The effect of this clinically is unknown. Diflunisal is not metabolized to salicylic acid. The parent compound is conjugated to glucuronide and excreted as such into the urine. In renal impairment the terminal elimination half-life increases from 10 hours to 115 hours when creatinine clearance falls below 2 ml/min. Gastrointestinal side effects are less common than with aspirin. Its use in metastatic bone pain has not been assessed.

Nonsteroidal Anti-Inflammatory Drugs (NSAID)

A non-steroidal anti-inflammatory drug modifies the inflammatory process and causes a reduction in local heat, swelling and/or stiffness. It also reduces or relieves pain, partly in consequence of its anti-inflammatory effect. It is not disease-specific and does not modify aspects of the disease other than inflammation.

Aspirin, introduced just before the turn of the century, was for many years the only non-steroidal anti-inflammatory drug (NSAID). Phenylbutazone was marketed in 1952, followed by indomethacin in 1964. Since then the number marketed has rapidly increased; and trebled between 1974 and 1980 (Table 7.7).

Like aspirin, all NSAID are analgesic and antipyretic, as well as anti-inflammatory. It would be correct therefore to style these agents non-steroidal anti-inflammatory *analgesics*. Common usage, however, still dictates the use of the word drug (NSAID). On the other hand, to refer to them simply as non-narcotic analgesics would disguise an important property, perhaps like calling Stork margarine [21]. In single-dose studies, NSAID demonstrate a plateau effect beyond which increasing amounts produce little or no additional relief. They are generally well tolerated by mouth, though in susceptible patients may, as with aspirin, produce gastric side effects. A patient who is unable to tolerate one NSAID may find another more acceptable. Most tend to constipate when taken regularly, though indomethacin and flurbiprofen may cause diarrhoea and mefenamic acid commonly does so.

Like aspirin, the other NSAID also interfere with clotting. They may cause bleeding in patients taking an oral anticoagulant by displacing the latter from its binding sites on the plasma proteins, and in those receiving chemotherapy. Ibuprofen, naproxen and tolmetin are less likely to interact with anticoagulants than other NSAID [22, 23].

The newer NSAID antagonize frusemide[1] in patients being treated for cardiac failure. The diuretic effect of frusemide is thought to be mediated at least in part by renal prostaglandins [24].

In general, even the new NSAID share the majority of aspirin's side effects. Gastric intolerance may be less, and occult bleeding is often within the normal range. Yet, because of its general overall efficacy, low toxicity and cheapness, aspirin remains, in our opinion, the anti-inflammatory drug of choice in cancer.

[1] furosemide (USA)

Table 7.7 Classification of non-steroidal anti-inflammatory drugs (NSAID)

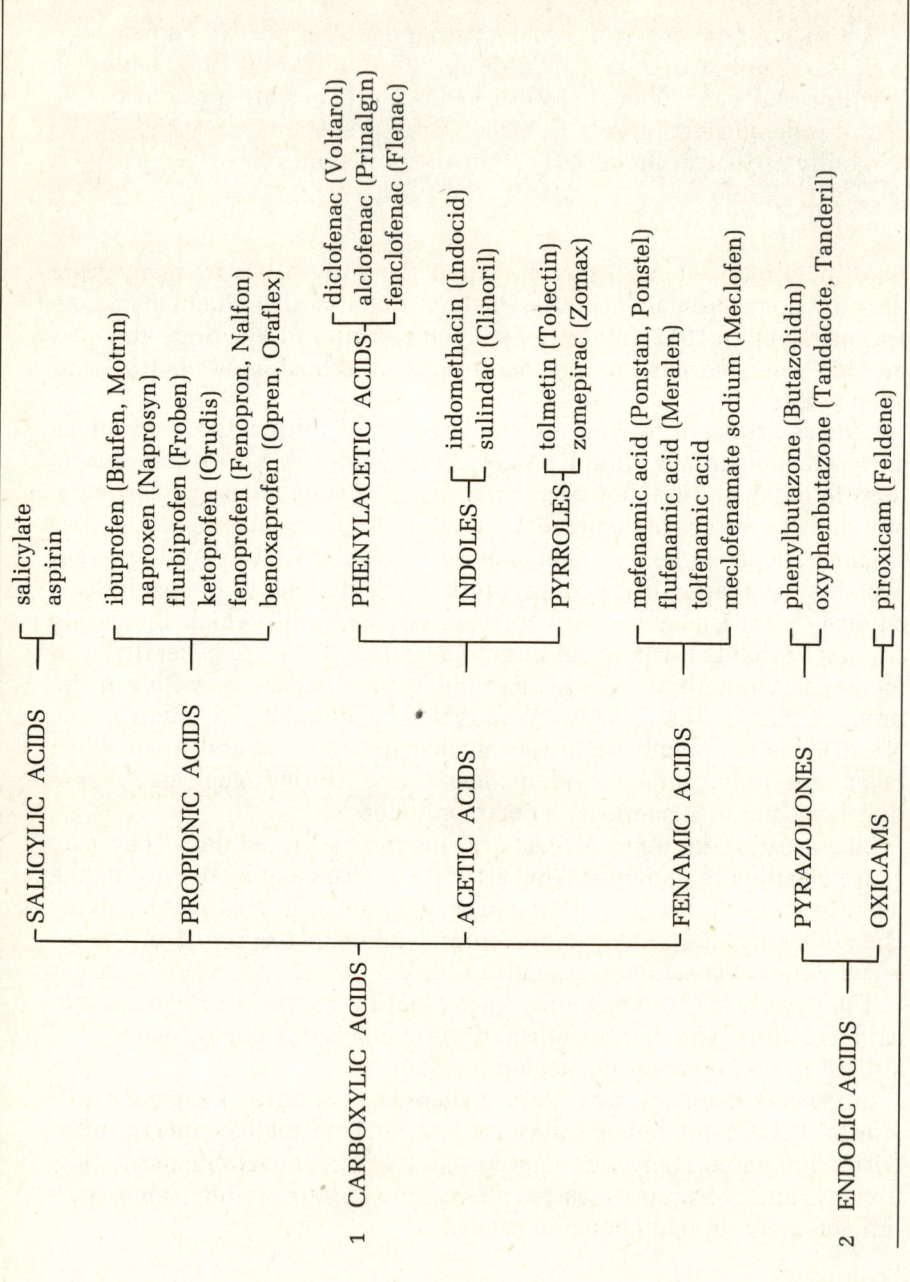

1 CARBOXYLIC ACIDS

SALICYLIC ACIDS — salicylate, aspirin

PROPIONIC ACIDS — ibuprofen (Brufen, Motrin), naproxen (Naprosyn), flurbiprofen (Froben), ketoprofen (Orudis), fenoprofen (Fenopron, Nalfon), benoxaprofen (Opren, Oraflex)

ACETIC ACIDS
  PHENYLACETIC ACIDS — diclofenac (Voltarol), alclofenac (Prinalgin), fenclofenac (Flenac)
  INDOLES — indomethacin (Indocid), sulindac (Clinoril)
  PYRROLES — tolmetin (Tolectin), zomepirac (Zomax)

FENAMIC ACIDS — mefenamic acid (Ponstan, Ponstel), flufenamic acid (Meralen), tolfenamic acid, meclofenamate sodium (Meclofen)

2 ENDOLIC ACIDS

PYRAZOLONES — phenylbutazone (Butazolidin), oxyphenbutazone (Tandacote, Tanderil)

OXICAMS — piroxicam (Feldene)

Mechanism of Action

The precise mode of action of NSAID is not known. During the last decade, the action of these drugs on prostaglandin (PG) synthesis has been extensively studied. All NSAID inhibit PG synthetase (PGS) activity and reduce the local concentration of PGs, some of which are known to be involved as mediators of the inflammatory process. There is, however, no close relationship between the effectiveness of a drug as a PGS inhibitor *in vitro* and its anti-inflammatory effect *in vivo*. Some compounds, including chlorpromazine and several of the tricyclic antidepressants, inhibit PG synthesis but are not anti-inflammatory [25] while a new drug, benzofen, has anti-inflammatory properties but is not a PGS inhibitor.

Further, the alkaline derivates of NSAID, for example, antipyrine and indoxole are almost as potent PGS inhibitors as their acidic counterparts, phenylbutazone and indomethacin, but have no real anti-inflammatory effect [26]. This may be a feature of plasma protein binding. Classical NSAID are weak acids with a pKa around 4 and have a high affinity for plasma proteins. Autoradiography has demonstrated that only the weak acid compounds concentrate in inflamed tissues, as well as in both gastric parietal cells and kidneys [27]. It seems likely that the plasma proteins, present in inflammatory oedema, act as carriers for the NSAID. Certainly the degree of protein binding correlates well with their anti-inflammatory potency. This would explain why *in vivo* these drugs only are anti-inflammatory, and also why gastric and renal side effects are not seen with other *in vitro* inhibitors of PGS such as chlorpromazine. The fact that NSAID are highly bound to plasma proteins may help to explain their effectiveness. Blood vessels in an inflamed area allow high molecular weight proteins to escape; this will enable NSAID to reach greater concentrations in sites of inflammation than in the extracellular fluid elsewhere. The acidic inflammatory environment causes dissociation of the NSAID from the plasma protein and the free molecules then penetrate the lipid membranes of neighbouring cells.

A few non-acidic compounds have, however, been shown to be anti-inflammatory *in vivo*, some being PGS inhibitors and others not. Some anti-inflammatory drugs are more selective than others with respect to inhibition of PGS. Indomethacin and the fenamates are relatively broad spectrum inhibitors, whereas phenylbutazone selectively inhibits PGE_2 and slightly *stimulates* the synthesis of PGF_2. Fenamates not only inhibit PG synthesis but also antagonize some of the effects of already synthesized PG, possibly by interfering with PG binding at their cellular receptor sites. A new compound MK-447 increases production of PGE and yet has definite *in vivo* anti-inflammatory properties [28]. MK-447, however, inhibits the production of the endoperoxide, PGG_2, which plays a pivotal role in inflammation.

In conclusion, it is clear that the mode of action of NSAID is complex.

Any simple global theory does not explain all the *in vivo* properties of these drugs. Too much attention to *in vitro* molar potency studies may result in a false view of the relative clinical value of NSAID.

Choice of NSAID
In rheumatoid arthritis and related arthropathies, it is accepted that considerable variation exists between patients both with respect to response and to tolerability. Even if a controlled trial shows that, overall, one drug is more efficacious than another, the 'better' drug may not be better for a given individual. This variability is particularly marked with the weaker propionic acid derivatives. As yet, no such variability has been reported in patients treated for bone pain in cancer, but that is not to say it does not exist.

Individual NSAID
Comments on individual NSAID are included for the following reasons:

Flurbiprofen	—alternate NSAID of choice at Sir Michael Sobell House, Oxford
Naproxen	—alternate NSAID of choice at The Connecticut Hospice
Zomepirac	—wider range of analgesic activity than other NSAID
Mefenamic acid	—broader mechanism of anti-prostaglandin action
Indomethacin	—used in several centres
Phenylbutazone	—historical perspective

Flurbiprofen*

Drug portrait
Flurbiprofen is a strong NSAID (Figure 7.8) with anti-inflammatory, antipyretic and analgesic properties. It is rapidly absorbed following oral administration, with peak plasma concentrations 90 minutes after a single dose. The plasma half-life is 4 hours. Flurbiprofen is excreted in the urine both as unchanged drug and a number of hydroxylated metabolites.

Flurbiprofen is best given twice daily [29]. It is used at Sir Michael Sobell House, Oxford, as the alternative NSAID of choice, commonly in patients who are receiving corticosteroid. In patients receiving 4-hourly morphine sulphate, it is easy to separate in time the administration of the NSAID from the corticosteroid. This eases compliance by reducing the number of tablets to be taken at any one time. It is also hoped that gastric irritation will be kept to a minimum. On the other hand, particularly in conjunction with corticosteroids, there is an increased likelihood of oedema. Flurbi-

* not yet available in the USA

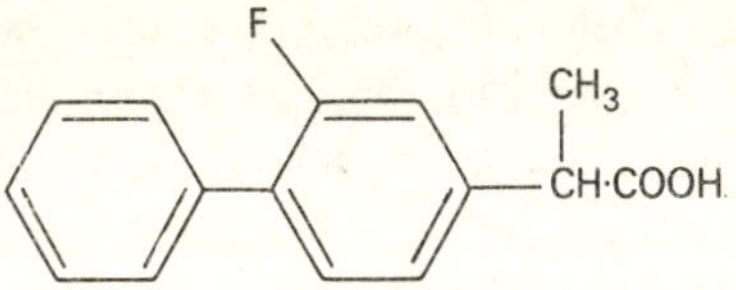

Figure 7.8 Chemical formula of flurbiprofen.

profen causes diarrhoea in some patients. The maximum effective dose in bone pain is not established. In a few patients receiving 100 mg t.i.d. or more, massive fluid retention has occurred. Sometimes this has not responded to diuretics, and it proved necessary to stop treatment. Currently, we use 100 mg b.i.d. or 50 mg t.i.d.

The manufacturer's literature places considerable emphasis on the extremely good showing of flurbiprofen as an *in vitro* inhibitor of PG synthesis (Table 7.8). However, as already stressed, *in vitro* and *in vivo*

Table 7.8 Relative molar potencies of some aspirin-like drugs for 50% inhibition of PGE_2 synthesis in vitro, potency of aspirin was taken as unity

Drug	Relative molar potency for 50% inhibition of PGE_2 synthesis
Flurbiprofen	5610
Indomethacin	257
Naproxen	45
Ibuprofen	22
Phenylbutazone	2.7
Aspirin	1.0
Salicylic acid	<0.02
Paracetamol[1]	<0.01

After Crook *et al*, 1976 [30]
[1] acetaminophen (USA)

are not the same, nor is *potency* synonymous with *efficacy*. The relatively poor showing of aspirin and phenylbutazone indicates that, although of interest, such studies are not a good guide to clinical efficacy. This means that it should not be assumed that flurbiprofen is, by definition, superior to the well tried drugs referred to above. The same paper which places aspirin low in the potency league table stresses that, in other tests, aspirin is unique in its superiority over other NSAID [30].

It is of interest to note that both indomethacin and flurbiprofen have been used in cases of instability of the detrusor of the urinary bladder. A number of PGs stimulate contraction of the human bladder muscle *in vitro*, PGF$_2$ being the most potent. Animal studies indicate that PGs are produced naturally by the detrusor and increase tone and spontaneous activity. In man, compared with a placebo, frequency, urgency and urge incontinence were all significantly reduced with flurbiprofen 50 mg t.i.d. [31]. Flurbiprofen was well tolerated by most patients. In an earlier study, indomethacin 100 mg b.i.d. produced headache and nausea in 60 per cent of cases [32]. We have also used flurbiprofen in the syndrome of pruritis and pain in *en cuirass* breast cancer (vide infra).

Naproxen

Drug portrait

Naproxen, a propionic acid derivative, is a NSAID with analgesic, anti-inflammatory and antipyretic actions (Figure 7.9). It is readily absorbed when given orally. Naproxen is also absorbed rectally but peak concentrations in plasma are achieved more slowly. The plasma half-life is 12 to 15 hours and it is extensively bound to plasma protein. Naproxen and its metabolites are almost entirely excreted in the urine. About 30 per cent of the drug undergoes demethylation and most of this is excreted as the glucuronide. The usual dosage interval is 12 hours.

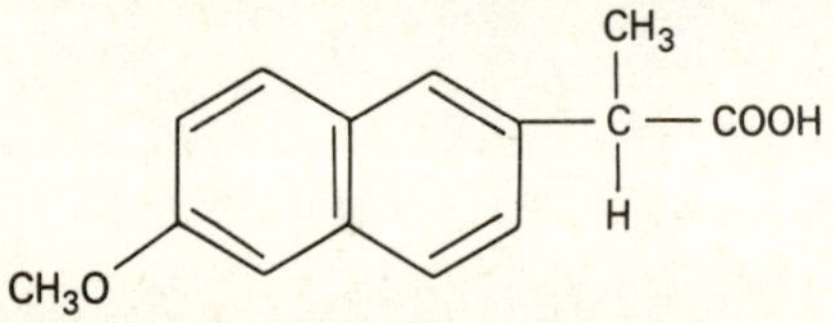

Figure 7.9 Chemical formula of naproxen.

Naproxen is the alternate NSAID of choice at The Connecticut Hospice, Branford. The longer half-life, about 14 hours, make twice-daily administration feasible. This provides adequate steady state plasma levels to maintain therapeutic efficacy [33]. Higher plasma levels can be obtained on a 6-hourly regimen to a maximum of 1375 mg/day, but whether this results in improved pain control has yet to be determined [34]. Given 12-hourly, plasma levels do not increase at doses greater than 500 mg twice daily, because of the rapid urinary excretion and the extent of plasma binding [35].

Recently a new formulation, naproxen sodium (Synflex), has been introduced. The sodium salt is heavier than the acid and 550 mg naproxen sodium is equivalent to 500 mg naproxen. Naproxen sodium appears to be an improved form for analgesic use. It provides more rapid absorption of naproxen, higher plasma levels, and earlier effect and probably better pain relief [34].

Zomepirac

Drug portrait
Zomepirac is a strong NSAID (Figure 7.10) with anti-inflammatory, antipyretic and analgesic properties. It has a wider range of analgesic activity than other NSAID, including aspirin. It is well absorbed when given by mouth reaching peak analgesic effect after 1 to 2 hours. There is a linear relationship between dose and plasma level with doses of 50 mg to 200 mg. The mean plasma half-life is 6 to 7 hours. The drug is excreted in the urine as the glucuronide and smaller amounts as the unchanged acid and hydroxyzomepirac with a trace of 4-chlorobenzoic acid [36].

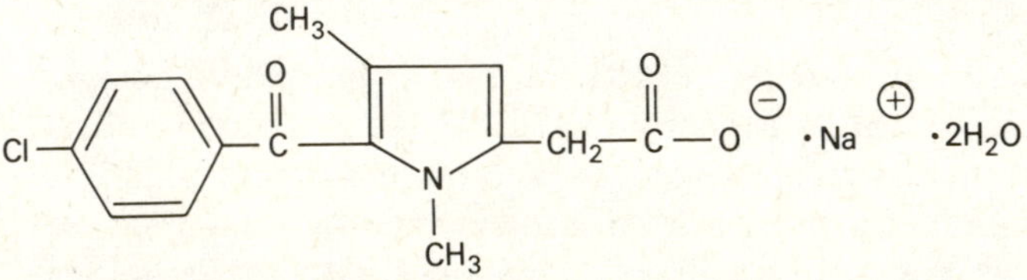

Figure 7.10 Chemical formula of zomepirac sodium dihydrate.

Zomepirac has been promoted as a useful non-narcotic analgesic. It has been suggested that zomepirac may inhibit PG formation within the CNS as well as acting locally. Zomepirac is rapidly and readily absorbed after oral administration and, like other NSAID, is highly protein bound. Zomepirac has a wider range of analgesic activity than other NSAID, including aspirin. The standard 100 mg dose is more effective than:

aspirin 650 mg [37],
dextropropoxyphene napsylate 100 mg-paracetamol 650 mg [38].

and at least as effective as:

APC-codeine 60 mg [39],
(APC = aspirin 454 mg-phenacetin 324 mg-caffeine 64 mg),
pentazocine 50 mg [40],
oxycodone-APC [41].

In one single dose study in cancer patients with *postoperative* pain, 100 mg of zomepirac by mouth was shown to be as effective as 16 mg IM morphine [42]. The relevance of this study to cancer pain *per se* remains in question. It is of interest to note that side effects, including drowsiness,

137

nausea and dry mouth, were roughly the same for both drugs. Sweating occurred more frequently after zomepirac.

Zomepirac works within 30 minutes of administration. Zomepirac appears to straddle the analgesic range of aspirin and the weak narcotics. It is recommended by the manufacturers in a dose of up to 600 mg daily, that is, 100 mg every 4 to 6 hours. In osteoarthritis, it has been used satisfactorily for periods of over 1 year [43]. It is, of course, expensive and, at present probably is indicated only in patients who cannot tolerate weak narcotic analgesics.

Mefenamic Acid

Drug portrait
Mefenamic acid, a derivative of fenamic acid, is a NSAID with anti-inflammatory, antipyretic and analgesic properties (Figure 7.11). Mefenamic acid displays central as well as peripheral analgesic action, by virtue of its capacity to inhibit cyclo-oxygenase. It is absorbed from the gastrointestinal tract and the plasma half-life is 4 to 6 hours. In man 20 per cent of the drug is excreted in the faeces, mainly as an unconjugated carboxyl metabolite. Other metabolites are excreted in the urine.

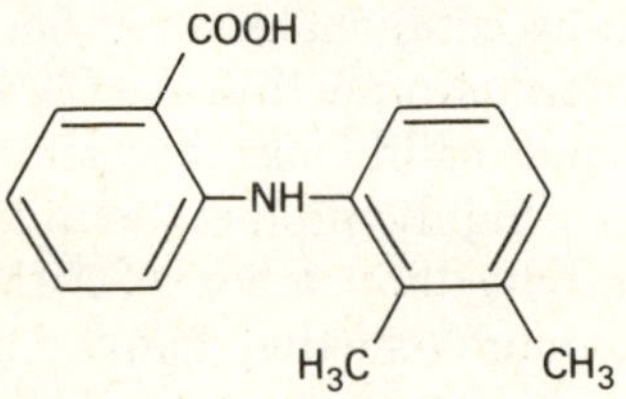

Figure 7.11 Chemical formula of mefenamic acid.

Mefenamic acid is the most commonly used fenamate. Peak plasma levels occur after 2 hours and the half-life is some 4 to 6 hours. The fenamates inhibit PGS and also block PG receptors in the cell wall [44]. The major gastrointestinal side effect is diarrhoea, which occurs in more than 10 per cent of patients. In America, its use is not recommended for more than 1 week because of the likelihood of more serious gastrointestinal effects and nephrotoxicity [45]. It has not been shown to be superior to aspirin and the anti-inflammatory potency is half that of phenylbutazone. In a few centres, mefenamic acid is used in conjunction with other NSAID, presumably in the belief that an additive effect will be obtained by virtue of the broader mechanism of action.

138

Indomethacin

Drug portrait

Indomethacin is a strong NSAID (Figure 7.12) with anti-inflammatory antipyretic and analgesic properties. It has central and peripheral effects. It is a potent inhibitor of the prostaglandin-forming cyclo-oxygenase. It is rapidly absorbed from the gastrointestinal tract, both when given orally and as a suppository. The plasma half-life is 2 hours. It is metabolized in the liver to inactive metabolites, and is excreted in the urine mainly as the glucuronide and, to a lesser extent, in the faeces.

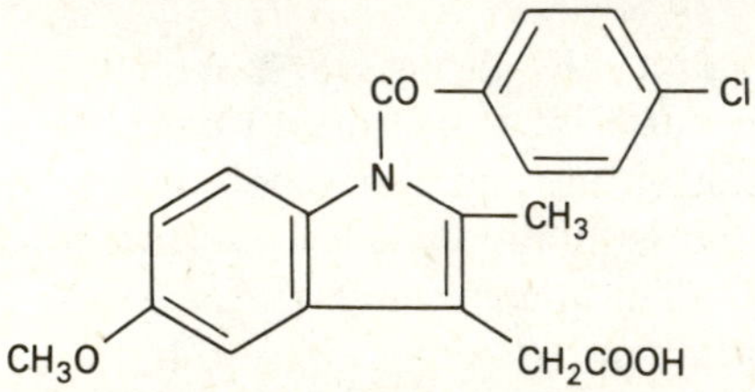

Figure 7.12 Chemical formula of indomethacin.

Indomethacin has been used at many centres as an adjunct to narcotic analgesics in the relief of severe bone pain, though controlled studies have not been undertaken. It is rapidly absorbed from the upper gastrointestinal tract and also from the rectum when given as a suppository. Indomethacin has a more prolonged action than its serum half-life of 2 hours would suggest. It is possible that there are two 'pools' of the drug. Degradation and excretion first takes place from the plasma pool, which is then replenished by indomethacin released from tissue stores.

In addition to inhibiting PG synthesis, indomethacin has been shown to exert anti-inflammatory effects in other ways. For example, in rats it interferes with the migration of leucocytes into inflammatory sites. It increases the intracellular concentration of cyclic AMP by inhibition of the enzyme phosphodiesterase. Among other things, cyclic AMP stabilizes lysosomal membranes in polymorphonuclear leucocytes and macrophages. Both these actions are likely to decrease the generation of the PG precursor, superoxide, and of hydroxyl radicals.

Gastrointestinal intolerance is the major complication of treatment with indomethacin. It has been known to produce almost every alimentary tract symptom from angular stomatitis to pruritis ani. Gastritis and gastric ulceration are perhaps the most common and certainly among the most important. Headache occurs in 50 per cent of patients when the total daily dose exceeds 100 mg. In cancer patients this may be masked if the patient is also receiving a narcotic. Other CNS effects are dizziness, drowsiness,

139

dysphoria (feeling of depersonalization), depression, confusional symptoms, hallucinations, seizures and syncope. In susceptible persons, these symptoms have occurred after ingestion of a single 25 mg dose. Like phenylbutazone, indomethacin can cause fluid retention and oedema.

In summary, indomethacin in a daily dose of 150 mg, is likely to be more toxic than soluble aspirin. The authors' preference lies with aspirin though we accept that indomethacin will prove both adequate and acceptable in many instances.

Phenylbutazone

Drug portrait
Phenylbutazone, a pyrazolone derivative, is a strong NSAID (Figure 7.13) with analgesic, antipyretic and anti-inflammatory properties. It is readily absorbed from the gastrointestinal tract, both when administered orally and per rectum. It is relatively slowly absorbed when administered intramuscularly. The plasma half-life is 50 to 100 hours. Phenylbutazone is almost completely metabolized in the liver and its metabolites slowly excreted in the urine. Oxyphenbutazone is a sodium-retaining metabolite with a half-life of several days. Recommended dosage interval is 6 hours.

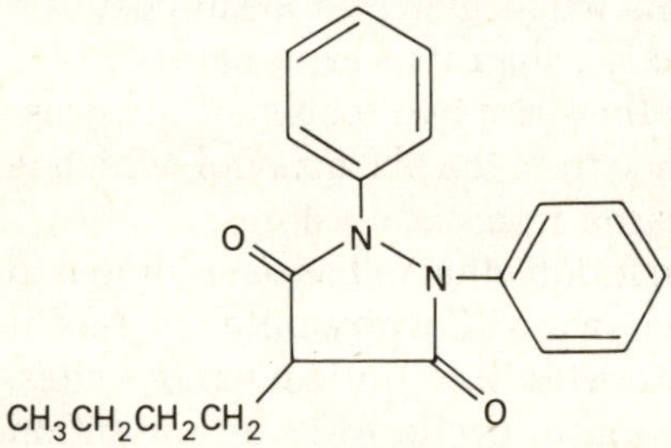

Figure 7.13 Chemical formula of phenylbutazone.

Phenylbutazone causes ankle oedema fairly commonly, particularly in patients who are hypoalbuminaemic. Ten years ago, phenylbutazone was used at most British hospices for bone pain. At the time, aspirin was overlooked. Further, the perceived alternative, indomethacin, tended to cause more gastrointestinal side effects. The possibility of leucopenia or pancytopenia was regarded as irrelevant in patients who were terminally ill. In recent years, with more patients living months rather than weeks, the matter is viewed differently. Moreover, fresh interest in aspirin *per se* and the advent of newer alternatives, such as flurbiprofen and naproxen means that the use of this more toxic choice is now unusual.

Pruritis and Pain in *En Cuirass* Breast Cancer

Each year, we see several patients with breast cancer who are experiencing a combination of pruritis and pain in association with *en cuirass* breast cancer.

Case History. A 73-year-old woman with recurrent breast cancer experienced pain in the affected area over the right breast and chest wall. At the time of referral, the symptoms had been present for about a year. Prior to referral several narcotic analgesics were tried but stopped because of vomiting. Several nerve blocks included a series of intrathecal blocks with either phenol or chlorocresol. After these, the pain was no better and she experienced in addition some weakness and discomfort in the right thigh. She became depressed and distressed by the lack of success. It was felt 'the major problem is psychogenic'. Two weeks after starting mianserin 10 mg t.i.d. she was noted to be generally better and eating well, but still in pain. When admitted to Sir Michael Sobell House, Oxford, the patient was taking only mianserin and a night time hypnotic (flurazepam). Treatment was started with Distalgesic* (dextropropoxyphene 32.5 mg, paracetamol 325 mg) two tablets 4-hourly and the mianserin was continued as a single 30 mg bedtime dose. A diuretic was prescribed in an attempt to reduce the oedema of the arm. As the Distalgesic helped only a little, flurbiprofen 100 mg t.i.d. was added after 48 hours. Within 2 to 3 days the chest wall and arm became almost completely pain and pruritis free, though the patient still had some intermittent thigh pain. Her mood improved and she became more active and completely independent. She was discharged after two weeks and, apart from a second short admission for other reasons, spent nearly two months at home essentially pain-free before she deteriorated rapidly and died, probably as a result of a cerebral metastasis.

Certain prostaglandins intensify both pain and pruritus [46]. The concurrence of both symptoms in patients with cutaneous metastases from breast cancer is, therefore, readily understandable. Although the relative and absolute intensities of pain and pruritis varies, much relief has been obtained in all patients with this syndrome following the prescription of a strong antiprostaglandin agent such as flurbiprofen or naproxen.

* 1 tablet Wygesic (USA) equivalent to 2 tablets Distalgesic (Britain)

Paracetamol (Acetaminophen)

Drug portrait

Paracetamol is a synthetic non-narcotic analgesic (Figure 7.14). It is also a pharmacologically active metabolite of both acetanilide and phenacetin. Like aspirin, it is antipyretic. Unlike aspirin, in most circumstances, it has no anti-inflammatory effect. As an analgesic it acts peripherally. It is mainly absorbed from the small intestine. Twenty-five per cent of subjects are slow absorbers. When sorbitol is included in the formulation, this figure drops to 10 per cent [47]. Drugs that delay gastric emptying delay the absorption of paracetamol. 500 to 650 mg is definitely more effective than 300 mg, but the effect of 1 g is not always clearly distinguishable from 500 mg and 650 mg. Within this range, it is equipotent with aspirin. Paracetamol is mostly excreted in the urine as sulphate or glucuronide. The metabolic pathways are saturable and, in overdosage, an intermediate metabolite causes acute hepatic necrosis which may be fatal. Paracetamol is *not* converted to aniline or paraphenetidin, toxic metabolites of acetanilide and phenacetin respectively. A single dose is effective for 4 to 6 hours.

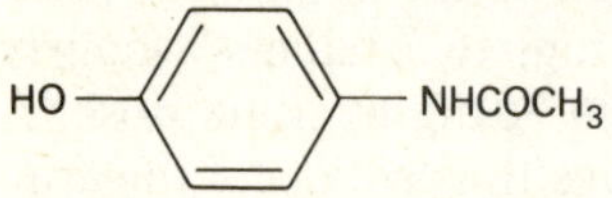

$$HO - \langle\!\!\!\rangle - NHCOCH_3$$

Figure 7.14 Chemical formula of paracetamol (acetaminophen).

Although paracetamol was known to have analgesic properties as long ago as 1893, it is less than 30 years since the introduction of 500 mg tablets in Britain. In 1963, paracetamol was added to the British Pharmacopoeia, since when its popularity as an over-the-counter analgesic has increased progressively. Currently it is as popular as aspirin. Aspirin is sometime thought to be stronger than paracetamol but, weight for weight, they are comparable in terms of both antipyretic and analgesic effects. The dose response curve for aspirin is, however, taller than for paracetamol. Moreover, in rheumatological conditions, the anti-inflammatory effect of higher doses of aspirin results in a much greater efficacy. On the other hand, in post-dental extraction pain, paracetamol appears to have an anti-inflammatory effect, and is more effective than aspirin in reducing both pain and swelling [48].

Studies indicate that a regular intake of 2 g of paracetamol per day may result in an increase in thrombotest times, necessitating a reduction in the dose of concurrently administered coumarin anticoagulants [49]. The underlying mechanism is not clear, but may relate to interference with the hepatic synthesis of factors II, VII, IX and X.

The other main distinguishing features of paracetamol are:

1 It can be taken by those hypersensitive to aspirin.
2 It is well tolerated by patients with peptic ulcers.
3 It does not affect plasma uric acid concentration.
4 It has no effect on platelet function.
5 Liquid preparations for children are stable.
6 Side effects are minor and minimal.

Paracetamol may be given by suppository. The bioavailability by this route varies from 68 to 88 per cent of that obtained after oral ingestion and the peak plasma concentration tends to be delayed. By mouth, the small differences in absorption observed between different products were overshadowed by individual variations [50]. The addition of sorbitol to the tablet formulation improves the rate of absorption from most slow absorbers. The precise mode of action remains conjectural. It may increase the rate of dissolution or it may stimulate gastric emptying. Sorbitol is not present in paracetamol BP but is included in certain British proprietary preparations, notably Panasorb, Panadeine Co., Solpadeine and Panadol Soluble.

Serious toxicity does not occur when paracetamol is used in therapeutic doses, that is, up to 1 g every 4 hours. Hepatotoxicity is caused by the formation in the hepatic parenchymal cell of a minor metabolite with high alkylating activity [3]. This binds covalently to cell constituents causing damage and necrosis. The small amount of this metabolite formed with therapeutic doses is rapidly detoxified by conjugation with reduced glutathione. With toxic doses glutathione is deleted and the excess metabolite is free to damage the cells. The smallest amount associated with a fatal outcome is said to be 18 g. Many have survived with doses of up to 25 g. Above this level, death is increasingly likely unless specific treatment is instituted, though survival has been reported after 75 g. Treatment consists of oral methionine or IV N-acetylcysteine, both of which are precursors of glutathione [3].

Nefopam

Drug portrait
Nefopam is a synthetic non-narcotic analgesic (Figure 7.15). It is the only member of a novel class of analgesics, the benzoxazocines. It is chemically related to orphenadrin and diphenhydramine. Unlike the latter, it is *not* an antihistamine. Its mechanism of action is not known. It does not cause respiratory depression, nor does it lessen opiate withdrawal signs. Its effects are not reversed by naloxone. It does not inhibit prostaglandin synthesis. It lowers normal body temperature but its action on fever has not been evaluated. It has anticholinergic and sympathomimetic activity which is not usually noticeable unless other drugs with these properties are taken at the same time. Nefopam can be given by mouth or by IM injection. The plasma concentration and the analgesic effect reach a peak after about 2 hours when given by mouth and about 1.5 hours after IM injection. The oral to parenteral potency ratio is about 1:3. The plasma half-life is about 4.5 hours. Nefopam is mostly excreted as an inactive metabolite in the urine.

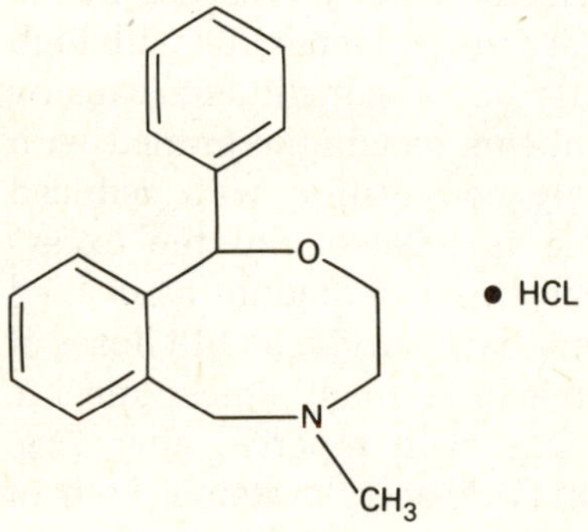

Figure 7.15 Chemical formula of nefopam.

Most clinical trials have been in patients with non-malignant pain. Intramuscularly, nefopam 15 mg is approximately equivalent to 50 mg of pethidine [51]. There is probably a low ceiling effect. In one study, nefopam 30 mg was no more effective than 15 mg, though it lasted longer and was associated with a higher frequency of adverse effects [52]. This ceiling effect may explain why reports of the potency ratio of nefopam to morphine vary between 1:1.66 and 1:3 [52, 53].

The main unwanted effects are insomnia and dryness of the mouth. Other reported unwanted effects include nausea, nervousness and light-headedness. Less frequently, vomiting, blurred vision, drowsiness, sweating, tachycardia and headache may occur. These effects are dose-related and transient, becoming less troublesome with continued treatment. Because of its anticholinergic action it should be used with caution in patients with glaucoma or urinary retention. Nefopam enhances motor neuron activity and patients with epilepsy should not take it. In dogs high doses of nefopam increased the hepatic toxicity of high doses of paracetamol. This effect was not observed at doses closer to those used in man, but, even so, it is probably wiser not to prescribe nefopam and paracetamol concurrently.

The place of nefopam in the relief of cancer pain is uncertain. It may prove to be a satisfactory alternative to the weak narcotics, but, for the moment, its use is not recommended. It is expensive. As yet, nefopam is not available in the USA.

References

1 Editorial. Analgesic nephropathy. *British Medical Journal* 1981; **282:** 339–340.

2 Temple AR. Acute and chronic effects of aspirin toxicity and their treatment. *Archives of Internal Medicine* 1981; **141:** 364–369.

3 Prescott LF. Hepatotoxicity of mild analgesics. *British Journal of Clinical Pharmacology* 1980; **10:** 373S–379S.

4 Morley J. Mode of action of aspirin in *Proceedings of the Aspirin Symposium* edited by Dale TLC. Ratleigh Printers, Rochford 1975, pp 19–22.

5 Ferreira S. Peripheral and central analgesia. *Abstracts 3rd World Congress on Pain*, Edinburgh 1981.

6 Leonards JR. Are all aspirins alike? *Australian and New Zealand Journal of Medicine* 1976; **6** (suppl. 1): 8–13.

7 Flower RJ, Moncada S and Vane JR. Analgesic antipyretics and anti-inflammatory agents; drugs employed in the treatment of gout in *The Pharmacological Basis of Therapeutics* (6th edition) edited by Gilman AG, Goodman LS and Gilman A. Macmillan, New York 1980, pp 682–728.

8 Galasko CSB. The development of skeletal metastases in *Bone Metastasis* edited by Weiss L and Gilbert HA. GK Hall, Boston, Mass. 1981, pp. 83–113.

9 Ferreira SH. Prostaglandins, aspirin-like drugs and analgesia. *Nature New Biology* 1972; **240:** 200–203.

10 Mundy GR and Spiro TP. The mechanism of bone metastasis and bone destruction by tumour cells in *Bone Metastasis* edited by Weiss L and Gilbert HA. GK Hall, Boston Mass. 1981, pp 64–82.

11 Miller DR. Combination use of nonsteroidal anti-inflammatory drugs. *Drug Intelligence and Clinical Pharmacy* 1981; **15:** 3–7.

12 Brooks PM. Clinical effects and interactions. Nonsteroidal anti-inflammatory drugs in *Clinical Pharmacology and Therapeutics* edited by Turner P. Macmillan, London 1980, pp 288–297.

13 Caruso I and Porro GB. Gastroscopic evaluation of anti-inflammatory agents. *British Medical Journal* 1980; **1:** 75–78.

14 Benson JA. Gastrointestinal reactions to drugs. *American Journal of Digestive Diseases* 1971; **16:** 357–362.

15 Editorial. Aspirin and the stomach. *British Medical Journal* 1981; **282:** 91–92.

16 Leonards JR. The influence of solubility on the rate of gastrointestinal absorption of aspirin. *Clinical Pharmacology and Therapeutics* 1963; **4:** 476–479.

17 Kweekel-De Vries WJ, Spierdijk J, Mattie H, Herman JMH. A new soluble acetylsalicylate derivative in the treatment of postoperative pain. *British Journal of Anaesthesia* 1974; **46:** 133–135.

18 Simon LS, Mills JA. Nonsteroidal anti-inflammatory drugs. Part I. *New England Journal of Medicine* 1981; **302:** 1179–1185.

19 Huskisson EC. Diflunisal—a new analgesic. *Practitioner* 1979; **222:** 415–418.

20 Brogden RW, Heel RC, Pakes GE, Speight TM and Avery GS. Diflunisal: a review of its pharmacological properties and therapeutic use in pain and musculoskeletal strains and sprains and pain in osteoarthritis. *Drugs* 1980; **19:** 84–106.

21 Huskisson EC. Editorial: what is an anti-inflammatory? *Rheumatology and Rehabilitation* 1978; **17:** 1–2.

22 Anonymous. Nonsteroidal anti-inflammatory drugs for rheumatoid arthritis. *The Medical Letter* 1980; **22:** 29–31.

23 Anonymous. Choosing a nonsteroidal anti-inflammatory drug. *Drug and Therapeutics Bulletin* 1981; **19:** 53–56.

24 Young Laiwah AC, Mactier RA. Antagonistic effect of nonsteroidal anti-inflammatory drugs on frusemide induced diuresis in cardiac failure. *British Medical Journal* 1981; **283:** 714.

25 Famaey JP. Recent developments about non-steroidal anti-inflammatory drugs and their mode of action. *General Pharmacology* 1978; **9:** 155–161.

26 Ham EA, Cirillo VJ, Zametti M, Shen TY and Kuehl FA. Studies on the mode of action of non-steroidal anti-inflammatory agents in *Prostaglandins in Cellular Biology* edited by Ramwell PW and Phariss BB. Plenum Press, New York 1972, pp. 345–352.

27 Brune K, Glatt M and Graf P. Mechanisms of action of anti-inflammatory drugs. *General Pharmacology* 1976; **7**: 27–33.

28 Kuehl FA, Humes JL, Egan RW, Ham EA, Beveridge GC and van Arman CG. Role of prostaglandin endoperoxide PGG_2 in inflammatory process. *Nature (London)* 1977; **265**: 170–173.

29 Kowanko IC, Pownall R, Knapp MS, Swannell AJ and Mahoney PGC. Circadian variations in the signs and symptoms of rheumatoid arthritis and in the therapeutic effectiveness of flurbiprofen at different times of day. *British Journal of Clinical Pharmacology* 1981; **11**: 477–484.

30 Crook D, Collins AJ, Bawn PA and Chan R. Effect of 'aspirin-like' drug therapy. Prostaglandin synthetase activity from human rheumatoid synovial microsomes. *Annals Rheumatic Diseases* 1976; **35**: 327–332.

31 Cardozo LD, Stanton SL, Robinson H and Hole D. Evaluation of flurbiprofen in detrusor instability. *British Medical Journal* 1980; **280**: 281–282.

32 Cardozo LD and Stanton SL. A comparison between bromocriptine and indomethacin in the treatment of detrusor instability. *Journal of Urology* 1980; **124**: 281–282

33 Segre EJ. Naproxen. *Clinics in Rheumatological Disease* 1979; **5**: 465–480.

34 Sevelius H, Runkel R, Segre E, Bloomfield SS. Bioavailability of naproxen sodium and its relationship to clinical analgesic effects. *British Journal Clinical Pharmacology* 1980, **10**: 259–263.

35 Simon LS, Mills JA. Nonsteroidal anti-inflammatory drugs. Part 2. *New England Journal of Medicine* 1980; **302**: 1237–1243.

36 Lewis JR. Zomepirac Sodium. A new non-addicting analgesic. *Journal of American Medical Association* 1981; **246**: 377–379.

37 Cooper SA. Efficacy of zomepirac in oral surgical pain. *Journal of Clinical Pharmacology* 1980; **20**: 230–242.

38 Cooper SA. Double-blind comparison of zomepirac sodim, propoxyphene/ acetaminophen, and placebo in the treatment of oral surgical pain. *Current Therapeutic Research* 1980; **28**: 630–638.

39 Baird WM and Turek D. Comparison of zomepirac, APC with codeine, codeine and placebo in the treatment of moderate and severe postoperative pain. *Journal of Clinical Pharmacology* 1980; **20**: 243–249.

40 de Andrade JR, Honig S, Ciccone WJ and Leffall L. Clinical comparison of zomepirac with pentazocine in the treatment of postoperative pain. *Journal of Clinical Pharmacology* 1980; **20:** 292–297.

41 Stambaugh JE, Tejada F and Trudnowski RJ. Double-blind comparison of zomepirac and oxycodone with APC in cancer pain. *Journal of Clinical Pharmacology* 1980; **20:** 261–270.

42 Wallenstein SL, Rogers A, Kaiko RF, Heidrich G and Houde RW. Relative analgesic potency of oral zomepirac and intramuscular morphine in cancer patients with postoperative pain. *Journal of Clinical Pharmacology* 1980; **20:** 250–258.

43 Honig S. Preliminary report: long-term safety of zomepirac. *Journal of Clinical Pharmacology* 1980; **20:** 392–396.

44 Tolman EL and Partridge R. Multiple sites of interaction between prostaglandins and nonsteroidal anti-inflammatory agents. *Prostaglandins* 1975; **9:** 349–359.

45 Abruzzo JL. Anti-inflammatory and antirheumatic drugs. *Annals of Internal Medicine* 1981; **94:** 270–271.

46 Editorial. Itch. *Lancet* 1980; **ii:** 568–569.

47 Gwilt JR. The absorption characteristics of paracetamol tablets in man. *Journal of Pharmacy and Pharmacology* 1963; **15:** 445–453.

48 Skjelbred P, Album B and Lokken P. Acetylsalicylic acid vs paracetamol: effects on postoperative course. *European Journal of Clinical Pharmacology* 1977; **12:** 257–264.

49 Boeijinga JJ, Boerstra EE, Ris P, Breimer DD and Jeletich-Bastiaanse A. Interaction between paracetamol and coumarin anticoagulants. *Lancet* 1982; **i:** 506.

50 Prescott LF and Nimmo J. Genetic inequivalence. Clinical observations. *Acta Pharmacologica (Kbh)* 1971; **29:** 288–303.

51 Tigerstedt I, Sepponen J, Tammisto T and Turunen M. Comparison of nefopam and pethidine in postoperative pain. *British Journal of Anaesthesia* 1977; **49:** 1133–1138.

52 Sunshine A and Laska E. Nefopam and morphine in man. *Clinical Pharmacology and Therapeutics* 1975; **18:** 530–534.

53 Beaver WT and Ferse GA. A comparison of the analgesic effect of intramuscular nefopam and morphine in patients with postoperative pain. *Journal of Clinical Pharmacology* 1977; **17:** 579–591.

Chapter Eight

Weak Narcotic Agonists

When aspirin or paracetamol* fail to relieve, a weak narcotic agonist should be used (Table 8.1). Most weak narcotics are prescribed in combination with aspirin or paracetamol. As non-narcotics and weak

Table 8.1 Weak narcotic agonists

codeine
dihydrocodeine
oxycodone†
dextropropoxyphene
ethoheptazine

† Oxycodone is available in Britain in Pro-ladone suppositories (as pectinate). It is not available in tablet form. It is available in the USA as tablets in combination with aspirin (Percodan) or acetaminophen (Percocet, Tylox) and as a syrup

narcotic agonists have different mechanisms of action, there can be no fundamental objection to the use of compound tablets. Combined use has been shown to produce an additive effect [1]. In Britain, however, the amount of codeine and dihydrocodeine in compound tablets is much less than is normally given when used alone (vide infra).

A number of trials have been undertaken in recent years comparing commonly used compound analgesic tablets. In one much quoted study in cancer patients [2], the results suggested that dextropropoxyphene and ethoheptazine are ineffectual when given by mouth in conjunction with

* acetaminophen (USA)

aspirin (Figure 8.1). Other studies (see page 160 and page 163) and clinical experience do not support this negative result. The following points should be noted:

1 Single-dose analgesic studies do not always predict the performance of a drug when taken repeatedly.
2 Drugs that are slowly absorbed will show up less well in single-dose studies.
3 Drugs with a prolonged plasma half-life cumulate when given repeatedly. This tends to enhance efficacy.
4 In this study, all preparations were given in standardized (double-blind) blue gelatin capsules. No information was offered concerning the bioavailability or the absorption characteristics of the drugs when given in this way.
5 The end-point (percentage of patients achieving 50 per cent relief) is perhaps not the best for patients experiencing a variety of pains associated with cancer.

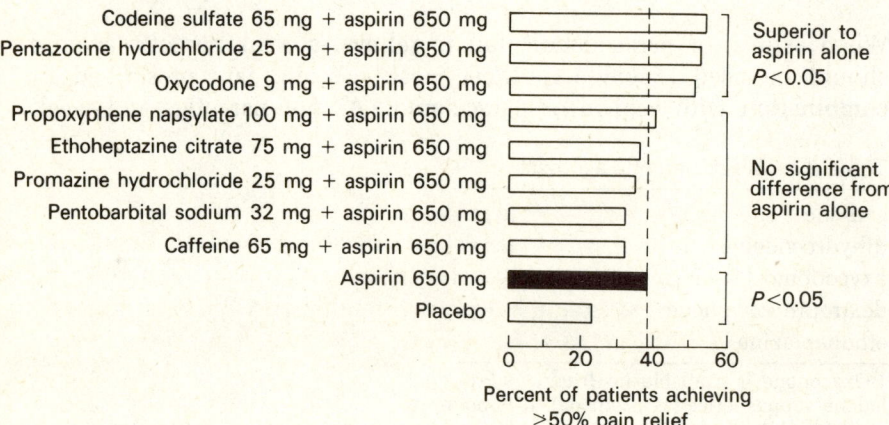

Figure 8.1 Comparative analgesic effect of placebo, aspirin alone, and aspirin combinations as indicated by the percentage of patients achieving more than 50 per cent relief of pain.
From Moertel et al, 1974 [2]

   In Chapter 6, we suggested that the weak narcotic agonists show a 'ceiling' effect in relation to analgesia. This is an oversimplification. Whereas agonist-antagonists like pentazocine and buprenorphine have a true ceiling effect, the maximum effective dose of the weak narcotic agonists is arbitrary. At higher doses there are progressively more side effects which outweigh the sometimes indistinct gains in terms of analgesic effect. The quantity of dextropropoxyphene and ethoheptazine in tablets such as Distalgesic* and Equagesic was chosen so that only a

* 1 tablet Wygesic (USA) equivalent to 2 tablets Distalgesic (Britain)

small minority of patients would experience nausea and vomiting when 2 tablets are taken. This adds a further constraint: the upper dose limit is set in practice by the number of tablets that a patient will readily accept. This is usually 2, sometimes 3 but almost never more.

In terms of efficacy, there is little to choose between the weak narcotics. Codeine and dihydrocodeine are more constipating. For this reason, Distalgesic (containing dextropropoxyphene 32.5 mg and paracetamol 325 mg) is preferred at most British hospices. It is important to change to something definitely stronger if a weak narcotic is inadequate when given regularly every 4 hours. Do not move sideways and try your luck with an alternative weak narcotic. Occasionally your luck will be in but usually the patient suffers—the alternative is either no better or worse. Generally, a stronger analgesic will mean either morphine (see Chapter 9) or an alternative strong narcotic agonist (see Chapter 14).

Codeine

> *Drug portrait*
> Codeine (methylmorphine) occurs naturally in opium and is closely related structurally to morphine (Figure 8.2). It is the parent weak narcotic analgesic, and is used for moderate pain in doses of 30 to 60 mg. It is well absorbed after administration by mouth or injection. It is O-demethylated to morphine and N-demethylated to norcodeine in the liver. These, together with codeine are excreted in the urine, partly as conjugates with glucuronic acid. Codeine has a linear dose-response curve when given IM in doses up to 360 mg. Higher doses have not been examined. The oral:parenteral potency ratio is said to be 2:3 [3]. The plasma half-life is 2.5 to 3 hours [4]. When used in adequate doses, the useful duration of effect is 4 to 6 hours. It has been suggested that codeine may exert its moderate analgesic effect through partial biotransformation to morphine [5].

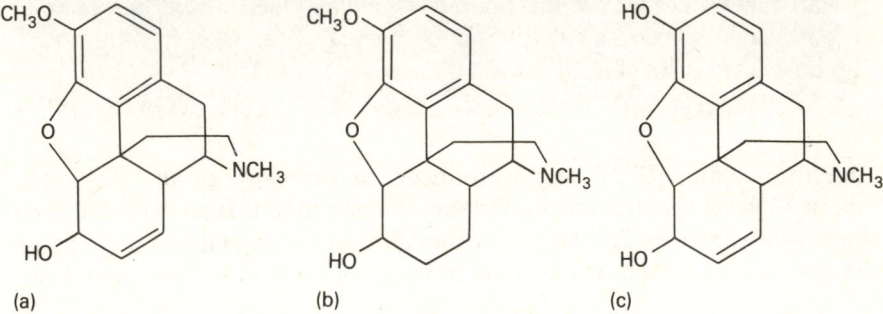

Figure 8.2 Chemical formulae of (a) codeine, (b) dihydrocodeine and (c) morphine.

Single-dose studies indicate that parenterally codeine is less than one-twelfth as potent as morphine [6] but between one-third and one-quarter as potent by mouth [7]. If this were true of repeated administration, it would mean that 60 mg of codeine was as potent as 15 to 20 mg of morphine by mouth. This is not so; the majority of patients poorly controlled on weak narcotics or weak narcotic-non-narcotic preparations are satisfactorily controlled on 10 mg of morphine sulphate 4-hourly. Parenteral codeine phosphate has no advantages over small oral doses of morphine sulphate.

In a single-dose study in patients with terminal cancer pain, it was not possible to distinguish between 32 mg of codeine and 650 mg aspirin, though both were better than a placebo [1]. When taken together, an additive effect was noted, lending support to the common practice of combining aspirin with codeine (Figure 8.3). It is, however, not always appreciated that the amount of codeine in, for example, a tablet of Codis* is only 8 mg (Table 8.2). As most patients take two tablets, this gives a total of 16 mg as a dose. Although it is held that such doses are 'homeopathic' some people assert that they notice a definite 'muzziness' when taking such tablets. One thing is certain though: when a patient transfers from 2 tablets of aspirin to 2 tablets of Codis, he increases his intake of aspirin from 600 mg to 1 g. It is possible therefore that codeine-aspirin tablets rely for their greater efficacy on the increased intake of aspirin rather than the addition of small amounts of codeine. Some other codeine preparations are listed in Tables 8.2 to 8.5. Codeine is of value as a cough sedative and as an antidiarrhoeal.

Dihydrocodeine

Drug portrait
Dihydrocodeine is a semisynthetic analgesic, related to codeine (Figure 8.2). It is a weak narcotic agonist used for moderate pain, with a potency perhaps one-third greater than codeine. The plasma half-life is 2.5 to 3 hours and it is metabolized along the same pathways as codeine. Duration of useful effect is 3 to 4 hours, consistently less than morphine.

Dihydrocodeine (DHC) was introduced in Germany as an antitussive about 70 years ago. Interest in its analgesic potential is more recent, dating back some 25 years (Table 8.6). Although it has been claimed to be twice as potent as codeine, some trials have reported it to be less potent [8].

---

* not available in the USA

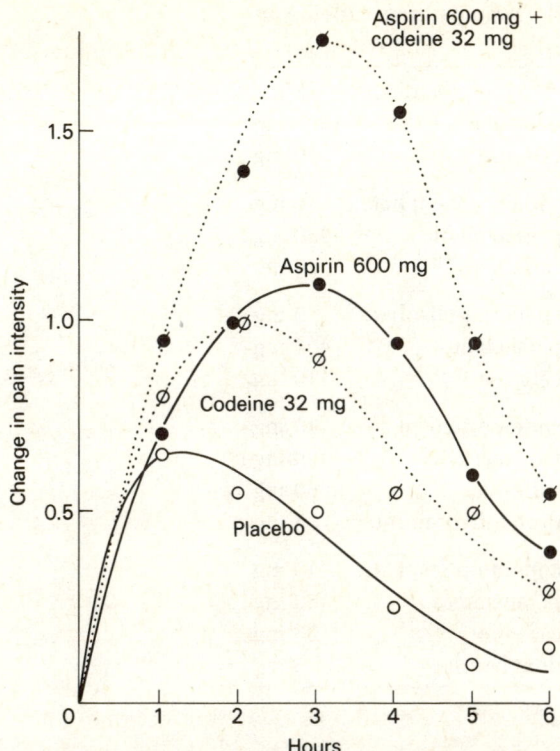

Figure 8.3 Time-effect curves for lactose placebo, aspirin 600 mg, codeine 32 mg and a combination of aspirin 600 mg and codeine 32 mg. Changes in pain intensity (ordinate) are plotted against time in hours (abscissa). Treatments were administered in a randomized order on a complete crossover basis to 11 patients with pain due to cancer. Nine of the patients repeated the crossover twice.
From Houde *et al*, 1966 [1]

Table 8.2   Codeine containing preparations in Britain

T	codeine phosphate		15 mg
			30 mg
			60 mg
T	Codis	codeine phosphate	8 mg
		soluble aspirin	500 mg
C	Neurodyne ⎫	codeine phosphate	8 mg
T	Panadeine ⎬	paracetamol	500 mg
T	Parake ⎭		
ET	Paracodol	codeine phosphate	8 mg
		paracetamol	500 mg

T = tablet; C = capsule; ET = effervescent tablet

153

Table 8.3 Codeine preparations containing caffeine in Britain†

T	Parahypon	codeine phosphate	5 mg
		paracetamol	500 mg
		caffeine	10 mg
T	Paralgin	codeine phosphate	6 mg
		paracetamol	450 mg
		caffeine	20 mg
T	Pardale	codeine phosphate	9 mg
		paracetamol	400 mg
		caffeine	10 mg
T	Pharmidone ⎫	codeine phosphate	10 mg
T	Propain ⎭	paracetamol	400 mg
		caffeine	50 mg
		diphenhydramine	5 mg
T	Syndol	codeine phosphate	10 mg
		paracetamol	450 mg
		caffeine	30 mg
		doxylamine	5 mg

† These are not recommended
T = tablet

Usually, the effect has been equal or slightly greater, on average by about one-third. It is suggested that the optimal *parenteral* dose is 30 mg [9]. At 60 mg IM pain relief is increased only slightly and morphine-like side effects become more evident. By mouth, if an oral to parenteral potency ratio of 1:3 is assumed, the optimal dose limit will be of the order of 90 to 120 mg. At all dose levels studied, the duration of relief is shorter with DHC than with morphine [10].

There appear to be no well-controlled clinical trials of *oral* DHC with other oral analgesics. A 60 mg dose of DHC *may* be as effective as 6 mg of morphine sulphate. As with codeine, a starting dose of morphine 10 mg 4-hourly is indicated for patients obtaining inadequate relief with DHC 60 mg. In a few, the dose may need to be increased rapidly to 20 mg.

In a study of 95 healthy volunteers, who took DHC 30 mg on 3 consecutive mornings after breakfast (compared with placebo taken in the same way a week later), nausea and dizziness occurred significantly more often in the 41 females than in the 54 male participants. The results also suggested that DHC might be more constipating in men than in women ($p = 0.064$) [1]. Whether these differences hold true for codeine, or indeed morphine, is not known.

Table 8.4   Oral preparations in the USA containing at least 30 mg codeine

T	Codeine phosphate		30 mg	
			60 mg	
T	Acetaco	codeine	30 mg	
		acetaminophen	325 mg	
T	Ascriptin with codeine No. 3	codeine	32.4 mg	
		aspirin	325 mg	
		magnesium-aluminium hydroxide	150 mg	
C	Bancap with codeine	codeine	32 mg	
		acetaminophen	300 mg	
		salicylamide	200 mg	
T, Sy	Capital with codeine	codeine	30 mg	
		acetaminophen	325 mg	
T	Empirin with codeine	codeine	30–60 mg	(Nos. 3–4)
		aspirin	325 mg	
T	Empracet with codeine	codeine	30–60 mg	(Nos. 3–4)
		acetaminophen	300 mg	
C	G-3	codeine	30 mg	
		acetaminophen	500 mg	
		butabarbital	15 mg	
C	Maxigesic	codeine	30 mg	
		acetaminophen	325 mg	
		promethazine	6.25 mg	
T	Phenaphen with codeine	codeine	30–60 mg	(Nos. 3–4)
		acetaminophen	325 mg	
T	Phenaphen–650 with codeine	codeine	30 mg	
		acetaminophen	650 mg	
T	SK–APAT with codeine	codeine	30–60 mg	(Nos. 495–497)
		acetaminophen	300 mg	
T, E	Tylenol with codeine	codeine	30–60 mg	(Nos. 3–4)
		acetaminophen	300 mg	

T = tablet; C = capsule; Sy = Syrup; E = elixir

155

Table 8.5 Preparations in the USA containing codeine and caffeine†

T	Emprazil – C	codeine phosphate	15 mg	
		pseudoephedrine	20 mg	
		phenacetin	150 mg	
		aspirin	200 mg	
		caffeine	30 mg	
T	Codalan No. 3	codeine	30 mg	
		acetaminophen	150 mg	
		salicylamide	210 mg	
		caffeine	30 mg	
C	Fiorinal with codeine No. 3	butalbital	50 mg	
		caffeine	40 mg	
		aspirin	200 mg	
		phenacetin	130 mg	
		codeine	30 mg	
T	Soma Co. with codeine	carisoprodol	200 mg	
		phenacetin	160 mg	
		caffeine	32 mg	
		codeine	16 mg	
T	Tabloid with codeine	aspirin	227 mg	
		phenacetin	162 mg	
		caffeine	32 mg	
		codeine	30–60 mg	(Nos. 3–4)

† These are not recommended
T = tablet; C = capsule

Table 8.6 Dyhydrocodeine-containing preparations

In Britain

T	DF.118	dihydrocodeine	30 mg
T	Onadox-118	dihydrocodeine tartrate	10 mg
		aspirin	300 mg
T	Paramol-118	dihydrocodeine tartrate	10 mg
		paracetamol	500 mg

In the USA

T	Synalgos-DC†	dihydrocodeine	16 mg
		promethazine	6.25 mg
		aspirin	194.4 mg
		phenacetin	162 mg
		caffeine	30 mg

† these are not recommended
T = tablet

Oxycodone

Drug portrait
Oxycodone (dihydro-hydroxycodeinone) is a semisynthetic mor-phine-like narcotic agonist (Figure 8.4). It is metabolized along the same pathways as codeine. Oxycodone *hydrochloride* acts for 3 to 5 hours when taken orally. Oxycodone *pectinate*, administered rec-tally or IM provides relief for 8 hours or more in most patients.

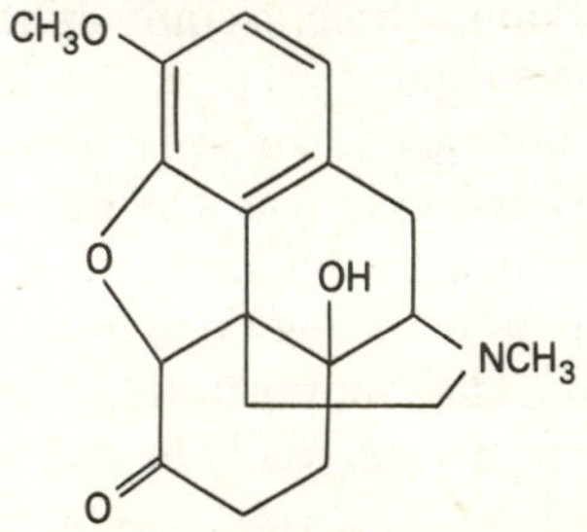

Figure 8.4 Chemical formula of oxycodone.

Until recently, oxycodone was available in the USA only in combination with other drugs. Thus although oxycodone could be characterized as a strong narcotic, possibly as potent as morphine [3], it has been used in the USA as a weak narcotic by virtue of the small content in available tablets. Dose increase has also been limited by aspirin toxicity.

Unfortunately, as the cancer progresses, patients tend to escalate the number of tablets ingested if not prescribed a strong narcotic to replace

Table 8.7 Oxycodone-containing preparations

In the USA			
Sy	—	oxycodone hydrochloride	1 mg/ml
T	Percodan	oxycodone hydrochloride	5 mg
		aspirin	225 mg
T	Percocet	oxycodone hydrochloride	5 mg
		acetaminophen	325 mg
C	Tylox	oxycodone hydrochloride	4.5 mg
		oxycodone terephthalate	0.38 mg
		acetaminophen	500 mg
In Britain			
Supp	Proladone	oxycodone pectinate	30 mg

T = tablet; C = capsule; Supp = suppository; Sy = syrup

the Percodan (Table 8.7). It is not uncommon for a patient to be admitted who, while awake, has been taking 2 to 3 Percodan tablets *every hour*, and who is suffering from salicylism. Such a patient may need 30 to 50 mg of oral morphine sulphate 4-hourly to match his previous narcotic intake. He may also need a lower dose of aspirin as a separate drug.

Oxycodone pectinate was first introduced to Britain about 25 years ago, initially as an injection and then in a suppository. The analgesic effect of oxycodone pectinate (Proladone) given IM or rectally lasts for 8 hours or more in most patients. If taken orally, oxycodone pectinate is hydrolyzed in the stomach and its effect lasts no longer than morphine. Each Proladone suppository contains 30 mg of oxycodone, which is equivalent to about 30 mg or orally administered morphine sulphate [12].

The main use of oxycodone suppositories in advanced cancer is as an alternative to narcotic injections. They may also have a place as a bedtime supplement to a regimen of oral morphine, reducing the need for a dose in the middle of the night (but *see* page 174). Some patients need two 30 mg suppositories to maintain analgesia overnight. The suppositories are small and better described as rectal tablets, so that two can easily be given together.

About 3 years ago, the production of oxycodone pectinate (Proladone) suppositories was stopped for economic reasons. In response to various representations, manufacture was restarted, but only as a 'special' product [13]. This means they are supplied only to order from a hospital pharmacy or local chemist. They are, however, held in stock by the manufacturers (Boots) and are available for immediate despatch.

Dextropropoxyphene

Drug portrait
Dextropropoxyphene is a synthetic analgesic structurally related to methadone (Figure 8.5). It is a weak narcotic agonist used for moderate pain and is readily absorbed from the gastrointestinal tract over a 2 to 3 hour period. Dextropropoxyphene injections are not available as they are painful and have a destructive effect on soft tissues and veins. Dextropropoxyphene is N-demethylated in the liver to yield norpropoxyphene which has substantially less central depressant effect. Dextropropoxyphene has a half-life of 6 to 12 hours, whereas that of norpropoxyphene is 30 to 36 hours. The latter is slowly excreted in the urine.

Dextropropoxyphene is known as propoxyphene in the USA. Weight for weight, it is said to be equal to codeine in analgesic effect. Its laevorota-

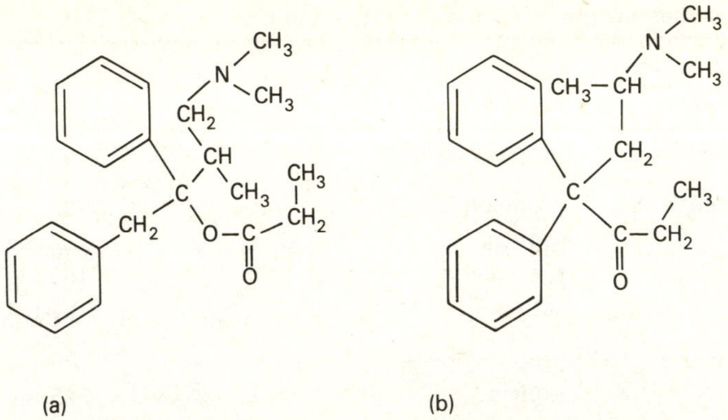

(a)   (b)

Figure 8.5 Chemical formulae of (a) dextropropoxyphene and (b) methadone.

Table 8.8 Dextropropoxyphene-containing preparations in Britain

C	Doloxene	dextropropoxyphene napsylate	100 mg
C	Depronal SA	dextropropoxyphene hydrochloride	150 mg
T	Napsalgesic	dextropropoxyphene napsylate†	50 mg
		aspirin	500 mg
T	Dolasan	dextropropoxyphene napsylate†	100 mg
		aspirin	325 mg
C	Doloxene compound	dextropropoxyphene napsylate	100 mg
		aspirin	375 mg
		caffeine	30 mg
T	Distalgesic ⎤	dextropropoxyphene hydrochloride	32.5 mg
T	Cosalgesic ⎦	paracetamol	325 mg

† dextropropoxyphene napsylate 50 and 100 mg is equivalent to 32.5 and 65 mg of the hydrochloride
T = tablet; C = capsule

tory isomer, levopropoxyphene, is not an analgesic, and is marketed in the USA as a cough suppressant under the trade name, Novrad. In Britain, dextropropoxyphene is generally prescribed in combination with paracetamol (Distalgesic) (Table 8.8.), whereas in the USA it is used both alone (Darvon) and in combination (Wygesic) (Table 8.9).

Controversy continues concerning the benefit of the dextropropoxyphene component in Distalgesic. This relates to the equivocal results in single-dose studies [14]. Dextropropoxyphene, however, has a plasma elimination half-life of 6 to 12 hours. When given 6-hourly, the plasma concentration increases progressively and reaches a steady state after 2 to

Table 8.9 Propoxyphene-containing compounds in the USA

propoxyphene hydrochloride

C	Darvon HO2	propoxyphene	32 mg
C	Darvon HO3	propoxyphene	65 mg
C	Darvon Compound	propoxyphene	32 or 65 mg
		aspirin	227 mg
		phenacetin	162 mg
		caffeine	32.4 mg
C	Darvon ASA	propoxyphene	65 mg
		aspirin	325 mg
C	Propoxyphene USP	propoxyphene	65 mg
C	SK – 65	propoxyphene	65 mg
T	SK – 65 APAP	propoxyphene	65 mg
		acetaminophen	650 mg
C	SK – 65 Compound	propoxyphene	65 mg
		aspirin	227 mg
		phenacetin	162 mg
		caffeine	32.4 mg
C	Š – Paincet	propoxyphene	65 mg
		acetaminophen	650 mg
T	Wygesic	propoxyphene	65 mg
		acetaminophen	650 mg

propoxyphene napsylate†

T	Darvocet N – 50	propoxyphene napsylate	50 mg
		acetaminophen	325 mg
T	Darvocet N – 100	propoxyphene napsylate	100 mg
		acetaminophen	650 mg
T	Darvon N	propoxyphene napsylate	100 mg
Susp	Darvon N	propoxyphene napsylate	50 mg/5 ml
T	Darvon N with ASA	propoxyphene napsylate	100 mg
		aspirin	325 mg

† propoxyphene napsylate 50 and 100 mg is equivalent to 32.5 and 65 mg of the hydrochloride
T = tablet; C = capsule; Susp = suspension

3 days [15]. In other words, a single-dose study may be incapable of determining the true relative efficacy of dextropropoxyphene in a preparation such as Distalgesic. A double-blind controlled trial has recently been carried out in 31 patients who had been using Distalgesic for chronic pain for a mean duration of 2 years [16]. Each patient initially took either 2 tablets of Distalgesic or of paracetamol (500 mg $\times$ 2) 4 times a day for 1 week, and then changed to the other drug, the order of administration being determined by random allocation. Twenty-two patients preferred Distalgesic, 5 preferred paracetamol and 4 expressed no preference. The difference in favour of Distalgesic is highly significant (Chi-squared = 10.7; $p < 0.005$).

Generally, Distalgesic is a well-tolerated preparation (Table 8.10). In a few patients, both young and old, it causes unacceptable central effects,

Table 8.10   Facts about Distalgesic[1]

1	It is used extensively by patients with chronic arthritides.
2	Patients stop taking it if the condition ameliorates.
3	Despite the association of recurrent depression with rheumatoid arthritis, there are no documented cases of deliberate self-poisoning with Distalgesic by rheumatoid patients.
4	22/27 patients found Distalgesic (2 tablets) of greater benefit than paracetamol[2] (500 mg $\times$ 2).
5	It is used as the weak narcotic-non-narcotic analgesia of choice in most British hospices.

[1] 1 tablet Wygesic (USA) equivalent to 2 tablets Distalgesic (Britain)
[2] acetaminophen (USA)

notably, muzziness, lightheadedness, dysphoria and/or confusional symptoms. There is no way of predicting such patients. As with other narcotics, constipation is a common side effect, although usually not as troublesome as with codeine and DHC. Occasional patients will experience nausea and/or vomiting. Thus, as with all narcotic analgesics, when prescribed dextropropoxyphene, the patient should be advised who to contact and how in the event of unacceptable side effects. Comparable side effects occur with other dextropropoxyphene-containing preparations.

An important drug interaction has been reported in 3 patients [17]. They were also taking carbamazepine and complained of headache, dizziness, ataxia, nausea and tiredness. Combined use resulted in an increase of the plasma concentration of carbamazepine which accounted for the symptoms. Dextropropoxyphene is thought to inhibit the oxidation of carbamazepine [17].

It has also been reported that, when taken regularly, dextropropoxyphene may interfere with coumarin derivative anticoagulants. Up to

150 mg of dextropropoxyphene a day once or twice a week is safe, but the regular ingestion of 200 mg or more may require a reduction in the dose of the oral anticoagulant [18]. As paracetamol may also increase thrombo-test times, anticoagulated patients commencing dextropropoxyphene-paracetamol tablets should be closely monitored and the dose of anticoagulant reduced if necessary.

Ethoheptazine

Drug portrait
Ethoheptazine is structurally related to pethidine* (Figure 8.6) and is about one-third as potent. It is a weak narcotic analgesic used for moderate pain. It is readily absorbed from the gastrointestinal tract and peak blood concentrations are reached in an hour. The half-life is not known. It is extensively metabolized in the liver and the metabolites excreted in the urine. By injection, the duration of useful effect appears to be 5 to 7 hours, though orally it is used every 4 hours.

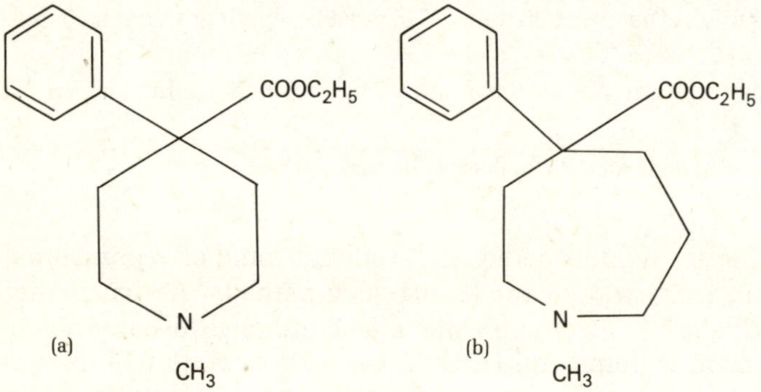

Figure 8.6 Chemical formulae of (a) pethidine and (b) ethoheptazine.

Ethoheptazine may be thought of as weak pethidine. Its basic structure comprises a heterocyclic ring of seven members, whereas pethidine, a piperidine, has six (Figure 8.6). Ethoheptazine is about one-third as potent [19]. Its half-life is not known. By injection, it is said to be longer acting than both pethidine and morphine; most patients requesting it at intervals of between 5 and 7 hours [20]. When first introduced, concern was expressed about cumulative CNS toxicity after several days to 3 weeks of regular administration. This took the form of nervousness, headache, dizziness, 'visual symptoms' and syncope [21]. Subsequently,

* meperidine (USA)

it was decided that these had been caused by an impurity in the original batch of medication. In contrast to pethidine, ethoheptazine does not cause lethargy in *rats*, does not produce morphine-like excitement in *cats*, and does not depress respiration until very high doses are administered [22].

Ethoheptazine has been used in doses of up to *500 mg every 4 hours* in patients with a variety of acute and chronic pains [20]. Two-thirds of those who received 250 mg 4-hourly experienced untoward side effects. As with the early parenteral studies, some patients developed toxic reaction after 1 to 3 weeks. On the other hand, two of the patients who received 500 mg 4-hourly did so for several weeks without toxicity. When the dose was reduced to 75 mg, any side effects were predominantly gastric, that is nausea and/or vomiting and epigastric discomfort.

As a result of this study [20], 50 mg of ethoheptazine base (75 mg of ethoheptazine citrate) has been adopted as the standard quantity per tablet. This gives a dose of 100 mg (citrate 150 mg) per dose of 2 tablets (Table 8.11).

Table 8.11 Ethoheptazine-containing preparations

T	Equagesic,	ethoheptazine citrate†	75 mg
	Meprogesic‡	meprobamate	150 mg
		aspirin	250 mg
T	Zactirin*	ethoheptazine citrate†	75 mg
		aspirin	325 mg
		calcium carbonate	97 mg
T	Zactipar*	ethoheptazine citrate†	75 mg
		paracetamol	400 mg

* not available in the USA
† ethoheptazine citrate 75 mg is equivalent to 50 mg of ethoheptazine base
‡ alternative brand name (USA)
T = tablet

It would seem, however, that there may be occasions when a higher dose could be used, in the absence of gastric intolerance, rather than necessarily change to oral morphine sulphate. The single-dose study of Moertel *et al* [2] almost certainly employed a suboptimal dose of ethoheptazine [23]. Further, an analgesic with a relatively long duration of action is likely to have a relatively long plasma half-life. This means that, with regular 4-hourly administration, the plasma concentration will rise substantially over the first few days, and result in progressively more relief—as probably happens in the case of dextropropoxyphene (though apparently not with dextromoramide,* *see* Chapter 14).

* not available in the USA

In the doses commonly used, ethoheptazine is as effective as codeine but, on a mg for mg basis, it is perhaps only one-third to one-fifth as potent. In the early studies, it was stated that ethoheptazine orally is more potent [20].

Compared with codeine, ethoheptazine is less constipating and causes less nausea. Drowsiness is unusual [20]. This makes ethoheptazine a more attractive drug than codeine in situations in which one wishes to avoid adverse alimentary and CNS effects. The ethoheptazine-containing preparation commonly used in Britain and the USA is Equagesic (Table 8.11). This also contains aspirin and meprobamate. Aspirin may itself cause gastritis and meprobamate, a mild anxiolytic and muscle relaxant, may cause drowsiness. When this occurs, it is usually transient and clears after 2 to 3 days. Occasionally, patients are hypersensitive to meprobamate and experience malaise or a skin rash after a few doses.

Pentazocine

Pentazocine, a weak agonist-antagonist is discussed in Chapter 15. We do *not* recommend its use for patients with cancer.

References

1 Houde RW, Wallenstein SL and Beaver WT. Evaluation of analgesics in patients with cancer pain in *Clinical Pharmacology. Section 6 of International Encyclopedia of Pharmacology and Therapeutics* edited by Lasagna L. Pergamon, Oxford and New York 1966.

2 Moertel CG, Ahmann DL, Taylor WF and Schwartau N. Relief of pain by oral medications. *Journal of the American Medical Association* 1974; **229:** 55–59.

3 Jaffe JH and Martin WR. Opioid analgesics and antagonists in *The pharmacological Basis of Therapeutics* edited by Goodman AG, Goodman LS and Gilman A. MacMillan, New York 1980, pp 494–534.

4 Kay DC, Gorodetzky CW and Martin WR. Comparative effects of codeine and morphine in man. *Journal of Pharmacology and Experimental Therapeutics* 1967; **156:** 101–106.

5 Findlay JWA, Jones EC, Butz RF and Welch RM. Plasma codeine and morphine concentrations after therapeutic oral doses of codeine-containing analgesics. *Clinical Pharmacology and Therapeutics* 1978; **24:** 60–68.

6 Lasagna L and Beecher KH. The analgesic effectiveness of codeine and meperidine (Demerol). *Journal of Pharmacology and Experimental Therapeutics* 1954; **112:** 306–311.

7 Eddy NB, Friebel H, Hahn K-J and Halbach H. Codeine and its alternatives for pain and cough relief. 1. *Bulletin of World Health Organization* 1968; **38:** 673–741.

8 Seed JC, Wallenstein SL, Houde RW, Belville JW. A comparison of the analgesic and respiratory effects of dihydrocodeine and morphine in man. *Archives of International Pharmacodynamics* 1958; **116:** 293–339.

9 Eddy NB, Halden H and Braenden OJ. *Bulletin of World Health Organization* 1956; **17:** 569–863.

10 Beecher HK, Gravenstein JS, Pederson DP and Smith GM. Analgesic effect and side effect liability of dihydrocodeine, codeine and morphine in man. *Federation Proceedings* 1957; **16:** 281.

11 Palmer RW, Eade OE, O'Shea PJ and Cuthbert MF. Incidence of unwanted effects of dihydrocodeine bitartrate in healthy volunteers. *Lancet* 1966; **ii:** 620–621.

12 Twycross RG. Relief of Pain in *Management of Terminal Disease*, edited by Saunders CM. Edward Arnold, London 1978; pp 65–92.

13 Anonymous. Oxycodone pectinate (Proladone) and other opiate suppositories. *Drug and Therapeutics Bulletin* 1979; **17:** 21–22.

14 Miller RR, Ferrigold A and Paxinos J. Propoxyphene hydrochloride. *Journal of the American Medical Association* 1970; **213:** 996–1006.

15 McLeod DC. Propoxyphenes—drug evaluation data. *Drug Intelligence and Clinical Pharmacy* 1972; **6:** 143–144.

16 Owen M and Hills LJ. How safe is dextropropoxyphene? *Medical Journal of Australia* 1980; **1:** 617–618.

17 Dam M and Christiansen J. Interaction of propoxyphene with carbamazepine. *Lancet* 1977; **ii:** 509.

18 Standing Advisory Committee for Haematology of the Royal College of Pathologists. Drug interaction with coumarin derivative anticoagulants. *British Medical Journal* 1982; **285:** 274–275.

19 Glessman JM and Seifter J. The analgesic activity of some phenylhexamethylenimine derivatives. *Journal of Pharmacology and Experimental Therapeutics* 1956; **116:** 23–24.

20 Grossman AJ, Golbey M, Gittinger WC and Batterman RC. Clinical effectiveness and safety of a new series of analgesic compounds. *Journal of the American Gerontology Society* 1956; **4:** 187–192.

21 Golbey M, Gittinger WC and Batterman RC. Analgesic potency of parenterally administered azocycloheptane derivatives in man. *Federation Proceedings* 1955; **14:** 344.

22 Seifter J, Eckfield DK, Letchack I, Gore EM and Glassman JM. Pharmacological properties of some azocycloheptane analgesics. *Federation Proceedings* 1954; **13**: 403.

23 Cass LJ, Frederick WS and Batholomey AF. Methods in evaluating ethoheptazine and ethoheptazine combined with aspirin. *Journal of the American Medical Association* 1958; **166**: 1829–1833.

Chapter Nine

Oral Morphine Sulphate

Morphine exists to be given, not merely to be withheld.

Drug portrait
Morphine is the main pharmacologically active constituent of opium
(Figure 9.1). It is a strong analgesic and is used primarily in severe
pain of acute and cancerous origin. Its effects are mediated by
specific opiate receptors, mainly within the CNS. Peripherally its
main action is on smooth muscle. It is readily absorbed by all routes
of administration. When given regularly by mouth it is about
one-third as potent as by SC or IM injection. The plasma half-life of
an oral dose is 2 to 2.5 hours; that of a parenteral dose about 1.5
hours. It is conjugated in the liver to form a glucuronide and
excreted by the kidneys. The duration of useful analgesia is 3 to 5
hours.

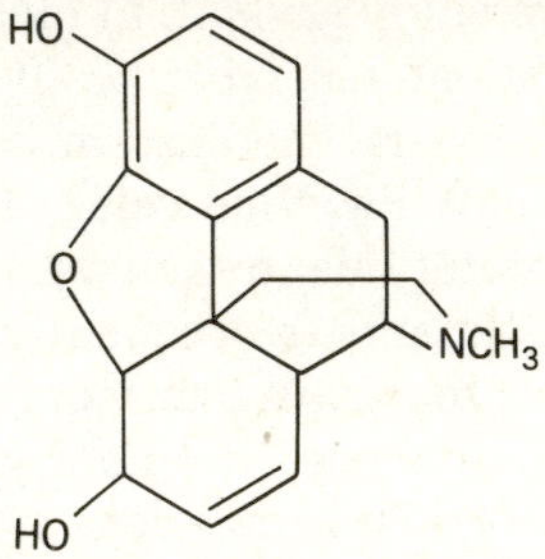

Figure 9.1 Chemical formula of morphine.

The use of morphine is indicated by intensity of pain not brevity of prognosis. This means that morphine should be prescribed when codeine (or alternative weak narcotic) fails to relieve. It is used as the strong narcotic analgesic of choice in most hospices, and is readily available as either morphine sulphate or hydrochloride. Their molecular weights are similar and they may be regarded as interchangeable. When given by mouth in simple aqueous solution, morphine is a versatile, reliable and safe drug.

Most centres in Britain and the USA use morphine sulphate. Commercially prepared morphine sulphate oral solution (Philips Roxane) is available in the USA. It comprises morphine sulphate 2 mg/ml in a bland unflavoured solution containing 10 per cent alcohol as preservative. In Canada, a comparable commercial preparation is manufactured containing morphine hydrochloride (M.O.S. Syrup). It is available in two strengths: 1 mg/ml and 5 mg/ml.

The use of morphine by mouth represents an evolutionary development from the age old use of opium to relieve severe pain. During the latter part of the 19th century morphine was increasingly substituted for opium following the extraction and purification of the main opium alkaloids.

Alkaloid An organic nitrogenous base, usually of vegetable origin, containing nitrogen as a component of a heterocyclic ring structure. (Examples—morphine, cocaine, atropine, nicotine.)

Although commonly given as an elixir, a simple solution of morphine sulphate in water is equally efficacious (*see* Chapter 11). The effective analgesic dose varies considerably, from as little as 2.5 mg to more than 500 mg every 4 hours (Figure 9.2). The majority of patients are satisfactorily controlled on doses of 30 mg or less.

Some two-thirds of each dose is absorbed [1], though because of first-pass metabolism by the liver the oral-parenteral potency ratio is of the order of 1:3. In the American literature a figure of 1:6 is generally quoted. This is based on a single-dose comparative study [2] and, in our experience, is incorrect. In other words, if a patient receiving orally administered morphine sulphate is changed to parenteral medication, a six-fold reduction in dose would result in renewed pain. Vice versa, a six-fold increase would lead to somnolence, respiratory depression and other untoward side effects. In American hospices, patients are frequently changed from unsatisfactory IM morphine regimens to a satisfactory oral one. This usually also includes a change from p.r.n. to a regular 4-hourly schedule [3]. In these circumstances, *the previous IM dose is doubled*: 'In clinical practice I generally double IM dose to determine PO dose, but

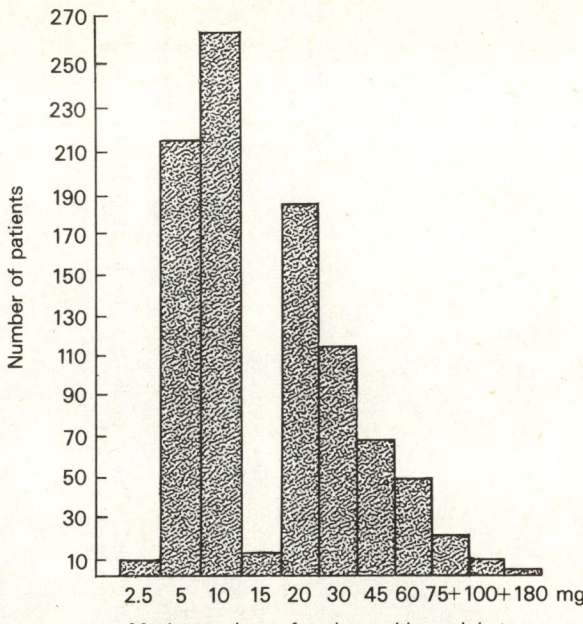

Figure 9.2 Histogram of maximum 4-hourly doses of orally administered morphine sulphate in 955 patients at St. Christopher's Hospice (1978–79). Median dose = 10 mg. Higher doses, up to 1200 mg, have been used occasionally by the authors.
Note: '75+' means 75, 80 or 90 mg, and '100+' means 100, 110 or 120 mg.

then adjust up or down according to pain assessment. When converting from PO to IM, I have often given one-third the dose and then increased the dose to one-half the oral if pain is still present' [4].

Choice of Starting Dose

The initial dose of morphine sulphate depends mainly on the patient's previous medication. Age and general condition are also important. For patients who have been taking a weak narcotic analgesic, either alone or in combination with a non-narcotic, a starting dose of 10 mg is generally appropriate. If the patient is elderly and frail, it is wise to begin with 5 mg (vide infra). For those who have been receiving an alternative strong narcotic, it is necessary to determine as closely as possible what the patient has been taking over a 24-hour period and convert, with the help of the Table of Oral Narcotic Analgesic Equivalents (Table 9.1), to 'morphine sulphate equivalents'. In patients with inadequate pain control, this dose should be increased by at least half and then divided into a convenient 4-hourly dose.

Unless the patient has been taking a narcotic agonist-antagonist such as pentazocine (Fortral, Talwin), the patient is advised to use his previous medication for 'topping up' as necessary over the first day or two until the

Table 9.1 Strong narcotic analgesics: approximate oral equivalents to morphine sulphate

Analgesic	Proprietary name	Potency ratio with morphine sulphate[1]		Duration of action (hours)[2]
pethidine/meperidine	Demerol	1/8	1/12[3]	2–3
dipipanone*	in Diconal	1/2	1/3	3–5
papaveretum	Omnopon, Pantopon	2/3	1/2	3–5
oxycodone**[4]	in Percodan ⎱ Percocet ⎰ Tylox (capsule)	1	2/3	3–5
dextromoramide*	Palfium	2[5]	1.5	2–4
methadone	Physeptone, Dolophine	3–4[6]	2–3	6–8
levorphanol	Dromoran, Levo-dromoran	5	3	4–6
phenazocine*	Narphen	5	3	4–6
hydromorphone**	Dilaudid	6	4	3–4

* not available in the USA
** not available in Britain

[1] Multiply dose of stated drug by the potency ratio to determine the equivalent dose of morphine sulphate.

[2] Dependent to a certain extent on dose, often longer lasting in very elderly and those with considerable liver dysfunction.

[3] Column of figures in italics refer to approximate potency ration with diamorphine (Heroin).

[4] Oxycodone is available in Britain only as oxycodone pectinate suppositories (q.v.).

[5] Dextromoramide single 5 mg dose is equivalent to morphine 15 mg (diamorphine 10 mg) in terms of peak effect but is generally shorter acting; overall potency rate adjusted accordingly.

[6] Methadone – single 5 mg dose is equivalent to morphine 7.5 mg (diamorphine 5 mg). It has a prolonged plasma half-life which leads to cumulation when given repeatedly. This means it is several times more potent when given regularly.

correct dose of morphine sulphate is determined. This prevents the patient becoming disillusioned and even more anxious should the starting dose prove woefully inadequate.

In the frail elderly patient, or patients with respiratory or hepatic failure, it is prudent to start on a dose which is likely to be suboptimal. This prevents distress in both patient and family, and non-compliance, should the patient on a higher dose become very sleepy, dizzy or confused. It is sometimes stated that it is best to start on a 'high' dose and then, when the pain is controlled, reduce to a lower maintenance level. Although this is reasonable for young patients in hospital, it is a recipe for disaster in the elderly and most of those being cared for at home. The analgesic effect of morphine is not an 'all or none' phenomenon. Thus, with rare exceptions, it is possible to choose a starting dose that is at least as effective as the previous medication, and usually more so.

Because of the gross difference in plasma half-lives, it is difficult to give even approximate equivalent doses for morphine and methadone. On the other hand, methadone is a useful alternative strong narcotic. This means that it is unlikely that there will be a need to change to morphine because of unrelieved pain. The only common reason for wishing to change is excessive drowsiness and confusional symptoms resulting from cumulation. In this circumstance, prescribing morphine sulphate in a ratio of 1:1 or 1:2 would be appropriate (see Chapter 14).

One other drug conversion may be difficult, namely, that from dextromoramide* (see Chapter 14). This is for several reasons, including the fact that many patients with severe pain take dextromoramide every 2 to 3 hours and sometimes hourly. Here there is a pyschological problem: if you have been taking medication every 1 to 2 hours and obtaining a fair measure of relief, it is difficult to accept that anything can and will last 4 hours. Moreover, dextromoramide appears to have a rapid onset of action and, if a patient has been taking his medication partly 'as required', he will experience worsening pain after the first dose of morphine, even if theoretically adequate, because of slower absorption. For someone with severe pain, this can be devastating to morale. The starting dose of morphine sulphate should therefore err on the side of generosity (Table 9.1). In addition, both at home and in hospital, the patient should be allowed to keep his dextromoramide tablets and to use them if he feels he needs them. Sometimes it is necessary to adopt a 3-hourly morphine regimen until the patient is reviewed the next day.

Adjustment of Dose
The patient should be advised to increase the dose by 50 per cent if the dose is not more effective than the previous medication or during the

---

* Not available in the USA

second day 'if the pain is not 90 per cent controlled', even if the patient feels moderately sleepy. Careful reassessment after 24 hours and again after 3 days is important. Ideally, reassessment should be by the doctor, though, when trained, can be carried out by a community nurse. Review at home, surgery (office) or outpatient clinic after 1 week is also necessary. In hospital, daily reassessment is, of course, feasible and therefore obligatory.

Most patients are well controlled on morphine sulphate in doses of between 10 and 30 mg every 4 hours (Figure 9.2). Although, if previously they have been taking an alternative strong narcotic, such as methadone, hydromorphone,** levorphanol or phenazocine,* the effective analgesic dose may be considerably higher. If the pain is not much relieved after one or two increments of 100 per cent (low starting dose) or 50 per cent (high starting dose) it is possible that the patient has a narcotic non-responsive pain (Table 9.2). In this circumstance, the use of a co-analgesic and non-drug measures should be considered (see Chapter 16). Alternatively it may indicate a higher than average psychological component to the pain, which will demand more time, more psychotherapeutic support, and probably the prescription of an anxiolytic or an antidepressant (Table 9.3).

Dose Increments
At lower doses, increments are generally greater in terms of percentage of previous dose than when adjusting a higher dose. For example:

2.5 mg→5 mg
5 mg→10 mg

are both 100 per cent increases. Whereas:

10 mg→15 mg
20 mg→30 mg
40 mg→60 mg

are 50 per cent increases, and:

30 mg→40 mg
60 mg→80 mg

are respectively, increases of 33 per cent and 25 per cent.

On occasion, we have seen satisfactory pain control on, say, 70 mg whereas 60 mg was inadequate. Generally however, we would *not* recommend such a small percentage increment, partly because experience indicates that it does not generally have such a marked effect. Increments

* not available in the USA
** not available in Britain

172

Table 9.2   Morphine unresponsive pains

Sedative response only: morphine should not be used
Tension headache
Postherpetic neuralgia
Dysaesthesia
Stabbing

Variable response: morphine best avoided
Gastric distension
Muscle spasm

Partial response: but morphine often necessary
Bone
Nerve compression
Activity precipitated (bone or nerve compression)
'Tenesmoid' (rectum or bladder)
Decubitus (superficial component)

Table 9.3   Incomplete relief with morphine sulphate†

1   Need to increase dose of morphine sulphate still further.
2   Patient has a morphine unresponsive pain (*see* Table 9.2).
3   Failure to use an appropriate co-analgesic (*see* Chapter 16).
4   Failure to use appropriate non-drug measures (*see* Chapters 4 and 5).
5   Activity precipitated pain (*see* Chapter 5).
6   Inability to increase dose further because of higher than average severity of unwanted side effects (*see* this Chapter).
7   Patient not interested in pain relief and therefore reluctant to cope with unwanted effects of treatment.
8   Poor compliance (because living alone, forgetful, etc.).
9   Non-resolution of anger, anxiety, fear (*see* Chapter 3).
10 Maladaptive psychological stance (*see* Expectations, Chapter 4).
11 Lack of time before patient dies.
12 Difficulty in swallowing medication, with loss through drooling and spluttering (*see* Chapter 12).
13 Vomiting, especially within 1 to 2 hours of taking medicine (*see* Chapter 12).

† It is assumed that the patient is being generally well cared for and that morphine sulphate is being administered regularly every 4 hours

tend to be more stereotyped at home as the scope for manoeuvre is limited: the patient has only one bottle of morphine sulphate solution, and not several 'stock' bottles as appertains in most hospices. At home, therefore, almost all increments will be 50 per cent in the first instance with the possibility of a second increment of 33 per cent before a new stronger supply of morphine sulphate is issued (that is, 10 ml→15 ml (50 per cent) →20 ml (33 per cent).

In general, in hospital we would recommend the following steps:

5→10→15→20→30→40→60→80→100→120→160→200→240→
280/300→320/360 mg.

A change from 20→25 mg and 40→50 mg are definitely *not* advised. Each adjustment takes time and, if an adjustment yields little or no benefit, time and confidence are lost.

Night Time

Although the rule when prescribing morphine sulphate is *every 4 hours around the clock*, there are occasions when it is possible to manage without an 0200 hour dose. If a patient is having good nights and

1 does not normally wake in the night to micturate;
2 is well controlled on a dose of between 5 and 60 mg of morphine sulphate.

it may be possible to go through the night with a large bedtime dose (± an hypnotic) (Figure 9.3). If the patient is happy to try, initially increase the bedtime dose by 50 per cent. If not successful, or only partly so, the dose should be increased further to double the daytime dose. With smaller doses, 10 mg or less, the bedtime dose should be doubled as the first step. Such a step may also be taken if the patient is not sleeping soundly and comfortably until 0200 hours. It is probably a better course of action than to add in an hypnotic *de novo* as there is less likelihood of morning drowsiness.

Many patients do, however, need a dose in the middle of the night. Patients at home should be advised to prepare their 0200 hours dose in advance. This can be done at the time of the bedtime dose and left in an easily accessible place by the bed. Thus, if the patient wakes and is drowsy, he does not have to measure an exact amount of morphine sulphate solution, he simply has to take it. Moreover, if he then wakes later, he does not have to wonder if he has had the 0200 hours dose; if the beaker/cup is empty—he has.

Other Than 4-Hourly

Apart from at night with some patients, there are times when it is appropriate to prescribe morphine sulphate other than every four hours.

1 *Initiation of treatment in the very elderly, particularly at home*
The potential for unwanted effects is obviously greater in the frail, elderly patient. It is sometimes wise to start with a *bedtime only* dose and to review the next morning. Depending on how the patient has fared, one may continue with the same regimen (using a less potent preparation during the day) or carefully introduce 2 or 3 daytime doses linked for convenience to meal times.

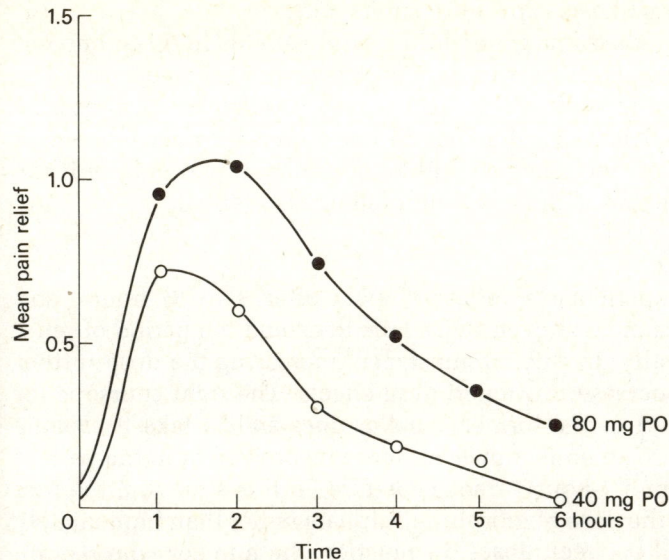

Figure 9.3 Time-effect curves for oral morphine sulphate. Those shown relate to the approximate mean upper and lower doses investigated in 25 cancer patients who received a series of *single* doses in random order. After 40 mg, a mean pain relief score of 0.5 or more is achieved for 2 hours; after 80 mg, for 4 hours. This explains why a double dose of morphine sulphate at night often obviates the need for an 0200 hour dose. The increased potential for drowsiness with the higher dose helps ensure a good night's rest.

After Houde *et al*, 1965 [2]

2   *Those with night pain only*

3   *Those with evening and night pain only*
A few patients fall into these categories and either a bedtime only regimen, or 1800 hours and bedtime, is appropriate. The reason for this is partly the effect of end-of-day fatigue on the patient's pain threshold and partly because of increasing anxiety as the patient begins to anticipate another bad night. In addition, some patients have pain which is made worse by lying down.

4   *Those who have occasional attacks of severe pain*
Some patients may be well controlled on a weak narcotic analgesic but fear a return of their previously intolerable pain. These are reassured by having a small supply of morphine sulphate 'in reserve'. The quantity need only be 200 ml but, if going on holiday, 500 ml may be more reassuring.

5   *The very elderly*
In a frail patient of over 80 years of age, a 6 or even 8-hourly regimen may be adequate.

6 *Extensive liver disease, especially in the elderly*
One proceeds along the same general lines with patients in this group but recognizes that drowsiness caused by cumulation may become a problem. If the patient is not in very severe pain it may be adequate to prescribe every 6 to 8 hours. Alternatively, after 24 hours on a 4-hourly regimen, a reduction in dose or frequency should be considered, particularly if the patient is pain-free and is drowsy, muddled or disoriented.

7 *Fast metabolizers*
A few patients experience a return of pain after 3 to 3½ hours, and increasing the dose once or even twice fails to extend the period of relief more than marginally. In this circumstance, increasing the dose further serves merely to increase unwanted drug effects. The right course is for the patient to revert to the former, smaller dose and to take it every 3 hours. A 3-hourly regimen is, however, more inconvenient to the patient and his family than a 4-hourly one. Therefore, in this situation, the first step is to increase the dose of morphine sulphate rather than immediately reduce the interval between doses. In practice, the number who require morphine 3-hourly is very small.

Unwanted Effects (Table 9.4)
Nausea and Vomiting
Unless a doctor is experienced in the use of oral morphine sulphate, it is best to prescribe an antiemetic routinely when starting on morphine therapy. If there is no pre-existing nausea or vomiting, the experienced

Table 9.4 Unwanted effects of morphine therapy

Early
Nausea and vomiting
Drowsiness
Dizziness/unsteadiness
Confusional symptoms — muddled thought
                                         disorientation
                                         hallucinations
Sweating

Continuing
Constipation
Nausea and vomiting
Inactivity drowsiness
Sweating

Late
Depression

doctor may decide not to prescribe an antiemetic automatically. This is particularly reasonable if the patient has been taking a weak narcotic or alternative strong narcotic analgesic for some time. In this situation, the patient may be issued with a small supply of haloperidol 1.5 mg tablets, to take one *statim* and then at bedtime for a week if he feels nauseated or vomits. Alternatively, prochlorperazine (Stemetil, Compazine) 5 mg tablets can be issued for, in the first instance, 8-hourly use. If there is no arrangement for close liaison and follow-up, it is better to prescribe prophylactically rather than risk non-compliance because of nausea and vomiting.

The likelihood of vomiting with morphine tends to lessen after a week or so. In some patients the antiemetic can be phased out after this time. However, if the patient experienced nausea or vomiting before starting morphine, the antiemetic should be continued. It is less common for patients taking 20 mg or more to manage without an antiemetic. This probably relates to morphine-induced gastric stasis. Metoclopramide, an antiemetic which enhances gastric emptying, is of value in those patients who continue to be troubled by nausea or vomiting despite the regular use of haloperidol or prochlorperazine. It should be noted that above a certain ill-defined dose, morphine blocks the gastric action of metoclopramide [5]. We have known patients benefit by its use when taking up to 100 mg of *oral* morphine sulphate. A trial of metoclopramide is, however, always worthwhile if delayed gastric emptying is thought to be a significant factor.

A mixture containing both morphine and a phenothiazine is best avoided, certainly to begin with, as an increase in morphine means an automatic increase in the phenothiazine. This increases the likelihood of drowsiness and anticholinergic effects, particularly when chlorpromazine (Largactil, Thorazine) is prescribed.

In advanced cancer, vomiting is frequently caused by several additive factors. When this is so, the above recommendations may prove inadequate.

Drowsiness
Most patients experience drowsiness initially. This is partly an effect of the drug itself and partly a result of being more comfortable, and able to relax and rest. Many patients have had poor nights for several weeks and are exhausted. They need to sleep more than normal to recuperate. Patients and their families should be warned that drowsiness may occur. However, provided it is not excessive and not associated with unsteadiness and confusional symptoms, the right thing to do is to press on knowing that it will clear after about 3 to 5 days on a steady dose. Possible reasons for persistent excessive drowsiness are shown in Table 9.5.

Table 9.5 Persistent excessive drowsiness

1 Is patient still recuperating from prolonged fatigue?
2 If the patient is completely comfortable, reduce the dose and review both drowsiness and pain control.
3 Is the patient on a psychotropic preparation, notably benzodiazepine (e.g. diazepam) or a phenothiazine (e.g. chlorpromazine)? Is it necessary? Can it be reduced or stopped?
4 If taking a phenothiazine as an antiemetic, can it be changed to haloperidol or metoclopramide?
5 Is the patient more ill than I thought?
6 If the patient is in hepatic or renal failure, try reducing the dose.
7 Is the patient cyanosed because of morphine exacerbated respiratory failure?
8 Could the patient have a cerebral secondary, unmasked by the intracranial pressure elevating effect of morphine?
9 If not agitated, or if cyanosed, consider using dexamphetamine 2.5 or 5 mg each morning (*see* Chapter 16).†

† This is only rarely necessary or appropriate

Confusional Symptoms

Those over 70 years of age should be warned that they may become muddled, dizzy and unsteady at times during the first few days of treatment but, unless very bad, they should persevere.

Dizziness and Unsteadiness

This may occur as a result of postural hypotension, particularly in the elderly. Patients over 70 years of age should be warned about the possibility. Sometimes because of this and for confusional symptoms, it is necessary to reduce the dose for 3 to 4 days before carefully increasing it again if the pain is still not fully controlled.

Constipation

Virtually all patients become constipated when taking morphine unless they:

1 have a colostomy,
2 have steatorrhoea,
3 take corrective dietary action.

Moreover, having a colostomy frequently is not sufficient to avoid what is the most serious unwanted effect of treatment with morphine or another strong narcotic. Patients may say that they have a laxative at home or that, if they get constipated, a dose of . . . 'soon puts me right.' It is necessary to explain that, in most people, the medicine they are about to start has a constipating effect and it is likely that the well-tried remedy will no longer work. A laxative should then be prescribed and the dose regulated carefully to achieve a satisfactory evacuation every one or two days.

When first seen, some patients have been on a narcotic analgesic for several weeks and may already be severely constipated or even impacted. Abdominal examination alone may demonstrate that the colon is full of faeces as far back as the caecum. If this is so, inpatient treatment is probably going to be necessary to sort it out.

In brief, unless the patient is over 80 years of age or gives a history of over-reaction to laxatives, treatment should be started immediately with both a softener and a colonic stimulant. A convenient preparation for most British patients is Dorbanex (Table 9.6). In America, a good choice is Peri-Colace (Table 9.7). Both contain a colonic stimulant and a faecal softener, and are available as a capsule or syrup.

Morphine slows peristalsis throughout the whole of the bowel (Table 9.8). Thus, if there is little or no response to Dorbanex *forte* 20 ml b.i.d. or Peri-Colace 8 capsules daily, it is necessary to add a 'small bowel flusher' in the form of a saline laxative (e.g. magnesium sulphate crystals 5 to 10 ml each morning with tea) or a non-absorbable sugar (e.g. lactulose 30 ml once or twice daily).

Review of laxative use at Sir Michael Sobell House shows that in the first week of treatment, half the patients who require a laxative also need rectal measures, that is, suppositories, enemas or manuals. This could be because the dose of Dorbanex is not yet optimal or it may be an indication of the size of the problem. The control of constipation is often more difficult than the control of pain.

The Urinary Tract

Morphine has an effect on the muscle of the urinary tract. The clinical significance of this is not clear. Experimentally, in animals urinary retention occurs with all species even with analgesic doses of morphine. In man, morphine contracts the vesical sphincter making it more difficult to pass urine. It also increases the tone of the detrusor muscle, which may give rise to urinary urgency. As the central depressant effect of morphine makes the patient less attentive to impulses from the bladder, the overall effect is a tendency to urinary retention [7].

Respiratory Depression

Respiratory depression is not generally of clinical importance; 10 mg of IM morphine sulphate raises the pCO_2 by about 5 mmHg [7]. This is the same as the usual nocturnal elevation of pCO_2 that occurs in the general population. In patients with *raised intracranial pressure*, however, elevation of the pCO_2 results in a reflex increase in pressure which may exacerbate or precipitate headache. Morphine should therefore be used with more care in patients with chronic obstructive airways disease,

179

Table 9.6 Guidelines for bowel management in patients on narcotics (Britain)†

1 Ask about patient's usual bowel habit and use of laxatives.
2 Do rectal examination if suspect faecal impaction or if diarrhoea/faecal incontinence (to exclude impaction with overflow).
3 Record bowel motions each day in 'bowel book'.
4 Encourage fluids generally, fruit juice, fruit and bran.
5 For patients on morphine, or alternative strong narcotic, prescribe:
    Dorbanex syrup 10 ml nocte
    (danthron 50 mg + softener).
6 If already on this and constipated, prescribe:
    Dorbanex *forte* syrup 10 ml nocte
    (danthron 150 mg + softener).
7 Adjust dose every 1 to 2 days, up to 20 ml of Dorbanex *forte* b.i.d., according to results.
8 If necessary, 'uncork' with the help of bisacodyl (Dulcolax) 10 mg suppository + glycerine suppository.
9 If suppositories are ineffective, administer a high phosphate enema, followed by a soap-sud enema (SSE) if no result.
10 Manually disimpact, if necessary.
11 If the maximum dose of Dorbanex *forte* is ineffective add:
    Epsom salts (magnesium sulphate crystals)
    $\frac{1}{2}$ to 2 teaspoons (2.5 to 10 ml) with early morning cup of tea.
12 If Dorbanex unpalatable/nauseating, consider use of:
    Dorbanex capsules (danthron 25 mg + softener)
    Normax capsules (danthron 50 mg + softener).
13 If Dorbanex/Normax cause recurrent abdominal cramps, change to a small bowel flusher:
    lactulose (Duphalac) syrup 30 to 40 ml b.i.d. to t.i.d.
    sodium picosulphate (Laxoberal) syrup 20 to 40 ml b.i.d. to t.i.d.
14 These should be used in preference to Dorbanex/Normax in patients with a history of irritable bowel syndrome (spastic colon) or of cramps with other colonic stimulants such as senna or in patients with ulcerative colitis.
15 Sometimes it is appropriate to optimize a patient's existing bowel regimen, rather than change automatically to Dorbanex.
16 Milpar (Milk of Magnesia + liquid paraffin) is a useful alternative for some patients.

† Based on experience at Sir Michael Sobell House, Oxford
Note: the dose of laxative should be decided by the physician. Close liaison with the nursing staff is imperative

Table 9.7 Guidelines for bowel management in patients on narcotics (USA)†

1 Ask about patient's usual bowel habit and use of laxatives.
2 Do rectal examination to check for faecal impaction.
3 Be aware that fluid stool, especially with incontinence, may mean faecal impaction.
4 Record bowel motions each day in the appropriate log.
5 Encourage fluids (i.e. water, prune juice) and foods that have a laxative effect if bowels do not move spontaneously.
6 For patients on morphine or alternative strong narcotic, prescribe: casanthranol 30 mg with docusate 100 mg (Peri-Colace) 1 capsule 1 to 4 times a day. Dose to be adjusted by nurse according to result.
7 If casanthranol with docusate causes abdominal cramps, change to docusate 100 mg alone 1 to 4 times daily.
8 If casanthranol with docusate 2 capsules q.i.d. is ineffective, give milk of magnesia and cascara suspension‡ 30 ml nocte *in addition*.
9 If no movement by next morning, manually assess location of stool in rectum. If good contact with rectal mucosa seems possible, use bisacodyl (Dulcolax) 10 mg suppository.
10 If suppository is not feasible or ineffective, administer oil retention enema and/or Fleets followed by soap-sud enema (SSE) if no result.
11 Manually disimpact if necessary.
12 If constipation persists, inform physician during daily rounds.
13 Wherever possible, strong patient preferences for bowel care should be honoured and requisite physician order sought.

† Based on those in use at The Connecticut Hospice
‡ Milk of magnesia and cascara suspension contains:
  25 ml milk of magnesia
  5 ml cascara aromatic fluid extract

Table 9.8 Morphine and the alimentary tract

Site	Delay (% of total)
Stomach Duodenum }	50
Small intestine	25
Large intestine	25

After Chapman et al, 1950 [6]

limited respiratory reserve and raised intracranial pressure. On the other hand, these conditions are *not* contraindications to the use of oral morphine sulphate in the terminally ill. In patients distressed by tachypnoea at rest, the prescription of morphine sulphate 5 to 10 mg every 4 hours may reduce the respiratory rate from 30 to 40/minute down to 20 to 25/minute. This makes the patient feel better and able to do more (*see* Chapter 13).

Interactions

Polypharmacy—the use of several drugs concurrently—is often necessary in patients with advanced cancer. Provided the physician is aware of the potential for interactions and the patient is reviewed after each drug innovation, it is unlikely that anything will go dangerously or irretrievably wrong. The sedative and respiratory depressant effects of morphine tend to be potentiated and prolonged by psychotropic drugs (e.g. phenothiazine, benzodiazepines, antidepressants) and alcohol. It is generally wise, therefore, to prescribe relatively small doses of psychotropic drugs initially (*see* Chapter 16). The effect of hypotensive drugs, phenothiazines and benzodiazepines on blood pressure is potentiated, and the cardiac effects of adrenergic β-blockers (e.g. propranolol, atenolol) may be enhanced.

Morphine Intolerance

Occasionally, a patient may experience one particular unwanted effect of morphine to such an extent that it is necessary to change to an alternative analgesic. The only relatively common form of intolerance is gastric (Table 9.9). In most patients, by temporarily reducing the dose of morphine (this may not be possible if the patient has very severe pain) and/or prescribing an appropriate 'antidote', it is possible to resolve the problem or reduce it to an acceptable level. In a few, it becomes clear that the situation is not improving and it is necessary to change to another strong narcotic. This should be as chemically distinct from morphine as possible in the hope that the alternative does not share the same disadvantage (*see* Chapter 14).

Instructions to Patients and Family

Advice about prescribing has also been given elsewhere (Chapter 17). Patients need to know they are receiving morphine. It should be presented as the next logical step within the framework of an explanation that there are only 2 basic analgesics, namely aspirin and morphine. Their previous medication can be explained in these terms, either as 'weak morphine' (if a weak narcotic agonist) or 'a synthetic or artificial morphine' (if an alternative strong narcotic). Morphine is, however, a negative emotive word. As with other such words (such as 'cancer' and 'dying') a qualifying

Table 9.9 Morphine intolerance

Type	Effects	Initial action	Comment
Gastric stasis	epigastric fullness, flatulence, anorexia, persistent nausea, intermittent vomiting	prescribe defoaming agent (e.g. Asilone 10 ml q.i.d.) + metoclopramide 10 mg 4-hourly	
Psychotomimetic	notably dysphoria and hallucinations	possibly prescribe haloperidol 3–5 mg nocte, chlorpromazine 10 mg t.i.d. or, if agitated, diazepam 5–10 mg nocte	If persists, change to chemically distinct narcotic†
Sedation	feels unacceptably 'drugged'	prescribe dexamphetamine 2.5–5 mg daily-b.i.d. in early part of day	
Vestibular stimulation	incapacitating movement-induced nausea and vomiting	prescribe cyclizine or dimenhydrinate 50–100 mg 4-hourly	Very rare. Try alternative narcotic† or methotrimeprazine§
Histamine release (a) Bronchial	bronchoconstriction → dyspnoea	administer antihistamine IV/IM (e.g. chlorpheniramine 5–10 mg) + bronchodilator	Very rare. Change to chemically distinct narcotic immediately†
(b) Cutaneous‡	pruritus	prescribe oral antihistamine (e.g. chlorpheniramine 4 mg b.i.d. and promethazine 25–50 mg nocte)	If does not settle after a few days or reappears when antihistamines stopped, prescribe an alternative narcotic†

† See Chapter 14
‡ A central neural component to narcotic-induced itching has been suggested (see page 217)
§ See Chapter 16

adjective or phrase does much to soften the initial negative impact: 'What we need to do is to get you sorted out with the help of *good old-fashioned morphine*.' Or: 'The best medicine for you is *liquid morphine*.' The patient will ask or wonder about addiction and tolerance and, at some stage, these concerns have to be faced and discussed (*see* Chapter 13). The use of a medication chart for the patient to work from is necessary (*see* Figure 17.4). Adequate follow-up for patients at home is essential (Table 9.10) (*see* Chapter 17).

Table 9.10 Physicians check list when prescribing morphine

---

1 Have I checked the Table of Analgesic Equivalents to determine the appropriate starting dose?
2 Do I need to prescribe a co-analgesic?
3 Have I prescribed an antiemetic?
4 Have I prescribed a laxative?
5 Have I written out the drug regimen in sufficient detail?
6 Have I warned about possible unwanted effects that might occur initially?
7 Have I explained what to do if the pain remains uncontrolled?
8 Have I made arrangements for follow-up after one, three and seven days – either by self or by trained community nurse?
9 Have I told the patient what to do if he needs help or advice before the next agreed follow-up?
10 Have I expressed confidence in my ability to improve the situation considerably, probably within a few days, certainly within one or two weeks?

Morphine on General Wards

In hospice units and in wards with 4-hourly medicine rounds, the administration of 4-hourly morphine should present few problems. Most wards, however, have only 4 drug rounds a day, at approximately 0700, 1300, 1700 and 2200 hours. These are commonly styled 0600, 1200/1400, 1800 and 2200. The standard British medicine chart/treatment sheet reflects this by having only 4 'boxes' per drug for the nurse to sign each day. In America, the usual hospital methods of charting drug administration do not clearly indicate at what time a regular drug was actually given. In addition somebody usually has to copy the physician's order from the order sheet to the cardex—another source of error. It is clear that, to a certain extent, special provision needs to be made to enable the patient to receive 4-hourly morphine.

A further difficulty is that the interval between the first drug round (0700) and the last (2200) is less than 16 hours. In practice, it is not uncommon to see a series of entries such as:

1   0725, 1125, 1550, 2130,
2   0725, 1125, 1525, 1925, 2350.

In the first, it proved impossible to give the third dose on time and the fourth has been delayed partly for convenience and partly to 'help the patient have a better night'. In the second example, the day staff have coped in an exemplary fashion with a highly individual drug regimen—until bedtime: 'Here is your night sedative Mr. Smith. You cannot have your morphine yet, you are not due. We'll bring that later . . .' The patient either fails to get to sleep because of unrelieved pain (or worry about the possibility) or complains bitterly when woken from a deep sleep by a nurse an hour or so later. In both instances, the comfort (and sleep) of the patient is put in jeopardy by a pharisaical attitude to the concept of 'every 4 hours'.

The following should be borne in mind:

1   It is important to make the 4-hourly regimen as easy to adhere to as possible.
2   As at home, so in hospital, the day is often less than 16 hours.
3   It is necessary, therefore, to catch up at some stages in the day. Generally, catching up is best done at 1000 hours. If 'time slippage' occurs by mistake or inevitably later in the day, catching up should be repeated at 2200 hours. This may mean that the interval between the 0600/on waking dose and the 1000 hour dose is less than 4 hours, sometimes less than 3, and similarly between the 1800 and bedtime doses. It is necessary, therefore, to advise nursing staff specifically on this point.
4   When catching up is practised, it is much easier for the nursing staff to administer 4-hourly medication. In fact, the only administration additional to the routine drug rounds is at 1000 hours. This is a time when the maximum number of nurses are available, and when the book keeping associated with the use of a Controlled Drug is most easy to complete.
5   Such a regimen, namely, on waking, 1000, 1400, 1800, bedtime (± middle of night), reflects outpatient recommendations. This makes the transition from hospital to home easier as the patient already knows the benefit of the regimen he is recommended to maintain.
6   It helps the nursing staff considerably if, on the medicine chart, the 'official' times of administration are included appropriately by the prescribing doctor (0200, 0600, 1000, 1400, 1800, 2200). This requires the use of 2 lines on charts which have only 4 boxes per drug for the nurse's signature (Figure 9.4).
7   It is necessary to check daily to ensure that doses have not been omitted through oversight or through the cumulative effect of time slippage. Both at Sir Michael Sobell House, Oxford and at The Connecticut Hospice a method of drug charting is used in which physician, nurse and pharmacist use the same sheet. In addition, the

MEDICINE SHEET

MONTH May 1982   DATE

DATE	DETAILS OF DRUG ADMINISTRATION	Time to be given	Signature of Prescribing Doctor	5 / 6	7 / 8			
5/5/82	MORPHINE (10 mg in 10 ml) P.O.	0200						
		0600						
	to take 10 ml 4 hourly	1000	*Morris*					
		1400						
		1800						
	* and 20 ml nocte	* 2200						
5/5/82	MORPHINE (10 mg in 10 ml) P.O.							
	to take 10 ml 2 hourly PRN		*Morris*					
5/5/82	HALOPERIDOL 1.5 mg tab. P.O.							
	nocte	2200	*Morris*					
5/5/82	DORBANEX SYRUP 10 ml P.O.							
	nocte	2200	*Morris*					

Figure 9.4 A suggested way of writing up a 4-hourly regimen on a medication chart that permits only 4 entries a day.

physician's order and the nurses' record of administration are in the same place. This system allows a rapid appraisal of the drugs the patient has actually received [8].

8   Most patients given a double dose at bedtime will sleep pain-free beyond 0200. The nursing staff should be advised to delay the middle of the night dose until about 0300 if the patient is sleeping soundly. On the other hand, if the patient wakes regularly at 0100 to micturate or because of pain, the 0200 dose should be given earlier.

9   Provision should be made for additional 'as required' morphine, in the event of breakthrough pain. Instructions must be clear: the use of 'as required' morphine does not mean that the next dose of regular morphine is omitted or delayed. If 'as required' morphine is needed several times a day, it is probably an indication that the regular dose needs to be adjusted upwards.

Postscript

And What About Driving?
Most patients requiring treatment with morphine are not fit to drive on account of their general poor state of health. From time to time, though, a patient asks, 'And can I drive, doctor?' This may be at the time morphine therapy is started. Alternatively, the patient may have improved since commencing morphine so that he begins to think about taking up some of

his former activities, including driving. In our opinion, the answer need not invariably be 'No!'

The following points must be borne in mind. Driving or being in charge of a vehicle when under the influence of a drug is an offence under the United Kingdom Road Traffic Act 1972. (Similar laws are in force in all countries and states.) Conviction carries an automatic penalty of disqualification from driving for 6 months. It is the driver's responsibility to know when he is unable to drive safely, but without guidance from his doctor he may not realize the danger until too late.

Drivers can be divided into three classes [9]:

1   vocational,
2   professional,
3   occasional.

Vocational drivers are those who drive all or most of their working day in heavy vehicles (HGV). Professional drivers include taxi drivers and commercial travellers. In the absence of formal testing to show that attention and reaction time are unimpaired, vocational drivers *must* be advised not to drive HGV. We would also include taxi drivers in this prohibition. But what of the patient who drives 20 to 30 miles to work each day? Or of the retired person who just wants to go 1 or 2 miles to the shops? The doctor must be aware that patients *will* drive if they want to unless specifically told not to.

Over the past 12 years, a significant number of our patients have driven. To date there have been no accidents. The following summarizes the advice given:

1   The medicines you are taking do *not* necessarily disqualify you from driving.
2   Some people's reaction time and general alertness are, however, affected when taking such medicines.
3   It is important, therefore, that you take the following precautions, particularly if you have not driven for some weeks because of ill health.

   (a)   Do not drive in the dark or when conditions are bad.
   (b)   Do not drink alcohol, however little, during the day.
   (c)   Choose a quiet time of the day, when the light is good.
   (d)   Chose an area where there are a number of quiet roads.
   (e)   Take a companion (husband, wife, friend).
   (f)   Drive for 10 to 15 minutes on quiet roads.
   (g)   If both you and your companion are happy with your attentiveness, reactions and general ability, then it is all right to drive for short distances.
   (h)   Do not exhaust yourself by long journeys.

As doctors, we must be aware that there is a legal requirement on every driver, as soon as he becomes aware of it, to report to the Licensing Centre any disability likely to make him now or in the future a danger when driving. Applicants for driving licences are also required to report such disabilities. Temporary disabilities unlikely to exceed 3 months are excluded. The obligation to notify the Licensing Authority falls on the patient, but he can only do this if his doctor advises him that he has a disability that is likely to affect his driving.

If the Licensing Centre becomes aware that a person holding a licence or applying for a licence has a disability it may require him to authorize his doctor to supply information about his disability to the Medical Adviser at the Centre. If he refuses he may be required to undergo medical examination by a nominated doctor or doctors.

In Britain, any doctor in doubt about the advice he should give his patient is invited to discuss the matter with the Medical Advisory Branch at the Driver and Vehicle Licensing Centre at Swansea (0792 42731). This is an answering service and the doctor leaves his name and telephone number. After these details have been checked, the doctor is telephoned back. There may be occasions when the doctor considers it necessary to take the initiative and notify the Licensing Centre of a patient's disability and its effect on his driving. Each case is a matter for the individual doctor's discretion.

Final Comment

Morphine sulphate by mouth is the best and the most versatile of the strong narcotic analgesics. It is still the strong analgesic of choice for cancer patients with severe pain. It is *not*, however, the panacea. Many factors will influence morphine requirements (Figure 9.5). It will often be used in conjunction with non-drug measures (*see* Chapters 4 and 5). In many patients, it is also necessary to prescribe a co-analgesic and other forms of adjuvant medication (*see* Chapter 16).

References

1 Twycross RG, Fry DE and Wills PD. The alimentary absorption of diamorphine and morphine in man as indicated by urinary excretion studies. *British Journal of Clinical Pharmacology* 1974; **1**: 491–494.

2 Houde RW, Wallenstein SL and Beaver WT. Clinical measurement of pain in *Analgetics* edited by de Stevens G. Academic Press, New York and London 1965, pp 75–122.

3 Lack SA. Pain control in terminal illness in *A Hospice Handbook*, edited by Hamilton MP and Reid HF, Eerdmanns, Grand Rapids 1980, pp 73–89.

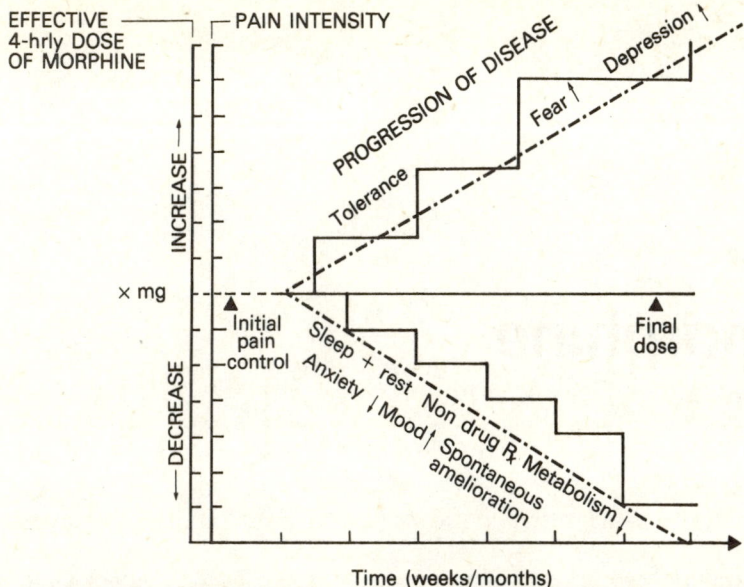

Figure 9.5 Factors influencing morphine requirements in cancer pain patients, assuming high standard of general care. ·—·—·— = intensity of pain. ———— = dose of morphine.

4 Scott JF. Personal communication.

5 Nimmo WS, Wilson J and Prescott LF. Narcotic analgesics and delayed gastric emptying during labour. *Lancet* 1975; **i**: 890–893

6 Chapman WP, Rowlands EW and Jones CM. Multiple-balloon kymographic recording of the comparative action of Demerol, morphine and placebos on the motility of the upper small intestine in man. *New England Journal of Medicine* 1950; **243**: 171–177.

7 Weinstock M. Site of action of narcotic analgesic drugs in peripheral tissues in *Narcotic Drugs. Biochemical Pharmacology* edited by Clouet D. Plenum Press, New York and London 1971, pp 394–407.

8 Cote L and Lack SA. *One Medication Record Shared by Physician, Nurse and Pharmacist.* Unpublished paper presented, American Society of Hospital Pharmacists Mid Year Clinical Meeting, New Orleans, Louisiana, 1981.

9 *Medical Aspects of Fitness to Drive* edited by Raffee A. Medical Commission on Accident Prevention, London 1978.

Chapter Ten

Diamorphine

Drug portrait
Diamorphine (diacetylmorphine, heroin) is a semisynthetic derivative of morphine (Figure 10.1) used primarily as a strong analgesic. Its effects are mediated by specific opiate receptors mainly within the CNS. Clinically its pharmacological profile is almost identical to that of morphine. Diamorphine is readily absorbed by all routes of administration. The oral to IM potency ratio is approximately 1:2.5. Given IV, it acts faster than morphine and causes less vomiting but more sedation. By mouth, because of relatively rapid *in vivo* deacetylation, diamorphine is essentially a pro-drug for morphine. The plasma half-life of diamorphine, and its pharmacologically active metabolites monoacetylmorphine and morphine, is comparable to that of morphine, that is, about 2 to 2.5 hours after oral administration and about 1.5 hours when given parenterally. After deacetylation to morphine, diamorphine is conjugated in the liver to form a glucuronide which is excreted by the kidneys (Figure 10.2). The duration of useful analgesia is 3 to 5 hours.

Diacetylmorphine was first prepared in 1874 by Wright at St. Mary's Hospital, London [1]. Initially it was largely ignored by the medical profession, but some 20 years later interest rapidly developed as a result of animal experiments conducted in Germany. Commercial production was started in 1898 by the Bayer Company who marketed the drug under the trade name of Heroin. It was used initially in a variety of respiratory

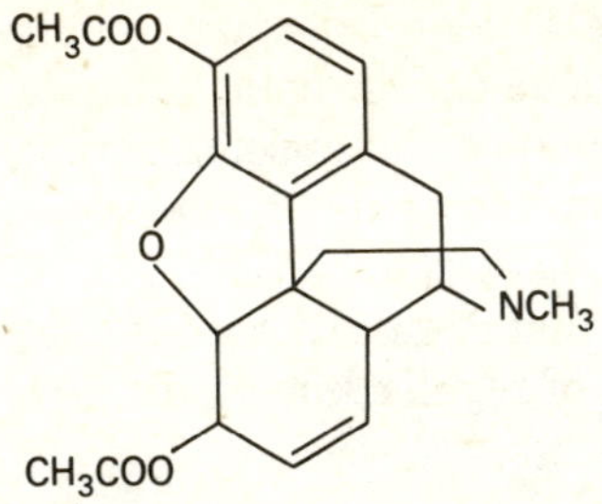

Figure 10.1 Molecular formula of diamorphine (diacetylmorphine).

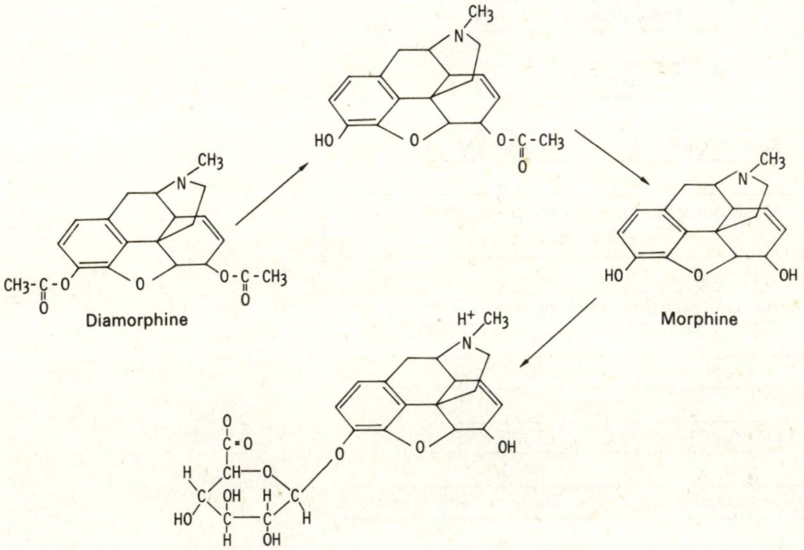

Figure 10.2 Metabolic pathway of diamorphine.

conditions, such as 'dyspnoea', pharyngitis, laryngitis, bronchitis, asthma and pulmonary tuberculosis. Later, hay fever, colds, coughs, pertussis and pneumonia were added to the advertisers' list of indications for its use. It was also recommended, in the USA, as a remedy for morphine dependence. Unfortunately, this only served to introduce diamorphine to the addict population of that country and resulted in increasing abuse.

Its reputation as a potent analgesic developed later. By then, its use in so wide a variety of respiratory conditions was falling into disfavour. Eventually, because of the increasing number of addicts, its medicinal use was banned in the USA in 1924. Since then all but a few countries have fallen into line with what subsequently became the policy of the League of Nations and, later, the World Health Organization. Diamorphine is still used in Britain as a strong analgesic to relieve severe acute pain. It is also used at a number of hospices and hospitals, and by some family practitioners, in preference to morphine to relieve cancer pain.

When given *intravenously*, diamorphine has an earlier onset of action, is more sedating, and causes less vomiting than morphine [2]. These are all properties which are desirable when seeking to relieve severe acute pain. On the other hand, there is no evidence that such differences exist after *oral* administration, or after several days of regular injections.

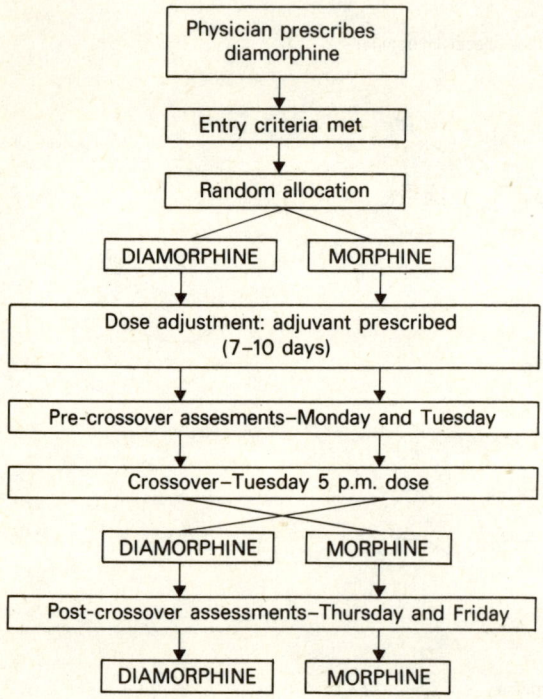

Figure 10.3 Flow diagram describing diamorphine–morphine trial.

A randomized controlled trial of oral diamorphine hydrochloride and morphine sulphate was undertaken in patients with far advanced cancer at St. Christopher's Hospice, London during the early 1970s [3]. The primary aim was to compare the incidence and severity of the side effects of the two preparations when prescribed regularly every 4 hours at the effective analgesic dose for each patient (Figure 10.3). Patients, stratified for sex, were randomly allocated to receive either diamorphine or morphine by mouth as first treatment. All the patients received a phenothiazine; other medication was prescribed when indicated clinically. A total of 699 patients of median age 67 years participated in the trial. Of these, 146 were well enough to crossover, but only 89 remained on an unchanged dose of 'diamorphine equivalent' and did not have their adjuvant medication modified during the 5-day period of observation. A potency ratio for orally administered diamorphine and morphine of 1.5:1 was assumed on the basis of a pilot trial.

In the 51 satisfactory female crossover patients, no statistically significant difference was noted in relation either to pain or the other symptoms evaluated. On the other hand, 38 satisfactory male crossover patients experienced significantly more pain ($p < 0.01$) and were significantly

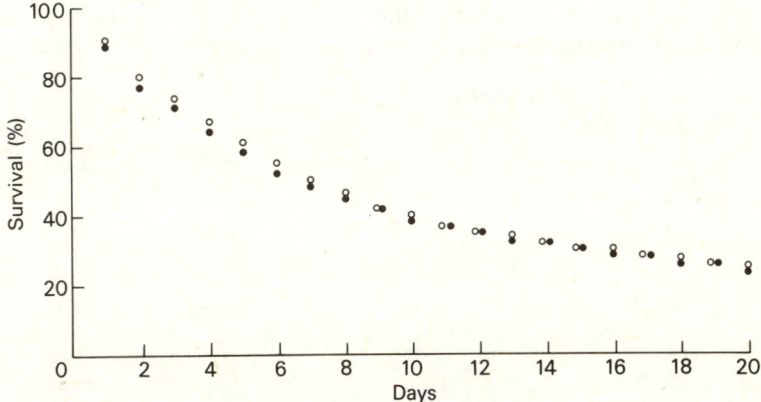

Figure 10.4 Graph plotting per cent survival for 350 diamorphine-receiving patients (open circles) and 349 morphine-receiving patients (filled circles). There is no difference between the two groups.

more depressed ($p < 0.02$) while receiving diamorphine. In these, the potency ratio of diamorphine to morphine was obviously less than 1.5:1. If this is allowed for, then the difference in mood is probably not significant. The patients who did not crossover appeared to do equally well on either drug (Figure 10.4).

It was concluded that, provided allowance is made for the difference in potency, diamorphine and morphine are equally efficacious when given in solution by mouth every 4 hours in individually optimized doses in association with a phenothiazine such as prochlorperazine or chlorpromazine.

In a parallel study of urinary excretion of morphine in patients receiving diamorphine or morphine regularly, the results indicated that while diamorphine is completely absorbed from the gastrointestinal tract, morphine is only some two-thirds absorbed [4]. This suggests that the potency ratio of orally administered diamorphine and morphine merely reflects the alimentary absorption ratio of the two preparations. This accords with the view of Way and his associates [5, 6], based largely on studies using organ homogenates from both animals and man, that diamorphine is deacetylated *in vivo* to 6-o-monoacetylmorphine and morphine so rapidly that it has only a transient pharmacological action of its own even after intravenous injection. In other words, by mouth, diamorphine is a pro-drug of morphine. It is better absorbed and therefore more potent. It is not, however, more efficacious.

Potency
Because diamorphine is deacetylated in solution, in the gastrointestinal tract, liver, plasma, and body tissues generally, its potency ratio with morphine will vary depending on the route of administration. Potency ratios have been determined for IM and PO routes. It is reasonable to suggest that IV, diamorphine may be even more potent (Figure 10.5). In

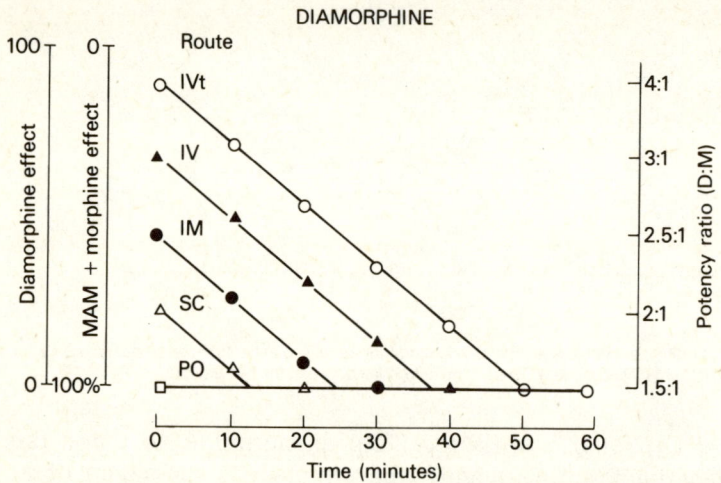

Figure 10.5 Diagram linking potency ratio of diamorphine: morphine to the route of administration of diamorphine, and showing the progressively shorter contribution made by diamorphine *per se* to its pharmacological effect as one moves from intraventricular (IVt) to the oral (PO) route.
Note: apart from the IM and PO potency ratios, the data in the figure are presumptive.
MAM = monoacetylmorphine.

this diagram, we have attempted to show not only the different potency ratios—actual or presumptive—but also the possible duration of an actual diamorphine effect, if any, when given by a particular route. In other words, the effect of diamorphine *per se* is much shorter than the total pharmacological effect of diamorphine. By whatever route, this includes contributions by the two active biotransformation products, monoacetylmorphine and morphine. The two definitely known potency ratios for diamorphine and morphine are [3, 7, 8]:

PO 1.5:1; IM 2–2.5:1.

Injections
It had been intended to do a similar trial of SC/IM morphine and diamorphine. Because diamorphine hydrochloride is far more soluble

194

than morphine sulphate, it proved very difficult to prepare indistinguish-able ampoules of morphine sulphate and diamorphine hydrochloride (Table 10.1). Further, as it has never been suggested that morphine is

Table 10.1 Solubility of morphine and diamorphine salts

Preparation	No. of ml water to dissolve 1 g at 25°C
Morphine	5000
Morphine hydrochloride	24
Morphine sulphate	21
Morphine tartrate	10
Morphine acetate	2.5
Diamorphine hydrochloride	1.6

Table 10.2 Volume of injection of equi-analgesic doses of diamorphine hydrochloride and morphine sulphate†

| Dose of drug (mg) | | Volume of injection (ml) | | |
diamorphine	morphine	diamorphine freeze-dried	morphine 15 mg/ml‡	30 mg/ml§
5	12.5	0.1	1	0.5
10	25	0.1	2	1
20	50	0.1	4	2
30	75	0.1	5	2.5
60	150	0.1	10	5
90	225	0.15	15	7.5
120	300	0.2	20	10

† Using a potency ratio of 2.5:1 [8]. If the potency ratio is taken to be 2:1 [7], the volumes given should be reduced by 1/5
‡ Maximum strength available in the USA
§ Maximum strength available in Britain

better than diamorphine, it was most unlikely that the trial would show anything except:

1 morphine and diamorphine are indistinguishable, or
2 diamorphine is better than morphine.

Both results would still leave diamorphine with the practical advantage of being much more soluble. An injection of diamorphine hydrochloride, available as a freeze-dried (lyophilized) pellet, need never exceed 0.2 ml (Table 10.2). In view of this, it was decided to abandon the trial and to recommend the continued use of diamorphine when injections were necessary [3].

Since then there has been considerable debate, particularly in the USA and Australia [9, 10] as to whether diamorphine is necessary for the management of pain in a proportion of patients with cancer. Data from Sir Michael Sobell House, Oxford, about injections of diamorphine hydrochloride are shown in Figure 10.6. If a 2 ml injection of morphine

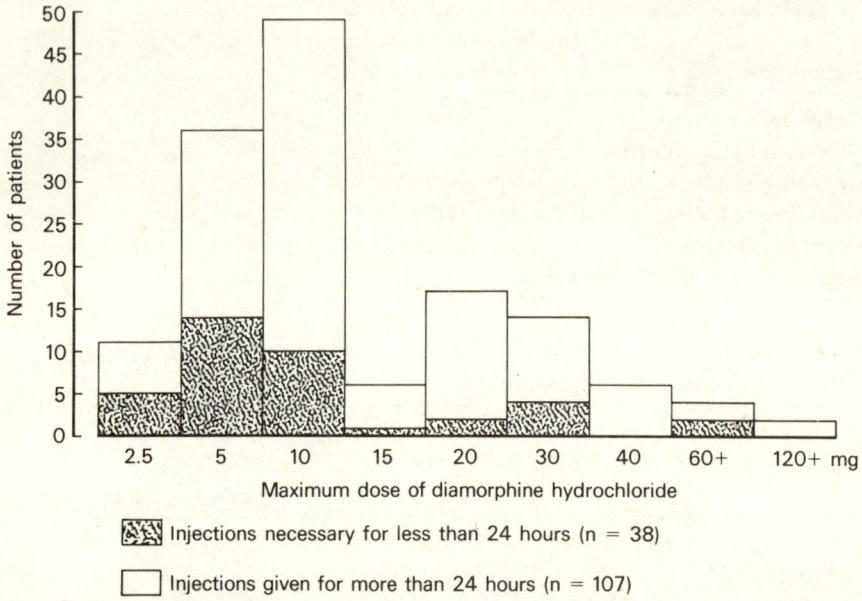

Injections necessary for less than 24 hours (n = 38)

Injections given for more than 24 hours (n = 107)

Figure 10.6 Histogram of maximum 4-hourly doses of IM or SC diamorphine hydrochloride in 145 patients at Sir Michael Sobell House (1978). Total number of patients admitted = 210; median dose = 10 mg.
Note: '60+' includes a patient who received 80 mg; '120+' includes one who received 140 mg.

sulphate is considered acceptable (3 ml with an antiemetic), then only those patients who received 30 mg of diamorphine or more 'needed' it; the rest could readily have received morphine instead. If a 1 ml (2 ml with an antiemetic) is considered the upper acceptable volume limit, all patients needing more than 10 mg would remain in the 'diamorphine necessary' group. Excluding patients who received diamorphine for less than 24 hours, this gives the percentage of patients at Sir Michael Sobell House 'needing' diamorphine as 9.5 using the 2 + 1 ml formula and 19 using the 1 + 1 ml formula.

Is 9.5 per cent sufficient to warrant the medical profession in countries without diamorphine to campaign for its reintroduction? Some feel the answer is 'yes' while others continue to say 'no'. For those who say 'yes', the following should be noted:

1   Hospices in North America are not campaigning for medicinal diamorphine; they are content to use morphine [11].

2 Syringe drivers for continuous SC infusion are now available (*See* Chapter 12).
3 Morphine acetate is almost as soluble as diamorphine and, if freeze-dried, could substitute readily for patients who 'need' diamorphine (*see* Chapter 12).
4 Hydromorphone hydrochloride (Dilaudid),** although half as soluble, is some 2 to 3 times more potent than diamorphine. The time-action characteristics of IM hydromorphone are comparable to those of diamorphine. This makes it an even more appropriate choice according to some [7]. As with morphine acetate, a freeze-dried preparation would be needed to maximize its benefits.

A first step in the right direction would, however, be the immediate introduction of an ampoule in the USA containing 30 mg of morphine sulphate in 1 ml (Table 10.2).

Stability of Diamorphine
Diamorphine in solution undergoes progressive hydrolysis first to 6-o-monoacetylmorphine and then to morphine itself. It is often stated that solutions of diamorphine hydrochloride should be freshly prepared, inferring that hydrolysis occurs rapidly. Using a similar mixture to the Diamorphine and Cocaine Elixir BPC, it has been demonstrated by thin layer chromatography that, at room temperature, it takes 8 weeks for a 10 per cent loss of diamorphine to occur ($t_{10\%}$ = 8 weeks) [12]. A number of factors were found to affect the $t_{10\%}$, namely ambient temperature, the content of alcohol and syrup, and also the presence or absence of a proprietary phenothiazine-containing syrup (Table 10.3). By contrast, freeze-dried diamorphine hydrochloride is, to all intents and purposes, completely stable [13].

A 10 per cent loss of diamorphine *per se* does not, however, mean a 10 per cent loss of analgesic effect. Monoacetylmorphine is equipotent with diamorphine [14]. There is, therefore, no loss of effect until monoacetyl-morphine is hydrolyzed to morphine. With added chlorpromazine or honey, morphine was first detected after about 7 weeks; in other mixtures, it was not detected in significant amounts for up to a year [12].

It would be of interest to assess the effect of alkalinity and heat on the mixture, both with and without previous exposure to simulated gastric fluid, for several hours in order to estimate the total effect of passage from the mouth through the upper intestinal tract and into the bloodstream. However, such an experiment would be of limited value. It is not known, for example, how much diamorphine is absorbed by the stomach, thus by-passing the alkaline medium of the small intestine, nor whether the alkaline medium of the latter so hastens absorption that further hydrolysis

** not available in Britain

Table 10.3   Approximate t_{10}% of various diamorphine and cocaine elixirs

Elixir	Temperature (°C)	$t_{10\%}$ (weeks)
Standard	22	8
Standard	4	>24
Standard	30	4
Standard	37	2
Double-strength alcohol (24%)	22	10
Half-strength alcohol (6%)	22	6
No syrup	22	10
Honey	22	6
Glucose	22	6
Prochlorperazine (1.25 mg/10 ml)	22	2
Chlorpromazine (6.25 mg/10 ml)†	22	2

† Half the recommended strength

is minimal. The fact that diamorphine by mouth begins to give relief after some 15 to 20 minutes suggests that some gastric absorption takes place.

References

1 Wright CRA. On the action of organic acids and their anhydrides on the natural alkaloids. *Journal of the Chemical Society* 1874; **12** (NS): 1031–1042.

2 Loan WB, Morrison JD, Dundee JW, Clarke RSJ. Hamilton RC and Brown SS. Studies of drugs given before anaesthesia. XVII: the natural and semi-synthetic opiates. *British Journal of Anaesthesia* 1969; **41:** 57–63.

3 Twycross RG. Choice of strong analgesic in terminal cancer: diamorphine or morphine? *Pain* 1977; **3:** 93–104.

4 Aherne GW, Piall EM and Twycross RG. Serum morphine concentration after oral administration of diamorphine hydrochloride and morphine sulphate. *British Journal of Clinical Pharmacology* 1979; **8:** 577–580.

5 Way EL, Kemp JW, Young JM and Grassetti DR. The pharmacologic effects of heroin in relationship to its rate of biotransformation. *Journal of Pharmacology and Experimental Therapeutics* 1960; **129:** 144–154.

6 Way EL, Young JM and Kemp JW. Metabolism of heroin and its pharmacologic implications. *Bulletin on Narcotics* 1965; **17**(1): 25–33.

7 Kaiko RF, Wallenstein SI, Rogers AG, Grabinski PY and Houde RW. Analgesic and mood effects of heroin and morphine in cancer patients with postoperative pain. *New England Journal of Medicine* 1981; **304:** 1501–1505.

8 Beaver WT, Schein PS and Hext M. Comparison of the analgesic effect of intramuscular heroin and morphine in patients with cancer pain. *Clinical Pharmacology and Therapeutics* 1981; **29:** 232.

9 Tattersall MHN. Pain: heroin versus morphine. *Medical Journal of Australia* 1981; **1:** 492.

10 Lasagna L. (Editorial) Heroin: a medical 'me-too'. *New England Journal of Medicine* 1981; **304:** 1539–1540.

11 Lack SA. Pain control in advanced cancer. The hospice approach. *American Urological Association Monograph Vol 1, Bladder Cancer*, edited by Benny WW and Prout GR. Williams and Wilkins, Baltimore and London 1982, *pp* 335–344.

12 Twycross RG. Diamorphine and Cocaine Elixir BPC 1973. *Pharmaceutical Journal* 1974; **212:** 153 and 159.

13 Lerner M and Mills A. Some modern aspects of heroin analysis. *Bulletin on Narcotics* 1963; **15**(1): 37–42.

14 Wright CI and Barbour FA. The respiratory effects of morphine, codeine and related substances. *Journal of Pharmacology and Experimental Therapeutics* 1935; **54:** 25–33.

Chapter Eleven

Brompton Cocktail

The Brompton Cocktail is a mixture containing morphine and cocaine in a vehicle of alcohol, syrup and chloroform water. It is a traditional British way of administering morphine by mouth to relieve pain or respiratory distress in patients with terminal disease. The first record of the combined use of morphine and cocaine appeared in the *British Medical Journal* in 1896 [1]. Because of the cost, the use of cocaine was discontinued the following year [2]. Some 30 years later, it was reintroduced by Roberts at the Brompton Hospital, who used a morphine-cocaine elixir as a post thoracotomy analgesic [3]. At other hospitals, similar elixirs were used in advanced malignant or terminal respiratory disease. These were known by a variety of names, such as *Mistura pro moribundo*, *Mistura pro euthanasia*, and *Mistura euphoriens*. It was not until 1952, when the Brompton Hospital produced its own supplement to the National Formulary, that the composition of a morphine-cocaine elixir appeared in print. In this it was called *Haustus E* and contained:

morphine hydrochloride	1/4 grain	(15 mg)
cocaine hydrochloride	1/6 grain	(10 mg)
alcohol 90%	30 minims	(2 ml)
syrup	60 minims	(4 ml)
chloroform water to	1/2 fl. oz.	(15 ml)

This was modification of the earlier formulation which contained gin and honey instead of alcohol and syrup. It appeared subsequently in Martindale [4] together with 3 variant formulations. In more recent years, diamorphine has commonly been used in Britain instead of morphine as the analgesic component in such elixirs, now generally known as the Brompton Cocktail.

There is a tendency to endow the Brompton Cocktail with mystical properties and to regard it as the panacea for terminal cancer pain. It does, however, contain 4 substances all of which may cause side effects. Not infrequently these have resulted in non-compliance by the patient. It is necessary to consider, therefore, whether such a mixture is a prerequisite of success or whether a simple solution of morphine (or diamorphine) is equally effective.

Cocaine

It is frequently stated that the addition of cocaine enhances the mood of the patient. On the other hand, the longer an opiate-cocaine elixir is administered, the greater is the likelihood of depression [5]. In a controlled trial at St. Christopher's Hospice, patients were treated with either morphine-cocaine (MC), diamorphine-cocaine (DC), morphine alone (MO) or diamorphine alone (DO) [6]. The dose of the opiate was adjusted as necessary to control pain; the dose of cocaine remained unaltered at 10 mg. After 2 weeks, patients receiving cocaine stopped taking it, and vice versa.

A total of 382 patients entered the trial, 144 males and 238 females, during the 13 months beginning September 1974. Patients in the 4 treatment groups were similar in terms of age (median = 67 years), sex primary cancer sites, and initial severity of pain. All the patients were prescribed other drugs concurrently. About two-thirds received chlorpromazine, usually 25 mg PO every 4 hours; compared with the DC group (67/95), significantly more of the DO group (85/97) were prescribed chlorpromazine ($p < 0.01$). There was no difference between the morphine groups (MC = 61/95; MO = 58/95). Compared with the DC and MC groups (57/190), significantly more of the DO and MO groups (80/192) received a glucocorticosteroid ($p < 0.02$). If those patients who began to receive corticosteroids before entering the trial are excluded, the difference is no longer significant; 15 patients were prescribed a corticosteroid de novo in the DC and MC groups compared with 20 in the DO and MO groups. Significantly more (42 per cent) of the non-cocaine-receiving patients survived for 2 weeks compared with those who received cocaine (32 per cent, $p < 0.05$; Figure 11.1).

A total of 61 patients crossed over, 17 males and 44 females; 29 from cocaine to no-cocaine and 32 in the reverse direction. Of these, 40 received diamorphine and 21 morphine ($p < 0.01$). During the period of observation 45 remained on a steady dose of diamorphine or morphine and no changes were made in adjuvant medication. Because of the small numbers, it was not possible to make a separate meaningful analysis of the

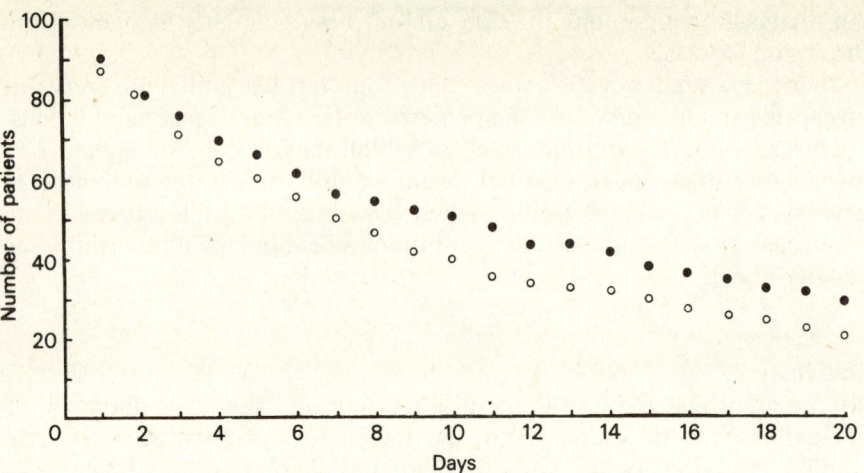

Figure 11.1 Survival chart for 192 patients not receiving cocaine (●) and 190 patients receiving cocaine (○). After 2 weeks, percentage surviving ● = 42, ○ = 32; $p < 0.05$.
From Twycross, 1979 [6]

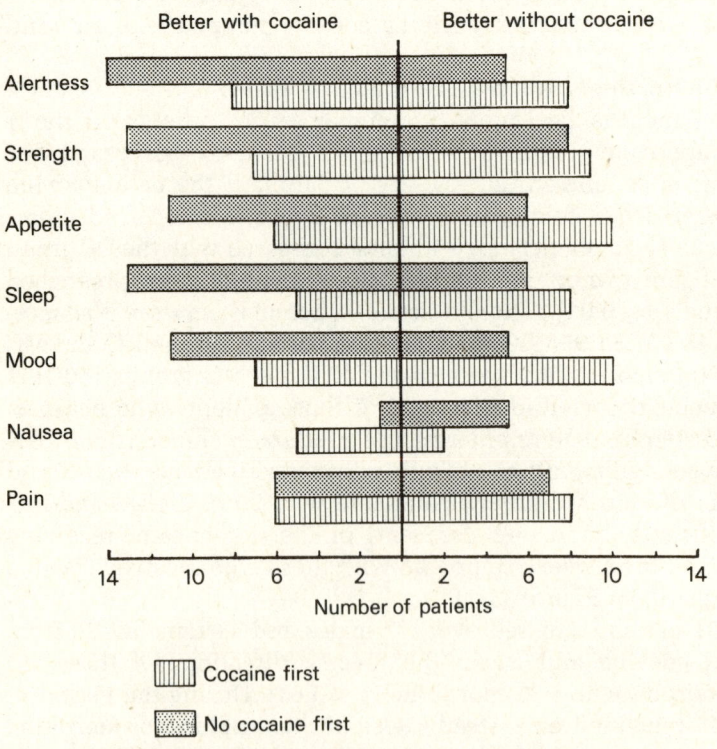

Figure 11.2 Non-parametric comparison of crossover effects. Ties excluded.
From Twycross, 1979 [6]

results from males or from morphine-receiving patients. The main analysis was, therefore, of all patients regardless of sex or opiate received. Separate analyses were made in relation to females and diamorphine-receiving crossover patients.

Non-parametric analysis suggested that patients who crossed from no-cocaine to with-cocaine benefited by the introduction of cocaine, whereas those crossing in the reverse direction fared equally well before and after crossover (Figure 11.2). Parametric analysis confirmed there was a difference in relation to alertness significant at the 0.05 probability level. An additional significant result was obtained when female patients were analyzed in relation to strength ($t = 2.45$, d.f. 33. $p < 0.05$). The trends in the male and in the morphine subgroups were in the same direction as those in the female and diamorphine-receiving patients, respectively.

The order of treatment effect suggests that, when cocaine is given in a small fixed dose, tolerance develops after a few days. Cocaine would thus be of benefit during the initial period of treatment with morphine or diamorphine, but thereafter would be relatively ineffective.

The survival data (Figure 11.1) suggest that non-prescription of cocaine does not shorten life. The difference seen between groups probably relates to the use or non-use of corticosteroids. Moreover, the proportions of non-cocaine patients and of with-cocaine patients well enough to crossover after 2 weeks were similar. This suggests that the absence of cocaine, at this stage, did not impair significantly the patients' mental and physical abilities.

The results of a second trial comparing the traditional Brompton Cocktail with morphine hydrochloride alone (i.e. no cocaine and alcohol) also failed to demonstrate measurable differences in relation to pain, nausea, drowsiness, and confusion [7]. On the other hand, many physicians have had experience of patients, usually elderly, who have become restless, agitated, confused or hallucinated when prescribed a morphine-cocaine mixture and whose symptoms have abated when the cocaine was withdrawn. In view of this, and the equivocal nature of the trial results, there is no longer justification for the routine concomitant prescription of cocaine. Our practice is to tell the patient that he may feel drowsy for 2 or 3 days when starting treatment but that, subsequently, the drowsiness will lessen. If the drowsiness persists, dexamphetamine 2.5 to 5 mg may be prescribed once or twice daily to determine whether a cerebral stimulant is of benefit. This is in fact only rarely necessary (see Chapter 16).

It is a matter of regret that since 1974 the British National Formulary (BNF) has included both morphine-cocaine and diamorphine-cocaine elixirs, as inclusion lends official blessing to the efficacy of such combinations. More regrettable is the inclusion of variant mixtures containing chlorpromazine. Given their respective doses, any stimulant action of cocaine will be antagonized by chlorpromazine.

In those hospices where cocaine is still administered with morphine (or diamorphine), most use 10 mg of cocaine hydrochloride as their standard dose. Occasional prescribers of the Brompton Cocktail sometimes use a higher dose of cocaine and, moreover, vary the dose of the opiate by varying the volume rather than the strength of the mixture. This means the dose of cocaine is increased in parallel with that of the opiate. It is perhaps not surprising that, at one centre known to us, hallucinations occur with the Brompton Cocktail. They occur to such an extent that patients are warned to expect them and are taught to accept them as the necessary price for pain relief.

Formulation

In 1972, a survey of more than 90 teaching and district general hospitals throughout the United Kingdom confirmed that opiate-cocaine elixirs were still in widespread use and demonstrated considerable variation in composition [8]. Differences existed both in the active constituents and in the vehicle in which they were dissolved. In addition to morphine or diamorphine, the majority include cocaine. A number also contained a phenothiazine (chlorpromazine or prochlorperazine) and, in some, morphine and diamorphine were both included. The variation in the vehicle was even greater; for example, the alcohol content ranged from 0 to 40 per cent and was frequently replaced by gin, whisky, or brandy. The syrup content varied from 0 to 50 per cent and honey was often substituted for sucrose. In the light of this, the introduction of standard diamorphine-cocaine and morphine-cocaine elixirs in the BNF is, in one sense, welcome.

Some patients, however, find the alcoholic 'bite' of the standard elixirs unpleasant. A few, usually with oral, pharyngeal or oesophageal carcinoma, may experience a marked *increase in pain* after taking the elixir due to the direct effect of alcohol on an *ulcerated area*. Patients with non-insulin-dependent diabetes treated with chlorpropamide may experience facial flushing (chlorpropamide-alcohol flushing) when prescribed a standard elixir. Many patients dislike the 'sickly' taste of the standard elixirs. There is much to be said for prescribing morphine sulphate or hydrochloride alone in water. If a patient dislikes the bitter taste of the morphine, orange or blackcurrant juice, or milk can be added at the time of administration. This is now current practice at an increasing number of hospices.

In the Canadian study [7], it was noticed that mixtures without alcohol tended to become cloudy after about a week because of the growth of yeast, fungi and bacteria. 0.75 ml of 98 per cent alcohol/10 ml of solution prevented this. It is possible that the removal of syrup would also have prevented this. In Britain, most pharmacists in fact use chloroform water as the vehicle for the morphine sulphate. This is antimicrobial. It is no longer available in the USA.

Conclusion

The Brompton Cocktail is, therefore, merely one way of prescribing oral morphine (or diamorphine). It is not the panacea nor does it possess mystical properties. To obtain maximum benefit, it must be used within the context of whole-person care. It is probably for this reason that the relief it gives is maximal in a hospice setting [9]. Whether a doctor prescribes the Brompton Cocktail or simply morphine sulphate in water will depend on personal inclination. It must be appreciated that each of the constituents may cause side effects, and enquiry must be made. These include an unpleasant taste in the mouth and a burning sensation in the throat. On the other hand, it is simpler for the pharmacist, cheaper for the patient, and easier for the doctor to adjust the dose of the opiate if a simple solution of morphine sulphate (or hydrochloride) is ordered.

Schlessinger's Solution

Schlessinger's Solution is a mixture of:

morphine sulphate	1 g
ethylmorphine	2 g
scopolamine hydrobromide	12 mg
distilled water to	50 ml

and is used in some parts of the USA. One millilitre contains 20 mg of morphine sulphate. Ethylmorphine is a weak narcotic like codeine (methylmorphine). Sometimes morphine sulphate is substituted for ethylmorphine making the solution considerably more potent.

The solution is very bitter and each dose (1, 2, 3 ml, etc.) is diluted with juice or water before administration. With a 1 ml dose, the amount of scopolamine (hyoscine) is relatively small ($240\,\mu g$) though will cause some anticholinergic effects in some patients. With a 3 ml or larger dose, there will be an increasing likelihood of unwanted effects such as dry mouth, urinary retention, disorientation and delirium. Although of interest historically, Schlessinger's Solution offers no advantage over a simple solution of morphine sulphate. By virtue of its concentration and the inclusion of scopolamine, it has a number of disadvantages. Its use is not recommended.

References

1 Snow H. Opium and cocaine in the treatment of cancerous disease. *British Medical Journal* 1896; **2**: 718–719.

2 Snow H. The opium-cocaine treatment of malignant disease. *British Medical Journal* 1897; **1**: 1019–1020.

3 Kerrane TA. The Brompton Cocktail. *Nursing Mirror* 1975; **140**: 59.

4 Martindale—The Extra Pharmacopoeia (24 edition). Pharmaceutical Press, London 1958, p 911.

5 Twycross RG and Wald SJ. Long-term use of diamorphine in advanced cancer in *Advances in Pain Research and Therapy, Vol. 1*, edited by Bonica JJ and Albe-Fessard D. Raven Press, New York 1976, pp 653–661.

6 Twycross RG. Effect of cocaine in the Brompton Cocktail in *Advances in Pain Research and Therapy, Vol. 3*, edited by Bonica JJ, Liebeskind JC and Albe-Fessard D. Raven Press, New York 1979, pp 927–932.

7 Melzack R, Mount BM and Gordon JM. The Brompton mixture versus morphine solution given orally: Effects on pain. *Canadian Medical Association Journal* 1979; **120**: 435–439.

8 Twycross RG. Unpublished data.

9 Melzack R, Ofiesh J G and Mount BM. The Brompton mixture: Effects on pain in cancer patients. *Canadian Medical Journal* 1976; **11**: 125–129.

Chapter Twelve

Morphine: Alternative Modes of Administration

Morphine Sulphate Tablets

Morphine Sulphate Tablets USP are a popular form of oral morphine in the USA, where slow release preparations (vide infra) are not yet available. They are formulated in 5 mg and 10 mg tablets which are small and easy to take provided the patient is able to swallow rapidly a mouthful of fluid. This is necessary because the pills crumble easily on contact with the buccal mucosa and are bitter to taste. Many patients with advanced cancer, weak and tending to have a dry mouth, find them unpleasant. The stronger patient, still at work, often prefers tablets as they are more convenient and more socially acceptable than a bottle of liquid medicine. The pharmacokinetics of morphine in simple tablet form are similar to those of morphine solution.

Controlled Release Morphine*

Some patients, especially if forgetful or partially sighted, are not able to cope with a 4-hourly regimen. In these, controlled release tablets containing 10, 30, 60 or 100 mg of morphine sulphate may be used. At present, only the 10 mg and 30 mg tablets are generally available. We have heard of conflicting opinions about controlled release tablets, ranging from 'no good at all' to 'very useful'. We therefore include an account of our initial experience with 10 and 30 mg tablets in selected patients at Sir Michael Sobell House.

Over a two-year period, 30 patients (18 female) of median age 76 years (range 48 to 93) were prescribed controlled release morphine sulphate

* not available in the USA

tables (CRM). Primary sites include large bowel 6, breast 5, stomach 3, prostate 3, myeloma 3, and bronchus 2. The majority of patients were changed from morphine sulphate in solution (MSS) while in hospital in preparation for discharge. On one occasion CRM was substituted because the patient disliked the liquid preparation. On another, a patient was prescribed CRM as she was known to be averse to taking any kind of tablets or medicine. Certainly she objected to 4-hourly medication. On 4 occasions, CRM was used *de novo* to provide a gentle induction to morphine therapy in elderly patients living at home, starting with a single 10 mg tablet at bedtime.

When changing from an established MSS regimen, a 1:1 ratio (mg for mg) was adopted, rounding up to the nearest 10 mg when necessary. Duration of treatment with CRM varied from 1 day to 5 months (median 3 weeks). The total daily dose ranged from 10 mg nocte to 60 mg twice daily (median 10 mg t.i.d.) and 3 received only a single dose each day at bedtime for night pain. Of the rest, 20 received CRM twice and 7 three times a day.

Those receiving other medication best administered with meals, such as corticosteroids, were given CRM three times a day (breakfast, tea and bedtime); as were those whose daily dose did not divide equally into two, that is, those needing 30 or 90 mg a day. The rest received CRM twice daily (breakfast and bedtime). Drugs such as benorylate and flurbiprofen, haloperidol and diazepam fitted readily into such regimens (Table 12.1). If nystatin was necessary, this was given more often, after meals and at bedtime.

Tablets were discontinued during the first week in 6 patients for the following reasons:

1 'the liquid was better' (after 1 dose in one patient),
2 became moribund (3 patients),
3 renewed pain (2 patients).

In the last two, the pain was increasing at the time of changeover. This related to leg ischaemia in one and to extension of the tumour through the sciatic foramen in the other. In the latter the change to CRM would not have been made if it had been appreciated that her pain had recurred and was getting rapidly more intense.

Reasons for discontinuing CRM in the remaining 24 patients were:

1 shortage of tablets (3 patients),
2 morphine no longer needed (4 patients),
3 moribund (7 patients),
4 renewed pain (10 patients).

Table 12.1   Examples of the more simple drug regimens possible with controlled release morphine sulphate tablets (CRM)

Patient 1:	CRM*	30 mg b.i.d.
	metoclopramide	10 mg b.i.d.
	dexamethasone	8 mg b.i.d.
	Moduretic	1 tab daily
	Mucaine	10 ml q.i.d.
	nystatin	2 ml q.i.d.
Patient 2:	CRM	10 mg b.i.d.
	haloperidol	0.5 mg b.i.d.
	diazepam	5 mg b.i.d.
	benorylate	10 ml b.i.d.
Patient 3:	CRM	10 mg b.i.d.
	dexamethasone	4 mg daily
	dioctyl forte	100 mg b.i.d.
	propantheline	15 mg nocte

* not available in the USA

Of the latter, 7 were changed back to MSS basically because they had been readmitted with little or no prospect of discharge. MSS was reintroduced when an increase in dose became necessary. With the other 3, it was felt that the greater flexibility of a 4-hourly regimen would help as renewed pain had not responded to one or two adjustments of the dose of CRM. Two of the 3 were not expected to go home; the third subsequently sustained a pathological fracture of a femur and, after surgical fixation, stopped taking morphine altogether.

We have continued to use CRM in selected patients (Table 12.2). Our experience continues to be mainly with 10 and 30 mg tablets. When we prescribe 60 and 100 mg tablets, we use them in exactly the same way. The availability of CRM has helped considerably in the management of a small though definite proportion of patients. When other medication does not need to be administered more than two or three times a day, the use of CRM means that a 4-hourly, or even q.i.d., regimen is not necessary.

Cautionary Note

There is evidence that doctors who find it difficult to use morphine sulphate 4-hourly do no better when prescribing CRM. There is the same need to adjust the dose, monitor unwanted effects and control constipation. Disillusion because of inadequate relief and non-compliance because of side effects are as common unless care is taken to establish a satisfactory regimen. Such attention to detail is as necessary with the use of CRM as with morphine sulphate in solution.

Table 12.2 Use of controlled release morphine (CRM) at Sir Michael Sobell House, Oxford

Criteria for use

1 Good pain relief on morphine sulphate in solution.
2 Anticipated difficulty in maintaining 4-hourly regimen when at home.
3 General reluctance by the patient to take more than a few tablets a day.
4 Strong dislike of liquid medicines.
5 Gentle induction to morphine therapy in the elderly.†
6 To overcome need for middle of the night dose† (taken at bedtime in addition to morphine sulphate solution).

Contraindications

1 Failure to maintain adequate relief despite upward adjustment of dose.
2 Patient not expected to go home.
3 'As required' use.
4 Relief of acute pain [1].

† We do not often use CRM in these ways, preferring alternative approaches (*see* pages 174 and 220)

Other iatrogenic abuses include the prescription of CRM on an 'as required' basis or 3 to 4-hourly. Of all the forms of morphine available, CRM is one that is *absolutely* contraindicated for 'as required' use, as the plasma morphine concentration does not reach its maximum level until 4 hours after administration (Figure 12.1). Its use 4-hourly indicates a failure to appreciate the pharmacokinetics of the preparation and is another example of the illogic that creeps in when doctors have to care for a dying cancer patient (Figure 12.2). The prescription of controlled release morphine tablets (*MST-Continus*) simply to avoid the use of the word 'morphine' is also to be deplored. The right use of morphine in any form requires a doctor who does not feel embarrassed or apologetic when prescribing it.

Morphine Suppositories

These are commercially available in Britain in a range of strengths: 10, 15, 20, 30 and 60 mg. Other strengths may be made according to the recommendations in the British Pharmaceutical Codex. In one patient at home, we used suppositories containing 150 mg of morphine sulphate. Although time-consuming, a pharmacist can make up morphine suppositories in countries where they are not commercially available. This is done at The Connecticut Hospice. Use of these suppositories avoids the equi-analgesic uncertainties associated with a change to an alternative strong narcotic suppository such as oxycodone or hydromorphone.**

** not available in Britain

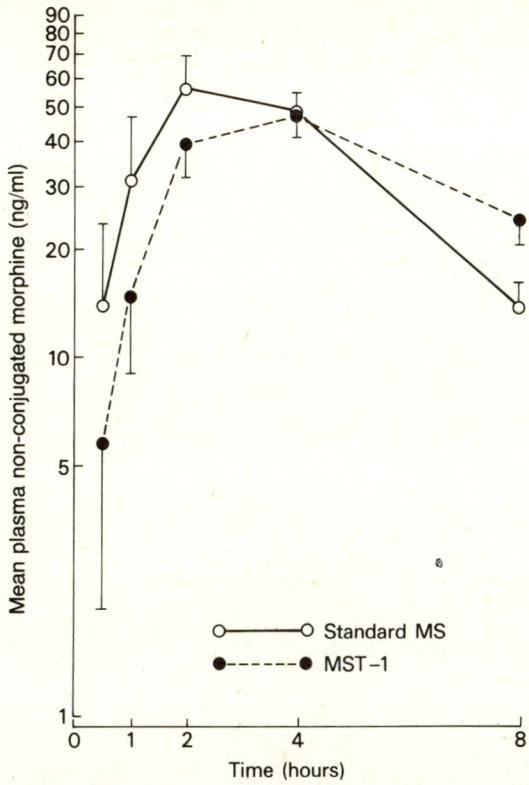

Figure 12.1 Mean plasma concentrations of non-conjugated morphine after a single oral dose of 20 mg morphine sulphate in solution or after two 10 mg controlled release morphine sulphate tablets (MST-1). From Hanks *et al*, 1981 [1]

The pharmacokinetics of rectally administered morphine sulphate have not been extensively studied. We recommend that the dose previously used by mouth is given per rectum.

Some hospices use suppositories as the formulation of choice when oral administration of morphine sulphate becomes difficult or impossible. Other centres claim that injections are easier to give and cause the patient no greater discomfort and sometimes less. Suppositories are particularly useful for patients at home (*see* Chapter 17).

Morphine by Injection

The use of diamorphine* parenterally was discussed in Chapter 10. In countries where this drug is not available, it is necessary to use morphine sulphate. It is regrettable that the maximum strength commercially available in the USA is only 15 mg in 1 ml (Table 12.3). As injected

* not available in the USA

Dr A B C Adams **EAST END SURGERY**
Dr D E Hicks **KINGSWORTH**
Dr Patricia Clifford **WILTS**
Dr J Fuller **Tel: 718863**

19 November 1981

Dr R G Twycross
Consultant Physician
Sir Michael Sobell House
The Churchill Hospital
Headington
Oxford

Dear Dr Twycross

re MRS KATRINA PAGE
    12 Eden Drive, Longworth, Wilts

Thank you for admitting the above patient with abdominal carcinomatosis, secondary to ca. gall bladder.

At present on four MST 1 every three hours, and Dalmane 50 mg nocte.

Yours sincerely

David E. Hicks

D E HICKS

Figure 12.2 Letter of referral from family practitioner demonstrating the *wrong* use of controlled release morphine sulphate tablets (MST-1). Names and addresses have been changed to preserve anonymity.

Table 12.3 Preparations of morphine sulphate for SC and IM use

Name	Strength
Morphine sulphate	8 mg, 10 mg, 15 mg/l ml (USP)
	10 mg, 5 mg, 30 mg (BP)
Cyclimorph 10*	10 mg morphine tartrate + cyclizine tartrate 50 mg/1 ml
Cyclimorph 15*	15 mg morphine tartrate + cyclizine tartrate 50 mg/1 ml
Duromorph*	microcrystalline morphine in aqueous suspension, 64 mg/1 ml

* not available in the USA

cyclizine stings, cyclimorph should be given only by deep intramuscular or intravenous routes.

A few doctors use Duromorph* to reduce the number of injections to 3/day. Duromorph is a microcrystalline suspension of morphine base and is equivalent to about 70 mg of morphine sulphate. It is not, however, equivalent to 70 mg of intramuscular morphine sulphate in terms of analgesic effect. This is presumably because more morphine is metabolized during its slow absorption into the system than after an injection of ordinary morphine sulphate. The manufacturers recommend that 1 ml of Duromorph (64 mg morphine) is used in place of 30 mg of ordinary morphine sulphate [2].

Some physicians, when prescribing injections for a moribund patient at home, give a relatively larger dose of diamorphine or morphine in the hope of providing relief for 6 hours. It is felt that, at this stage, a deleterious effect on the level of consciousness is a secondary consideration compared with the need for continued and continuous relief. It is obviously easier for a team comprising doctor, community nurse, hospice home care sister and family to cope with a 6-hourly regimen than a 4-hourly one. On the other hand, if a night nursing service can be arranged, 4-hourly injections are much easier to organize as the night nurse is responsible for 3 of the 6 daily injections.

Morphine by Infusion

To avoid the need for regular injections, of whatever volume, some centres administer morphine by infusion. There are three alternative approaches:

1   continuous subcutaneous infusion,
2   intermittent intravenous infusion,
3   continuous intravenous infusion.

Continuous Subcutaneous Infusion

Motor driven syringes, sometimes called 'syringe pumps', have been manufactured for many years, though it is only relatively recently that small portable models have been available. The syringe driver in Figure 12.3 has a battery with a running life of about 3 months. It is calibrated in mm/hour, rather than ml/hour, to allow different types of syringes to be used. The rate switch and starting button are flush with the surface and cannot be accidentally operated. Adjustment is made with a screwdriver. It is often possible to leave a subcutaneous needle in situ for weeks. The use of the syringe driver in terminal cancer patients has been pioneered in Britain by Russell [3], who uses it extensively for home care when oral medication is difficult or impossible. Other drugs such as metoclopramide and haloperidol are added as necessary. In Britain, diamorphine

* not available in the USA

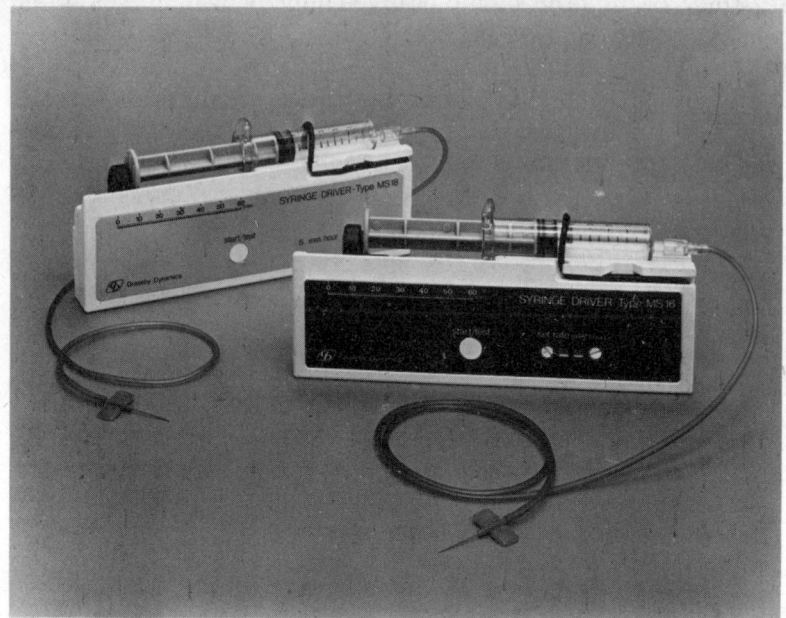

Figure 12.3 Graseby Dynamics syringe drivers. MS16 is a portable, battery-operated, variable speed syringe driver which allows the infusion SC or IV of small volumes over periods ranging from 30 minutes to 50 hours. MS18 is a fixed speed syringe driver. It is cheaper than MS16, but lacks versatility. We recommend the use of MS16 for the administration of morphine, at least initially.
Photograph by courtesy of Graseby Dynamics Ltd.

hydrochloride is generally used instead of morphine sulphate. The principles of use are, however, the same (Table 12.4).

Although theoretically an attractive approach, in practice the use of a syringe driver for home care is not always trouble-free. Moreover, the regular district nurses do not handle them. This means that a *daily* visit by the hospice nurse is necessary and, if anything goes wrong, it requires a second visit. The number of patients that a home care sister can help look after is reduced considerably if the syringe driver is widely used.

Intermittent Intravenous Infusion
This method is sometimes used for patients with a continuous IV infusion, again to avoid repeated IM or SC injections. It is rare for a hospice patient to have a continuous IV infusion. Intermittent IV infusion is possible using a Gordh or Butterfly needle. Postoperative studies have shown, however, that continuous IV infusion is more efficacious and has fewer unwanted effects than intermittent administration [4–6]. A few have had successful experience with intravenous demand analgesia. In one hospital, morphine or pethidine[1] was used in a motor syringe that

[1] meperidine (USA)

214

Table 12.4 Continuous diamorphine infusion using a Graseby Dynamics portable syringe driver†

Continuous subcutaneous infusion of diamorphine obviates the need for 4-hourly injections when oral administration of opiates is no longer possible.

Indications

Relief of severe pain with:
1   Nausea and vomiting.
2   Difficulty with swallowing.

Advantages
1   Even analgesia – no peaks or troughs.
2   Reloaded only once in 24 hours.
3   Comfort and confidence – no repeated injections.
4   Mobility.
5   Less nausea and vomiting.

The Machine

Graseby Dynamics MS 16 Portable Syringe Driver

Measures: 166 × 53 × 33 mm
Weighs: 175 g
Battery driven: PP3 alkaline 9v, running life approximately 3 months.
Catheter 60 cm and Butterfly needle.
Fabric shoulder holster.

Method
1   Estimate 4-hourly requirement as if given IM.
2   Give one loading '4-hourly dose' SC/IM to raise plasma concentration.
3   24-hour requirement = previous 4-hourly dose ×6.
4   Dissolve 24-hour requirement in 10 ml water and load syringe.
5   Connect to and fill cannula.
6   Insert Butterfly cannula subcutaneously in upper abdomen or above breast and tape with Micropore.
7   Load syringe in driver and start motor.
8   Always use at rate 2 mm/hour, equivalent to approximately 10 ml/24 hours.
9   Place in case and shoulder holster.
10 Recharge every 24 hours.

Note: The Butterfly cannula needs changing on average every three weeks

† Adapted from Michael Sobell House, Mount Vernon Hospital, Northwood, Middlesex with permission

could be triggered by the patient to deliver a fixed volume into an IV infusion each time the machine was activated. In 9 cancer patients with a prognosis of a few weeks and troublesome pain, IV demand analgesia resulted in more satisfactory pain control and a reduced daily narcotic intake when compared with the previously used SC and IM routes [7].

Continuous Intravenous Infusion

This method is useful for patients who have an IV infusion. However, as few dying patients want or need continuous parenteral hydration and nutrition, it is not recommended that an infusion is set up for the sole purpose of administering morphine or other strong narcotic. There is a report of this method in a series of 8 children, aged 3 to 16 years, who had been admitted to hospital with unrelieved severe pain [8]. Five had leukaemia, 2 sarcoma and 1 a lymphoma. The causes of pain included osseous metastasis, nerve pressure and cellulitis. In 2, there was associated severe vomiting. In 1 patient, bruising at injection sites precipitated the change to infusion.

The initial constant infusion dose was based on the pain medication given in the preceding 24 hours. For example, those who had received intermittent IV morphine sulphate during the previous 24-hour period, received the same total daily dose over the first 24 hours when given as a continuous infusion. The dose was subsequently increased or decreased as required to achieve complete relief of pain as judged by the physician and nurse, and also by the parent(s) and patient, the aim being to give the minimum effective dose. All the patients achieved satisfactory pain control. The dose of morphine ranged from 0.8 to 80 mg/hour; the median dose was 2 to 4 mg/hour (Table 12.5). Six developed drowsiness, though this was usually mild and did not prevent interaction with family or staff. In 3 the respiratory rate decreased to about 10/minute. Continuous infusion was necessary for 1 to 16 days. One child required repeated dose increments; the others did not until within a day or so of death. Since this report was published, the hospital in question has modified its approach; continuous SC infusion is now preferred [9]. In adults [10], dose escalation did not occur when morphine sulphate was given by continuous IV infusion *for up to 10 weeks.*

Extradural and Intrathecal Morphine

It has been demonstrated that the intrathecal injection of a narcotic produces analgesia mediated by morphine receptors in the dorsal horn of the spinal cord [11]. This effect can also be produced by injection of β-endorphin [12]. Extradural injection of morphine produces a similar but smaller effect, presumably because less of the drug reaches the receptor sites. Many of the early reports were uncontrolled and tended to over-emphasize the relief obtained and under-report the incidence of side

Table 12.5   Efficacy of continuous infusion morphine sulphate

Patient	Duration of infusion (days)	Dose mg/hr	Dose mg/kg/hr	Pain control	Additional medications
1	16	0.5–16.0	0.2–0.76	Complete	hydroxyzine
2	3	2.2–3.0	0.11–0.15	Complete	–
3	3	1.0–2.5	0.04–0.10	Complete	–
4	3	5.0–14.0	0.05–0.15	Complete	–
	1.5	2.5–10.0	0.03–0.11	Complete	–
5	3	0.8–1.5	0.04–0.07	Adequate	–
6	5	2.0–5.0	0.03–0.06	Complete	chlorpromazine
7	12	2.0–0.0	0.04–0.0	Adequate	–
8	1	50.0–80.0	1.67–2.67	Adequate	–

From Miser et al, 1980 [8]

effects, including potentially fatal respiratory depression. This has been observed to occur some 8 to 12 hours after intrathecal injection [13]. The time intervals between injection and respiratory depression suggest that the effect may be a function of CSF flow. Because of the possibility of delayed respiratory depression, some anaesthetists regard intrathecal morphine as too dangerous to use. Others reported late side effects including itching, sweating and vomiting. All are abolished by intravenous naloxone without loss of analgesic effect. A central enkephalinergic component to narcotic-associated itching has, therefore, been invoked. Intraspinal narcotics consistently induce itching in the distribution of the trigeminal nerve. One observer suggests that this phenomenon is neural in origin, the result of a spinal reflex transmitted through a medullary itch centre associated with the spinal nucleus of the trigeminal nerve [14].

Two controlled trials of extradural morphine have been published. Both were undertaken in gynaecological postoperative patients. In the first, normal saline alone was compared with 2 or 5 mg of added morphine sulphate [15]. In the second, 10 mg was compared when given by extradural or IM routes [16]. The results of the first showed that morphine, at either dose, was better than a placebo, but did not always give satisfactory relief. In the second, there were no statistically significant differences in the early period after administration. Though when doses were compared after 24 hours, it was found that the extradural group had only required an extra 6.7 mg of morphine on average, compared with 18.8 mg in the IM group.

One group have used a modified Infusaid reservoir infusion pump in series with a silastic epidural catheter [17]. This has a 50 ml percutaneously rechargeable reservoir with a preset continuous infusion of morphine. The reservoir is recharged after about 5 weeks. It is hoped that this approach will reduce the likelihood of sepsis around the catheter and the possibility of meningitis. The incidence of this type of complication is, however, very low if an antiseptic such as povidone-iodine is used [18].

Experience with extradural morphine in cancer patients is accruing. It has been used for up to 4 months in some patients [18]. Extradural morphine provides effective, segmented analgesia with minimal side effects since there is no effect on sensory, motor or efferent sympathetic pathways. It is effective for constant aching pain (transmitted in the palaeospinothalamic tract) but is relatively ineffective in relieving neuralgic pain particularly if stabbing in nature (transmitted by the neospinothalamic tract) [19, 20]. Duration of relief varies but is usually sufficiently prolonged to avoid the need for a further injection while there is risk of cumulative systemic effects. Only one centre has reported that tolerance is a problem [21].

Morphine sulphate in a *preservative-free* solution with normal saline or 10 per cent dextrose is most commonly used [22]. Two mg in 5 to 10 ml is the recommended starting dose. Side effects occur infrequently. Concurrent administration of a narcotic systemically is inadvisable. There is need for the extradural catheter to be inserted accurately at the level of the pain, preferably with radiographic confirmation of the position. Nursing the patient in a head-up position to prevent cephalad spread of the injected solution and avoiding mixing local anaesthetic and morphine are other safeguards [22]. Patients should always be observed in hospital for several hours after the introduction of a catheter.

The use of extradural morphine is still in its infancy. The early enthusiastic reports were uncontrolled and largely impressionistic. There is still much to be discovered about its optimum use. Its limitation in relation to neuralgic cancer pain certainly reduces its potential.

Morphine Acetate

Organic morphine salts are more soluble than inorganic ones (*see* Table 10.2, page 195). Morphine tartrate is twice and acetate ten times more soluble than hydrochloride and sulphate. Morphine acetate is, unfortunately, unstable in solution and the resultant free morphine is virtually insoluble in water. Similarly, although 100 mg of morphine tartrate will, in theory, dissolve in 1 ml, in practice it is generally less soluble because of the partial dissociation of morphine from tartaric acid.

The use of freeze-dried (lyophilized) preparations would circumvent this problem, and offers a way round the difficulty of large volume injections in cachectic patients in countries where diamorphine is not available for medical use. Morphine acetate has a solubility in water, at room temperature, of 1 g in 2.5 ml. For the occasional patient who requires, for example, 120 mg of diamorphine hydrochloride, 240 to

300 mg of morphine would be needed. As 400 mg of morphine acetate dissolves in 1 ml, the volume of injection will only rarely exceed this amount if this salt of morphine is used.

Nepenthe*

At one time Nepenthe was a standardized alcoholic tincture of opium [23]. In recent years, it has been reformulated [24]. *Nepenthe oral solution* still contains anhydrous morphine 0.84 per cent but only 0.05 per cent of this derives from opium tincture; the rest is morphine (Table 12.6). This is equivalent to almost 1.2 per cent morphine *sulphate*. Nepenthe is usually diluted and given as a 10 per cent solution. Thus, 10 ml of 10 per cent Nepenthe contains the equivalent of approximately 12 mg of morphine sulphate. Stronger solutions can also be prepared. As Nepenthe has no advantage over morphine sulphate, its use is not recommended.

Table 12.6 The changing face of Nepenthe

Source	Description
Martindale: The Extra Pharmacopoeia, 26th Edition 1972 [23]	'A liquid preparation of *opium* with added morphine containing the equivalent of 0.84% of anhydrous morphine.'
Martindale: The Extra Pharmacopoeia, 27th Edition 1977 [24]	'Oral solution. Contains anhydrous morphine 0.84% (0.05% from papaveretum and 0.79% from morphine hydrochloride).'

Nepenthe is often prescribed with aspirin. It is not always appreciated that this must be dispensed separately, and the two 300 mg aspirin tablets added at the time of administration. If the aspirin is dissolved in Nepenthe by the pharmacy, hydrolysis occurs with the formation of the less potent salicylic acid. Patients have been supplied with such a mixture and have noted that 'the new medicine is not so good as the first lot'. Reverting to separately prescribed Nepenthe and soluble aspirin has resulted in a return to the former satisfactory pain relief.

Opium

Opium contains a variable mixture of about 25 alkaloids, including morphine 9 to 17 per cent, noscapine 2 to 9 per cent, codeine 0.3 to 4 per

* not available in the USA

cent, and smaller proportions of thebaine, narceine, papaverine and hydrocotarnine. Pharmaceutical opium powder is standardized to contain some 10 per cent of morphine by weight. In some countries concentrated opium (papaveretum) is available. This contains 50 per cent morphine together with the other opium alkaloids (vide infra).

The weight of morphine in these preparations denotes the content of morphine *base*. In other circumstances, morphine content refers to the weight of morphine *salt* (sulphate, hydrochloride, etc.). To allow a better comparison with morphine sulphate, it is necessary to adjust the morphine content of opium upwards by some 40 to 50 per cent. Thus 10 mg of papaveretum is equivalent to 5 mg of morphine base, which is approximately equivalent to 7 mg of morphine sulphate.

Powdered Opium

This is used in opium and belladonna suppositories (B & O Supprette, USA). Two strengths are available containing either 30 or 60 mg of powdered opium and 15 mg of belladonna. (The latter is approximately equivalent to 0.2 mg of atropine-hyoscine). The data sheet states that 'the belladonna counteracts the undesirable effects of ureteral spasm and increased gastrointestinal muscle tone induced by morphine'. As far as we know, this has not been objectively evaluated. At The Connecticut Hospice these suppositories are used for rectal tenesmoid pain, particularly if associated with spasmodic exacerbations. Generally, however, ordinary morphine sulphate suppositories should be used if rectal administration is indicated.

Papaveretum

A number of preparations containing concentrated opium are available in both Great Britain and the USA:

papaveretum tablets 10 mg (Omnopon, Britain)
papaveretum injections 20 mg/1 ml (Omnopon, Britain; Pantopon, USA)
aspirin (500 mg) and papaveretum (10 mg) tablets (Britain)

There is no place for papaveretum injections; morphine or diamorphine* should be used instead. We sometimes use papaveretum tablets as a gentle induction into morphine therapy, partly to see the effect—both good and bad—in an elderly patient who is at home with little support and no longer controlled on a weaker narcotic analgesic. Usually, after a few test doses, the patient is put onto a 4-hourly oral morphine sulphate regimen.

The aspirin and papaveretum tablets are of interest for two reasons. The first is that, although the tablets are large, they are effervescent and relatively easy to take. The second is that they do not come under the

* not available in the USA

Controlled Drugs regulations. Each tablet contains 10 mg papaveretum, equivalent to 5 mg of anhydrous morphine. As each tablet weighs over 2.5 g, the anyhdrous morphine equivalent content is less than 0.2 per cent. The preparation is therefore exempt from Controlled Drugs regulations. A tablet containing the same quality of papaveretum but weighing less would not be. There are no other advantages to be gained by its use. The disadvantages are those common to fixed drug combinations. Accordingly, the use of these tablets is not recommended.

The aspirin-opium (A & O) tablets available in parts of India contain *powdered* opium, not papaveretum. The opium content (30 mg) is only 10 per cent morphine, equivalent to some 4 mg of morphine sulphate.

References

1 Hanks GW, Rose NM, Aherne GW and Piall EM. Analgesic effect of morphine tablets. *Lancet* 1981; **i:** 732–733.

2 Rabinovitch J. Personal communication.

3 Russell PSG. Analgesia in terminal malignant disease. *British Medical Journal* 1979; **1:** 1561.

4 Church JJ. Continuous narcotic infusion for relief of postoperative pain. *British Medical Journal* 1979; **1:** 977–979.

5 Nayman J. Measurement and control of postoperative pain. *Annals of Royal College of Surgeons of England* 1979; **61:** 419–426.

6 Rutter PC, Murphy F and Dudley HAF. Morphine: controlled trial of different methods of administration for postoperative pain relief. *British Medical Journal* 1980; **280:** 12–13.

7 Keeri-Szanto M. Demand analgesia for the relief of pain problems in 'terminal' illness. *Anaesthesiology Review* 1976; **3:** 19–21.

8 Miser AW, Miser JS and Clark BS. Continuous intravenous infusion of morphine sulphate for control of severe pain in children with terminal malignancy. *Journal of Paediatrics* 1980; **96:** 930–932.

9 Miser AW. Personal communication.

10 Holmes AH. Morphine IV infusion for chronic pain. *Drug Intelligence and Clinical Pharmacology* 1978; **12:** 556–557.

11 Bullingham RES, McQuay HJ and Moore RA. Extradural and intrathecal narcotics in *Recent Advances in Anaesthetics and Analgesics, Vol 14*, edited by Atkinson RS and Langton-Hewer C. Churchill-Livingstone, London and Edinburgh 1982, pp 141–156.

12 Oyama T, Jin T, Yamaya R, Ling N and Guillemin R. Profound analgesic effects of β-endorphin in man. *Lancet* 1980; **i:** 122–124.

13 Davies GK, Tolhurst-Cleaver CL and James TL. Respiratory depression after intrathecal narcotics. *Anesthesia* 1980; **35:** 1080–1083.

14 Scott PV and Fischer HBJ. Intraspinal opiates and itching: a new reflex? *British Medical Journal* 1982; **284:** 1015–1016.

15 McClure JH, Chambers WA, Moore E and Scott DB. Epidural morphine for postoperative pain. *Lancet* 1980; **i:** 975–976.

16 Chambers WA, Sinclair CJ and Scott DB. Extradural morphine for pain after surgery. *British Journal of Anaesthesia* 1981; **53:** 921–925.

17 Coombs DW, Saunders RL, Gaylor MS, Pagean MG, Leith MG and Schairberger C. Continuous epidural analgesia via implanted morphine reservoir. *Lancet* 1981; **ii:** 425–426.

18 *Peridurale opiat-analgesie,* edited by Zenz M. Gustav Fischer Verlag, Stuttgart and New York, 1981.

19 Magora F, Olswant D, Eimeryl D, Shurr J, Katzenelson R, Cotev S and Davidson JT. Observations on extradural morphine in various pain conditions. *British Journal of Anaesthesia* 1980; **52:** 247–251.

20 Howard RP, Milne LA and Williams NE. Epidural morphine in terminal cancer. *Anaesthesia* 1981; **36:** 51–53.

21 Ventafridda V, Figliuzzi M. Tamburini M, Gori E, Parolaro D and Sala M. Clinical observations on analgesia elicited by intrathecal morphine in cancer patients in *Advances in Pain Research and Therapy, Vol. 3,* edited by Bonica JJ. Liebeskind JC and Albe-Fessard DG, Raven Press, New York 1979, pp 559–565.

22 Mehta M. Chronic pain in *Recent Advances in Anaesthetics and Analgesics, Vol 14,* edited by Atkinson RS and Langton-Hewer C. Churchill-Livingstone, London and Edinburgh 1982, pp 157–177.

23 *Martindale–The Extra-Pharmacopoeia, 26th edition.* The Pharmaceutical Press 1972, p. 1128.

24 *Martindale–The Extra-Pharmacopoeia, 27th edition.* The Pharmaceutical Press 1977, p. 973.

Chapter Thirteen

Myths About Morphine

The use of morphine in the management of pain in cancer is often restricted because of misconceptions about possible deleterious side effects. Often deeply ingrained in the minds of both doctors and nurses, these misconceptions overstate the potential for harm. The more common myths are examined in this chapter.

'Morphine Is Dangerous As It Depresses Respiration'
The mechanism of morphine-induced respiratory depression is believed to be a reduction in the ability of the brain stem respiratory centres to respond to increases in arterial pCO_2 [1]. Clinically significant respiratory depression is rarely seen in patients with severe pain due to malignant disease even when receiving large doses of morphine. This is because pain and emotional stress are a powerful antagonist to narcotic-induced respiratory depression. In a study of 20 cancer patients of median age 58 years, all of whom were taking 30 mg or more of morphine sulphate by mouth every 4 hours to control pain, the respiratory rates were all >12/minute when resting [2]. Twelve of the patients had a history of chronic bronchitis and 7 had carcinoma of the bronchus. All pCO_2 values except one were below the upper limit of the normal range (45 mmHg). Seven patients were hypoxic (pO_2 < 80 mmHg) but in only one was this signifi-cant. These results support clinical experience.

On the other hand, respiratory failure has been reported in a 76-year-old man with a pleural mesothelioma. He required morphine sulphate 90 mg by mouth every 4 hours to control severe chest pain [3]. After a successful thoracic intrathecal nerve block with chlorocresol, respiratory failure was induced by doses of oral morphine sulphate at the same level as those used without trouble before the block, and also by substantially smaller doses (Figure 13.1). This indicates the need for caution in those with limited respiratory reserve if the level of pain is dramatically altered as a result of non-drug measures. Oral morphine sulphate is a safe analgesic for chronic cancer pain, even in those with pre-existing respiratory disease. This is provided the drug is carefully titrated against the pain in the individual patient.

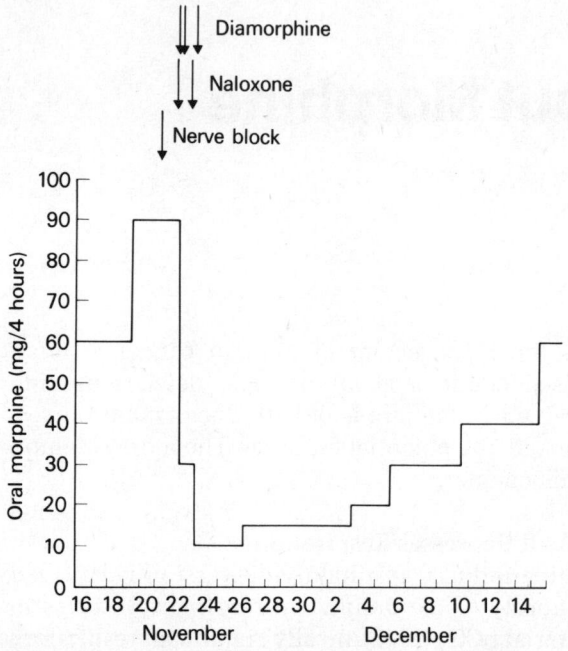

Figure 13.1 Narcotic requirements in a 76-year-old man with a pleural mesothelioma before and after intrathecal chlorocresol nerve block.

'Morphine Is So Poorly Absorbed By Mouth That It Is Ineffective By This Route'

Morphine sulphate is the strong analgesic of choice at most hospices and is being used increasingly at other centres. Experience has shown it to be the most versatile, reliable and safe strong narcotic analgesic that is readily available. In a series of 89 cancer patients who were receiving either morphine sulphate or diamorphine hydrochloride* regularly by mouth, a highly significant positive correlation was found to exist, for both drugs, between the dose administered and the serum concentration (Figure 13.2) [4]. Four-hourly doses ranged from 2.5 to 90 mg. Since the study was completed, higher oral doses of morphine sulphate have been

* not available in the USA

224

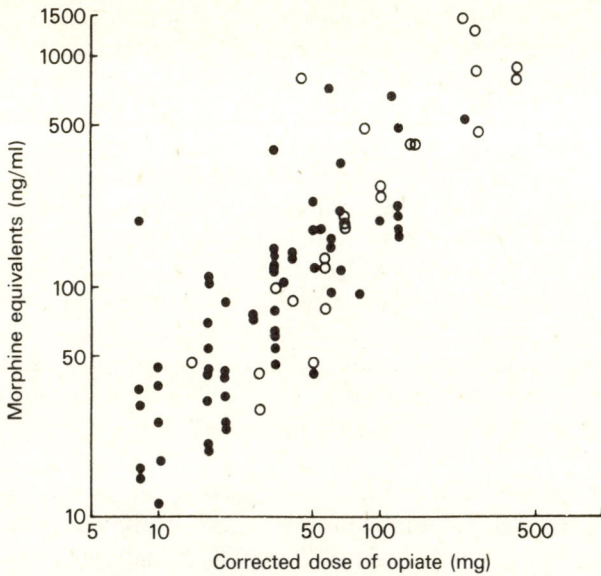

Figure 13.2 Plasma morphine concentration (non-conjugated) in 89 cancer patients receiving either morphine sulphate or diamorphine hydrochloride every 4 hours by mouth. Dose expressed in terms of morphine base. Patients receiving diamorphine = ● and those receiving morphine = ○.

        Diamorphine (●), $y = 26.98 + 2.35x$, $r = 0.661$, $n = 65$, $t = 7.0$, $P < 0.001$
        Morphine   (○), $y = 78.89 + 2.52x$, $r = 0.751$, $n = 24$, $t = 5.3$, $P < 0.001$
        All Data $y = 27.55 + 2.64x$, $r = 0.785$, $n = 89$, $t = 11.9$, $P < 0.001$
        From Aherne *et al*, 1979 [4]

used when indicated. Prior to this, patients had been changed to parenteral medication if 60 mg of oral morphine sulphate did not give relief. Doses of up to 700 mg 4-hourly have been used with good effect at one hospital [5] though, apart from at bedtime, we have rarely used more than 300 mg. Part of the problem in administering oral morphine is a lack of understanding by nurses and doctors about oral-parenteral analgesic equivalents (*see* page 168). Nurses feel uncomfortable administering such 'large doses' of morphine [6], but if there is a clear grasp of how oral narcotics work this particular myth can be overcome.

'Morphine Only Alters A Patient's Response To His Pain'

It is frequently stated that narcotic analgesics do not erase the patient's perception of pain but change his affective interpretation of it. In other words, he is still aware of the pain but its quality is less distressing. Sometimes this is so but in *narcotic-responsive pain* the goal of treatment is total relief from pain. This is usually possible if the analgesic is given prophylactically in a dose adjusted to individual need. The danger of believing that morphine *only* alters a patient's response to his pain is that the doctor, unaware that morphine can usually erase the pain, will fail to

225

increase the drug and provide adequate analgesia. With pains that are non-responsive to morphine (see Table 9.2, page 173) the patient continues to complain of pain and continues to be distressed by it.

'Morphine Induces Euphoria'

It is often stated that the use of morphine induces a state of euphoria. This is not so. Euphoria is rarely seen in cancer patients receiving morphine. Patients with unrelieved pain are understandably dysphoric. Relief of pain with morphine or other narcotic analgesic results in a return to a more normal affect. This is not euphoria. Indeed, data from St. Christopher's Hospice indicates that the longer a patient takes a narcotic analgesic the greater the likelihood that he will become depressed and need concurrent antidepressant treatment [7].

The belief that narcotics commonly cause euphoria may derive from the writings and experiences of literary figures, such as de Quincy and Coleridge, and to the unqualified transfer of the results of studies on drug addicts to non-addicts. Evidence from volunteer studies and clinical experience both indicate that this belief is unfounded [8]. In patients with far advanced cancer, morphine, diamorphine and other narcotics do not cause euphoria.

'Morphine Is Addictive'

Although the term drug addiction has been replaced officially by drug dependence, unofficially it continues to be used. Drug dependence is currently defined as:

> 'A state, psychic and sometimes also physical, resulting from the interaction between a living organism and a drug, characterized by behavioural and other responses that always include a compulsion to take the drug on a continuous or periodic basis in order to experience its psychic effects, and sometimes to avoid the discomfort of its absence. Tolerance may or may not be present' [9].

This is a broader definition than that of 1964, which emphasized the need for both tolerance and an early development of physical dependence in addition to strong psychological (psychic) dependence [10]. The term drug dependence closely approximates to the popular conception of addiction—a compulsion or overpowering drive to take the drug in order to experience its psychological effects.

Recently the Boston Collaborative Drug Surveillance Programme examined the files of nearly 12,000 medical inpatients who had received medicinal narcotics, so as to determine the incidence of narcotic addiction. There were only 4 cases of reasonably well documented dependence in patients with no history of addiction. The dependence was considered major in only one instance. The drugs implicated were pethidine[1] in 2 patients, Percodan (oxycodone and aspirin) in 1 and hydromorphone** in 1 [11.].

Although the authors did not define addiction, their conclusion coincides with the hospice experience. The development of addiction in the popular sense is rare in medical patients with no history of addiction, despite the widespread use of narcotic drugs in hospitals. Furthermore, iatrogenically produced addiction does not feature in two recent reports on drug dependence prepared for the World Health Organization [12, 13].

We suspect that many of our patients are *physically* dependent and, if no longer needed for pain control, advise a gradual reduction of the dose of narcotic after more than 4 weeks of use (vide infra). However, we do not see psychological dependence—the craving and compulsion to take the drug for its psychic effects.

Occasionally, a patient is admitted who appears to be addicted, demanding 'an injection' every 2 or 3 hours. Typically such a patient has a long history of poor pain control and for several weeks will have been receiving fairly regular (4-hourly as required) but inadequate injections of one or more narcotic analgesics.

In this situation, given time, it is usually possible to control the pain adequately, prevent the clock-watching and demanding behaviour, and eventually change progressively to an oral preparation. But even here, in the terms of the WHO definition, it cannot be said that the patient is addicted. He is not demanding the narcotic in order to experience its psychological effect but to be relieved from pain for at least an hour or two.

More difficult to deal with is the rare patient, usually young, who was a 'street addict' before becoming ill. Usually one of two errors will be made. On the one hand his pain is discounted by the professional staff and requests for narcotics resisted; 'after all he is an addict'. At the other extreme the patient is treated as a non-addict patient and allowed to escalate his narcotic intake far beyond reasonable estimates of what is needed to control his pain. This is one situation in which the patient's statements about what hurts must be carefully balanced by the judgement of the experienced hospice doctor (Table 13.1).

'Tolerance To Morphine Develops Very Rapidly'

Many doctors are reluctant to use strong narcotic analgesics, particularly morphine and diamorphine, because they assume that the medication will eventually become ineffective as a result of tolerance. This is understandable as little information has been available concerning the long-term effects of narcotic analgesics when administered regularly to

[1] meperidine (USA)
** not available in Britain

Table 13.1 Guidelines for helping the patient who was narcotic-dependent (a 'street addict') before becoming ill

1 Patient should be under the care of an *experienced* hospice doctor, well able to make a reasonable estimate of narcotic requirements (amount, route and frequency) for the pain commonly associated with the extent of the patient's disease.

2 Patient should be under the care and observation of an *experienced* hospice nurse, well able to identify non-verbal signs of pain, who can advise less experienced members of the nursing team and upgrade their judgement.

3 Narcotics should be prescribed by one doctor only.

4 Clear statements must be in the nursing plan about what to do when the patient requests top-up or breakthrough narcotic medications.

5 It must be clearly recognized that most hospice staff are *unaccustomed* to dealing with narcotic-dependent patients. Outside advice can be very helpful in achieving a successful synthesis between methods of hospice pain control and those of drug dependency units.

6 Change the patient from parenteral to oral and rectal narcotics as soon as confidence has been established. This immediately breaks the association with the street ritual of injecting drugs, and establishes a new link between drugs and pain control. This also gives the doctor a clear basis of distinction when discussing the issue with the patient:
    'I am prepared to increase your oral morphine at 6 pm and 10 pm because I am sure this will stop you waking in pain at 3 o'clock in the morning.'
    'I will give you an extra supply of oral morphine when you go home for the day on Saturday because the extra activity may well exacerbate the pain.'
    'I will not give you injectable morphine to take home because it is not necessary for your pain control, and because of the difficulties you have had with that in the past.'

relieve persistent pain. The lack of data resulted in predictions being made on the basis of animal and human volunteer studies. In these studies the emphasis was on *inducing* tolerance and physical dependence as rapidly as possible by using maximum tolerated doses. This is not comparable to administering the drugs in doses and at intervals found in a clinical regimen. Thus, although such studies are useful in predicting abuse liability, they are largely irrelevant to clinical practice.

To allow predictions to be made on the basis of clinical experience, the notes of 500 patients admitted consecutively to St. Christopher's Hospice were reviewed [14]. A total of 205 patients received diamorphine regularly for at least 1 week. By grouping the patients according to survival

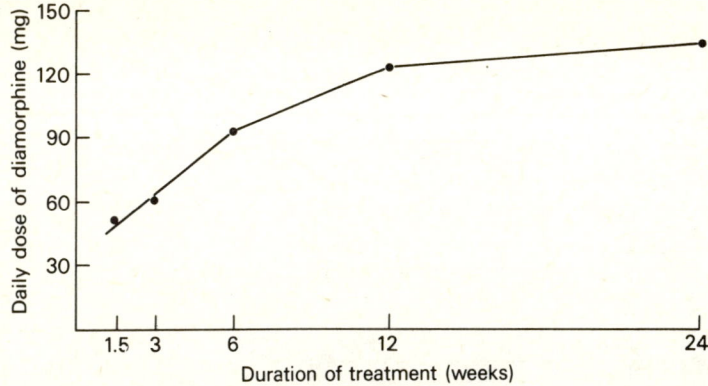

Figure 13.3 205 patients admitted consecutively with advanced cancer were grouped according to survival following the start of treatment with diamorphine; group median final daily dose of diamorphine is shown plotted against group median duration of treatment.
From Twycross, 1974 [14]

after commencing diamorphine, it was demonstrated that the longer the duration of treatment the slower the rate of rise in dose (Figure 13.3). In a second review [7], 115 patients who had received diamorphine regularly for at least 12 weeks were selected from approximately 3,000 patients admitted over 7 years. Dose-time charts were prepared. Visual analysis indicated that in many there was an initial phase when the dose was increased several times within 1 or 2 weeks, followed by a prolonged phase when the dose was increased less often or not at all (Figure 13.4). It was also clearly demonstrated that the longer a patient survived after prescription of diamorphine, the greater the likelihood of a reduction in dose.

Dose reductions were made on a trial and error basis in patients who had improved generally over a number of weeks and who had had no recent episodes of 'breakthrough' pain. Reductions were also made after successful intrathecal nerve blocks in 5 patients and after chemotherapy or irradiation in several others. Nine of the 115 patients stopped receiving diamorphine. Three never required any again but the other 6 did when severe pain recurred; 4 after more than 4 months and 2 after about 3 weeks.

In summary, it was demonstrated that the longer the duration of treatment with diamorphine:

1 the slower the rate of rise in dose,
2 the longer the periods without a dose increase,
3 the greater the likelihood of a dose reduction,
4 the greater the likelihood of stopping medication.

Thus, when used as part of the pattern of total care, diamorphine may be used for long periods without concern about tolerance. Although

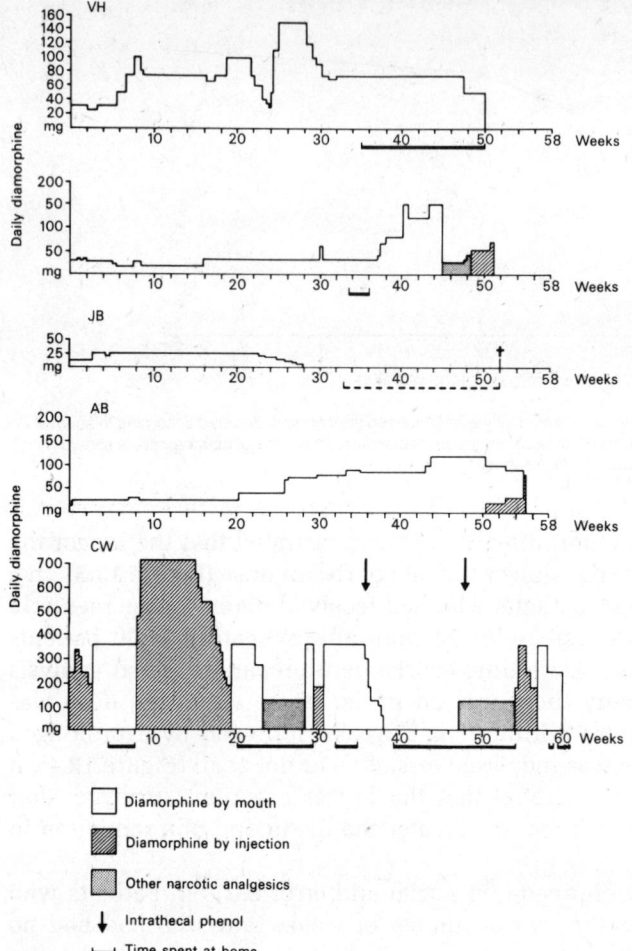

Figure 13.4 Dose time charts of 5 patients with advanced cancer. VH, VE, and AB received diamorphine up to the time of death; CW is still alive.
From Twycross and Wald, 1976 [7]

physical dependence almost certainly develops in most patients after several weeks of continuous treatment, this does not prevent an appropriate downward adjustment of dose.

We have not as yet analyzed the notes of a comparable group of patients receiving morphine. In fact, as diamorphine by mouth is but a pro-drug for morphine (*see* Chapter 10), it is difficult to imagine that a similar review could demonstrate anything except the same conclusions. Certainly, our experience with morphine since 1974 has not suggested anything else. Figures 13.5 to 13.7 summarize the morphine requirements of 12 patients, alive at the end of 1980. All had been receiving morphine for at least 6 months and, then or since, have completed at least one year of such treatment [15]. Experience with methadone, levorphanol, and phenazocine* suggests that the natural history of their long-term use in cancer patients is also similar to that of diamorphine.

'If A Cancer Patient Is Given Morphine, He Is Going To Die Soon'
'Morphine Has Been Prescribed, The Doctors Have Given Up'
Unfortunately, these remarks are frequently true in the context in which they are made. All too often, patients are denied satisfactory pain relief as the doctor muddles from one ineffective analgesic to another. In the 1980s a radiotherapist can still lament 'pain control is frequently poorly executed and often there is delay in exhibiting analgesics of the right calibre because of the fear of addiction' [16]. Only when moribund is the patient allowed the benefit of a strong analgesic such as morphine. In these circumstances, near to death, exhausted and demoralized, the use of morphine (usually parenteral) often appears to precipitate the patient's death. However, the use of oral morphine *earlier* when the patient is relatively well, but troubled by pain, should not carry the same connotation (Figure 13.8). There is plenty of circumstantial evidence to show that patients whose pain is relieved, albeit with morphine, do better than those whose rest and nutrition continues to be disturbed by continued pain.

'If A Patient Has Morphine At Home, It Will Get Stolen'
'Patients Will Use The Morphine To Commit Suicide'
The authors know of only one recorded instance of a patient's supply of morphine sulphate being misappropriated by another person. A patient who was short of money sold his 'Brompton Mixture' to a group of heroin addicts who found the mixture cheaper and longer lasting in its effects [17]. We know of no patient whose morphine was stolen by family, friends or intruders. We also know of no example of self-poisoning by a cancer patient in which the agent used was a solution of morphine sulphate. The incidence of suicide in cancer patients is, in any case, not above that of the general population; an overdose of tablets or non-drug method maybe but, so far, never morphine sulphate.

'A Kind of Living Death'
Many doctors and nurses have a markedly negative attitude towards the medicinal use of morphine. As one doctor wrote [18]:

'What about the inoperable cancer patient who may not die for months or a year, and yet who is suffering agonies from chronic pain . . .? Is a

* not available in the USA

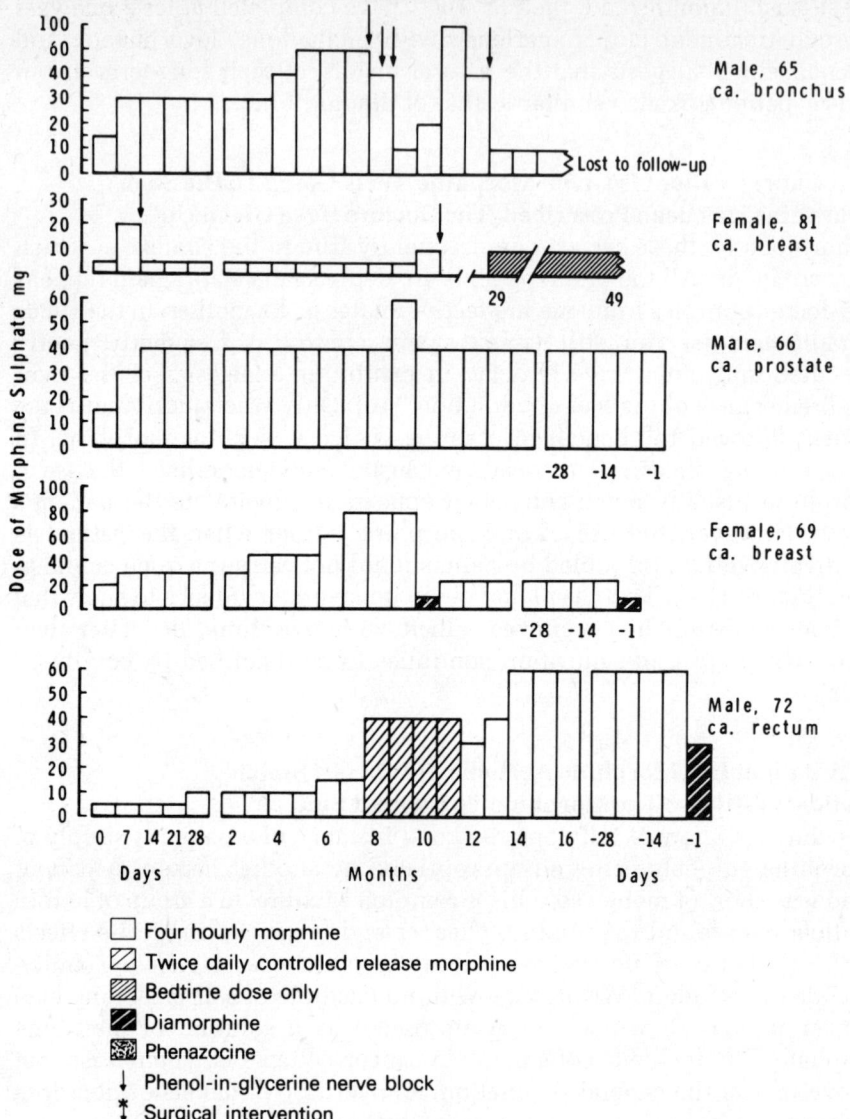

Figure 13.5 Dose-time charts of 5 patients who received oral morphine sulphate for more than 1 year. Requirements recorded at 7-day intervals for first month, monthly thereafter. Requirements during final month also recorded at 7-day intervals (−28 days = four weeks before death); final dose recorded relates to day before death.

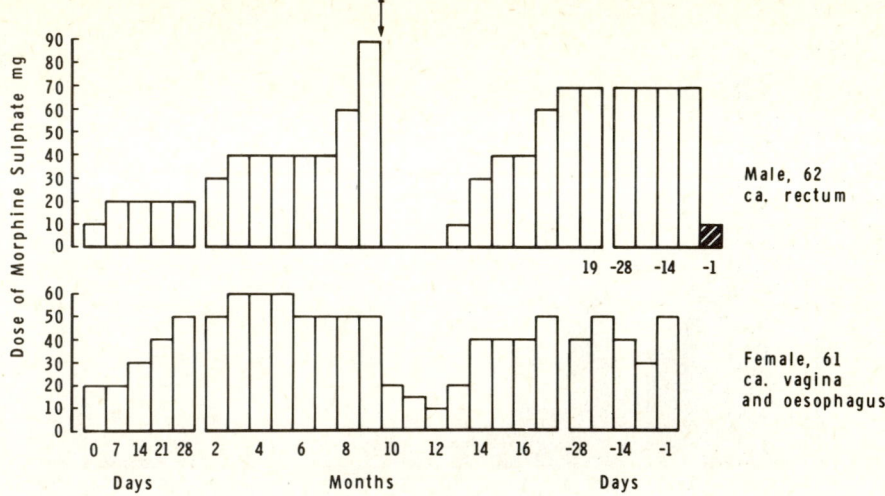

Figure 13.6 Dose-time charts of 2 patients who received oral morphine sulphate for more than 1 year. Explanation and key as for Figure 13.5. Surgical intervention in 62-year-old male: open thoracic spinothalamic tractotomy.

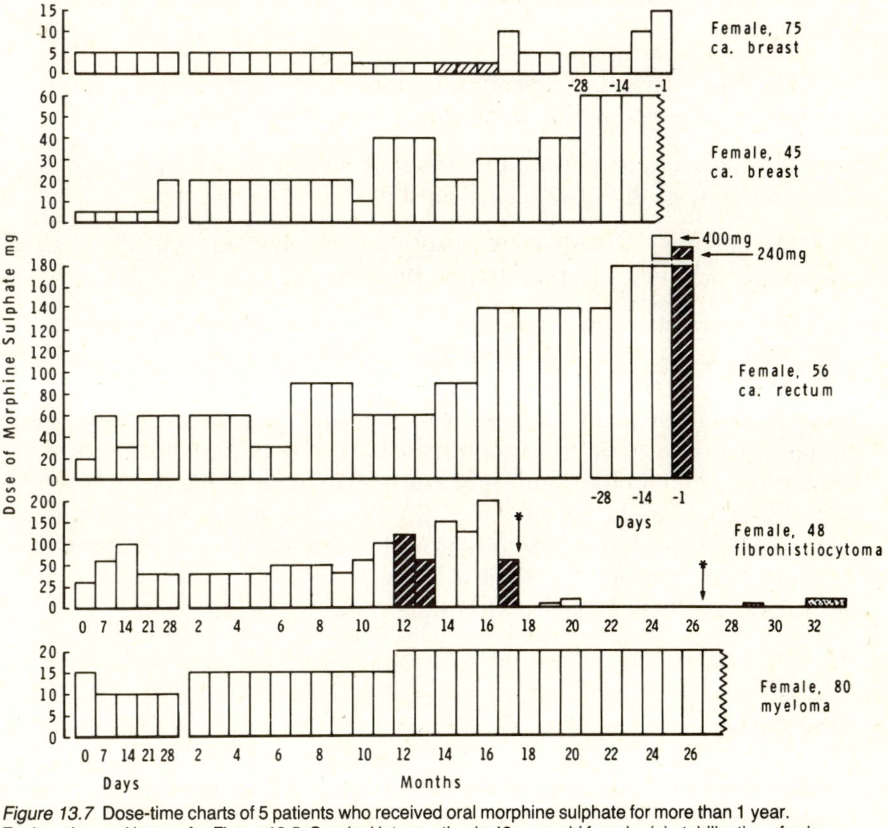

Figure 13.7 Dose-time charts of 5 patients who received oral morphine sulphate for more than 1 year. Explanation and key as for Figure 13.5. Surgical intervention in 48-year-old female: (a) stabilization of spine with Harrington's rods; (b) spinal cord transection.

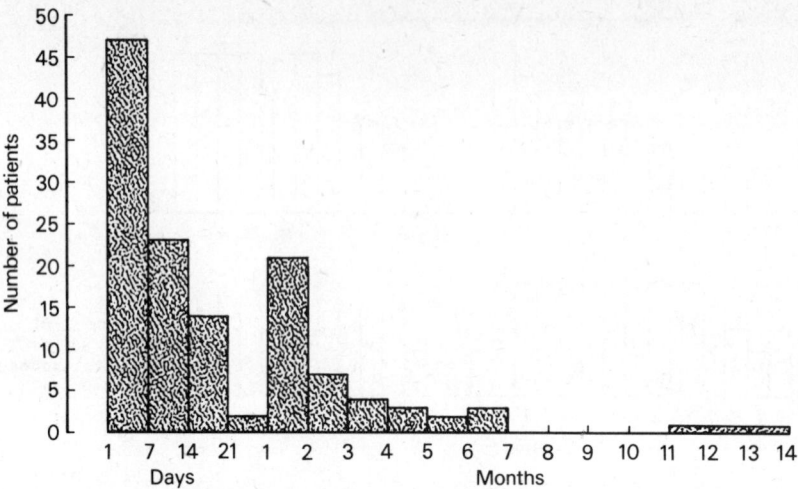

Figure 13.8 Histogram showing survival after commencing treatment with morphine sulphate in 129 patients admitted to Sir Michael Sobell House, Oxford, in 1978. As some patients received morphine for several weeks before referral to Sobell House, the data understates the survival in these patients. Median duration of treatment = 13 days 33 per cent of patients survived for more than 4 weeks; 12 per cent for more than 3 months.

doctor then justified in prescribing such drugs when he knows full well he will be sentencing his patient to a kind of living death?'

And although they might not express it so succinctly, many doctors still share the view of the physician who said [19]:

'I try to postpone giving morphia until the very end and am best pleased if the first dose of morphia is also the last.'

These views stem from ignorance about and misunderstanding of the correct use of morphine in cancer patients with pain. Indeed, the patients who are truly sentenced to 'a kind of living death' are the ones who are not prescribed an adequate analgesic regimen, like one man who was bed-ridden because of pain for 2 months. His wife then found him crawling around the room on his hands and knees searching for his gun which she had hidden for fear he would shoot himself. The correct use of morphine, unless delayed until the patient is almost moribund, enables the patient to live a far more normal life than otherwise would be possible. A visit to any good hospice will demonstrate the truth of this statement.

References

1 Swerdlow M. General analgesics used in pain relief: Pharmacology. *British Journal of Anaesthesia* 1967; **39**: 399–712.

2 Walsh TD, Baxter R, Bowman K and Leber B. High-dose morphine and respiratory function in chronic cancer pain. *Pain* 1981; Suppl. 1: 39.

3 Hanks GW, Twycross RG, and Lloyd JW. Unexpected complication of successful nerve block. *British Journal of Anaesthesia* 1980; **36:** 37–39.

4 Aherne GW, Piall EM, and Twycross RG. Serum morphine concentration after oral administration of diamorphine hydrochloride and morphine sulphate. *British Journal of Clinical Pharmacology* 1979; **8:** 577–580.

5 Bolund C. Personal communication.

6 McCaffery M. How to relieve your patient's pain fast and effectively with oral analgesics. *Nursing* 1980; **10:** 58–63.

7 Twycross RG and Wald SJ. Long-term use of diamorphine in advanced cancer in *Advances in Pain Research and Therapy, Vol. 1*, edited by Bonica JJ and Albe-Fessard DG. Raven Press, New York 1976, pp 653–661.

8 Twycross RG. *Studies on the use of diamorphine in advanced malignant disease.* DM Thesis, Oxford University 1976.

9 Expert Committee on Drug Dependence. *16th Report; Technical Report Series No. 407.* WHO Geneva 1979.

10 Expert Committee on Drug Dependence. *13th Report; Technical Report Series No. 287.* WHO Geneva 1964.

11 Porter J and Jick H. Addiction rare in patients treated with narcotics. *New England Journal of Medicine* 1980; **302:** 123.

12 WHO Expert Committee on Drug Dependence. *19th Report; Technical Report Series No. 526.* WHO Geneva 1973.

13 WHO Expert Committee on Drug Dependence. *20th Report; Technical Report Series No. 551.* WHO Geneva 1974.

14 Twycross RG. Clinical experience with diamorphine in advanced malignant disease. *International Journal of Clinical Pharmacology, Therapy and Toxicology* 1974; **9:** 184–198.

15 Twycross RG and Trueman T. Unpublished observations.

16 Neal FE. The patient with lung cancer in *The Dying Patient*, edited by Wilkes E. MTP Press, Lancaster 1982, pp 135–152.

17 Fischbeck KH, Mata M, D'Aquisto and Caronna JJ. Brompton mixture taken intravenously by a heroin addict. *Western Journal of Medicine* 1980; **133:** 80.

18 Bunyard P. Intractable pain—how treatable is it? *World Medicine* 1971; Dec. 1: 17.

19 Anonymous in *Postal Symposium No. 1: Management of Terminal Illness.* Smith and Nephew Pharmaceuticals 1972, p 29.

Chapter Fourteen

Alternative Strong Narcotic Agonists

In the majority of patients, morphine sulphate will be both efficacious and acceptable. There are, however, occasions when it is more appropriate to rationalize an existing narcotic regimen rather than change to morphine sulphate. Further, those patients who experience marked persistent intolerance to morphine need an alternative strong narcotic. It is necessary, therefore, to be familiar with a number of different strong narcotics. In this chapter, pethidine[1] and methadone will be discussed in some depth. The former because of its widespread misuse and the latter because, in a number of centres, it is the strong narcotic of choice.

It is possible to classify morphine-like drugs in a number of ways. As we saw in Chapter 6, the most basic classification relates to potency-efficacy and divides narcotics arbitrarily into weak and strong. An alternative classification is based on the agonist-antagonist potential of each narcotic in relation to morphine (*see* Chapter 15). This is important in situations where a patient may have access to more than one narcotic, or where a second drug is supplied for occasional 'as required' use. In this chapter, we consider a third way, namely, by chemical structure (Table 14.1).

If a patient appears to have persistent intolerance to morphine, an alternative that is chemically distinct should be used in the hope that this does not cause the same unwanted effect. Choice depends to a certain extent on the age of the patient and the dose of morphine that requires substitution (Table 14.2). In an elderly patient one would avoid levorphanol and methadone (vide infra). For a patient receiving more than

[1] meperidine (USA)

Table 14.1   Classification of narcotic analgesics according to chemical structure

1   Naturally occurring (opium alkaloid)
    codeine ⎫
    morphine ⎭   extracted from opium

2   Semisynthetic (opiates)
    dihydrocodeine
    oxycodone ⎫   obtained by relatively simple
    diamorphine* ⎬   structural modifications of the
    hydromorphone** ⎬   morphine or codeine molecule
    oxymorphone** ⎭
    buprenorphine

3   Synthetic (opioids)
    Morphinans ⎫
    pentazocine
    phenazocine*
    levorphanol

    Phenylpiperidines
    pethidine[1]   synthetic compounds with structural
    anileridine ⎬   resemblance to the whole or to a
    alphaprodine   part of the morphine molecule
    fentanyl

    Diphenylpropylamines
    dextropropoxyphene
    dipipanone*
    dextromoramide*
    methadone ⎭

* not available in the USA
** not available in Britain
[1] meperidine (USA)

30 mg of morphine sulphate 4-hourly, one might use phenazocine† or hydromorphone; for a patient receiving less, dipipanone, dextro-moramide or, in the USA, pethidine (meperidine).

Case History. A 48-year-old woman with far advanced breast cancer vomited intermittently when taking morphine sulphate in solution 30 mg 4-hourly. Cyclizine 50 mg 4-hourly and haloperidol 5 mg nocte helped much of the time but it was necessary to reduce intake to avoid exacerbating the vomiting. Metoclopramide did not help. Changing to phenazocine 5 mg 4-hourly maintained relief and the intermittent attacks of nausea and vomiting cleared up. She looked better and began to eat well.

Table 14.2 Strong narcotic analgesics: approximate oral equivalents to morphine sulphate

Analgesic	Proprietary name	Potency ratio with morphine sulphate[1]		Duration of action (hours)[2]
pethidine/meperidine	Demerol	1/8	1/12[3]	2–3
dipipanone*	in Diconal	1/2	1/3	3–5
papaveretum	Omnopon, Pantopon	2/3	1/2	3–5
oxycodone***[4]	in Percodan	1	2/3	3–5
	Percocet			
	Tylox (capsule)			
dextromoramide*	Palfium	(2)[5]	1.5	2–4
methadone	Physeptone, Dolophine	(3–4)[6]	2–3	6–8
levorphanol	Dromoran, Levo-dromoran	5	3	4–6
phenazocine*	Narphen	5	3	4–6
hydromorphone**	Dilaudid	6	4	3–4

* not available in the USA
** not available in Britain

[1] Multiply dose of stated drug by the potency ratio to determine the equivalent dose of morphine sulphate.

[2] Dependent to a certain extent on dose, often longer lasting in very elderly and those with considerable liver dysfunction.

[3] Column of figures in italics refer to approximate potency ratio with diamorphine (Heroin).

[4] Oxycodone is available in Britain only as oxycodone pectinate suppositories (q.v.).

[5] Dextromoramide single 5 mg dose is equivalent to morphine 15 mg (diamorphine 10 mg) in terms of peak effect but is generally shorter acting; overall potency rate adjusted accordingly.

[6] Methadone – single 5 mg dose is equivalent to morphine 7.5 mg (diamorphine 5 mg). It has a prolonged plasma half-life which leads to cumulation when given repeatedly. This means it is several times more potent when given regularly.

Case History. A man of 54 with widespread prostatic cancer began to itch when morphine sulphate 10 mg was prescribed. The itching cleared within 24 hours of changing to levorphanol 1.5 to 3 mg 4-hourly.

Pethidine

Drug portrait

Pethidine (meperidine; Demerol) is a synthetic narcotic analgesic (Figure 14.1). Despite substantial structural differences, its effects are generally similar to those of morphine. It also has atropine-like effects. Its central effects are mediated via CNS morphine receptors; peripherally it acts directly on smooth muscle. It is absorbed from all routes of administration, and is about one-third as potent by mouth as by SC or IM injection. The plasma half-life of a parenteral dose is about 3 to 4 hours. It is about one-eighth as potent as morphine. It cannot relieve such severe pain as morphine but in higher doses is considerably more effective than codeine. Pethidine is metabolized initially by hydrolysis or N-demethylation and then by conjugation. It is generally shorter acting than morphine, useful analgesia lasting some 2 to 4 hours.

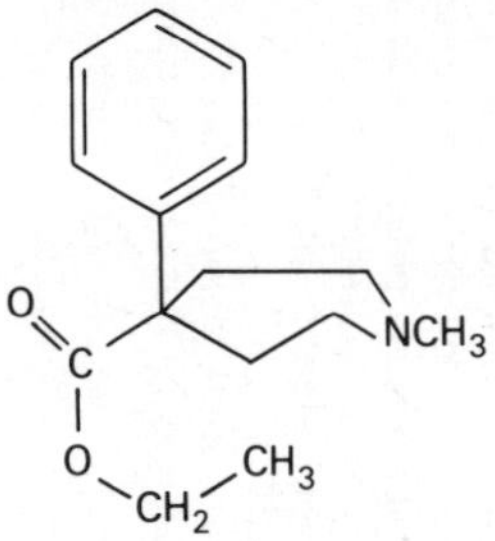

Figure 14.1 Chemical formula of pethidine (meperidine).

Pethidine differs from morphine in a number of ways (Table 14.3). It causes vomiting about as often as morphine. Equi-analgesic doses depress the respiratory centre to the same extent. Like morphine it may cause sedation.

Peak plasma concentrations are obtained after 1 to 2 hours after oral ingestion. Absorption from the alimentary canal is more variable than with morphine, making it a less reliable oral analgesic. It is generally shorter acting than morphine, useful analgesia lasting 2 to 4 hours. Pethidine is hydrolyzed to pethidinic acid which, in turn, is partially

Table 14.3 Pethidine[1] differs from morphine

1 Shorter duration of action
2 Ceiling effect
3 Not antitussive
4 Less constipating
5 Less smooth muscle spasm (e.g. biliary tract, sphincter of Oddi)
6 Pupils not constricted
7 Atropine-like side effects
8 Metabolism→norpethidine[1] overdose causes tremors, twitching, convulsions:
9 Interactions with phenobarbitone, chlorpromazine, monoamine oxidase inhibitors

[1] meperidine, normeperidine (USA)

conjugated. It is also N-demethylated to norpethidine which may then be hydrolyzed to norpethidinic acid and conjugated. About one-third of administered pethidine can be accounted for in the urine as N-demethylated derivatives. Little is excreted unchanged, though the amount is increased if the urine is acid.

Used correctly, pethidine can be an alternative to morphine for patients with an analgesic narcotic requirement of 30 mg or less morphine sulphate 4-hourly. Unfortunately, pethidine is often prescribed with little regard for its pharmacokinetics. Careful attention must be paid to analgesic equivalence (Table 14.2) and it usually needs to be given every 2 to 3 hours because of the short duration of its action. An order for 4- to 6-hourly administration condemns the average patient to intermittent pain for 12 out of every 24 hours.

It is difficult to persuade a patient to take more than 200 mg pethidine 3-hourly because of the number of tablets required. This is not such a problem in the patient who cannot take morphine and who is strongly motivated by the prospect of pain relief without unacceptable side effects. However, with pethidine the incidence of unwanted CNS effects, namely, tremor, twitching, agitation and convulsions, increases considerably at doses above 200 to 300 mg 3-hourly. These are caused by cumulation of the toxic metabolite, norpethidine. The norpethidine phenomenon together with compliance difficulties means that there is, in practice, a ceiling to pethidine's efficacy. In this way it resembles a weak rather than a strong narcotic. It is not a complete alternative to morphine.

Uses and Contraindications

Pethidine may be used as an alternative to morphine for the relief of severe acute pain and chronic cancer pain when the narcotic requirement is not above average. Pethidine is also commonly used for obstetric analgesia because of its shorter duration of action. It is often used in preference to morphine to relieve biliary colic because it causes less biliary tract spasm.

1   It is *not* used as an antidiarrhoeal.
2   It is *not* used as an antitussive.

Pethidine should not be given to patients with impaired renal function because of the likelihood of irritability, twitching and convulsions caused by cumulation of norpethidine [1]. Phenobarbitone and chlorpromazine enhance the production of norpethidine [2, 3].

Case History. A 42-year-old man who had osteogenic sarcoma of the sacrum received paracetamol[1] 650 mg PO and pethidine 150 mg IM every 2 to 3 hours. Plasma biochemistry indicated mild renal insufficiency. He gradually became more agitated and confused, and had two episodes of seizures. By then, he had received a total of 63 doses of pethidine. After the second seizure, the plasma pethidine concentration was 0.14 g/ml and the norpethidine concentration 0.67 g/ml, giving a norpethidine/pethidine ratio of 4.8:1. Pethidine therapy was discontinued and levorphanol and phenytoin were started. The seizures did not recur [1].

Case History. A 25-year-old woman with chronic renal failure received pethidine 75 mg IM about every 3 hours for deep painful ulcers on her legs. She also received azathioprine, imipramine, diazepam, haloperidol, and prednisolone. After 2 weeks of pethidine therapy she became very irritable and began to twitch. Her pethidine level was 0.28 g/ml and norpethidine level 1.8 g/ml, with a norpethidine/pethidine ratio of 6.4:1. Pethidine was discontinued and morphine started. Other drug treatment was unchanged. The twitching and irritability subsided over the course of the next 2 days [1].

Pethidine should not be given to a patient receiving a monoamine oxidase inhibitor, as this may cause respiratory depression, restlessness, hypotension, and even coma. This possibly relates to inhibition of the hepatic enzyme that demethylates pethidine.

Precautions

Adverse effects are similar to morphine. Like morphine, pethidine should be used with caution in patients with acute asthma, chronic obstructive airways disease, limited respiratory reserve, raised intracranial pressure, hepatic failure, myxoedema, cardiogenic or hypovolaemic shock. Extra care is necessary when it is given IV. Physical dependence occurs both in addicts and in patients following repeated regular use over several weeks. In these circumstances, as with morphine, treatment should be curtailed

[1] acetaminophen (USA)

gradually over several days rather than abruptly. Withdrawal symptoms tend to develop more rapidly, are generally not so intense and are shorter in duration than with morphine.

Dose Regimen
For acute severe pain, 100 to 150 mg IM repeated every 2 to 3 hours as necessary. It may be given IV in doses of 50 to 100 mg. The solution is irritant and should not be given SC. If used in terminal cancer, doses of 100 to 300 mg PO every 2 to 3 hours may be necessary to achieve adequate relief (Tables 14.2, 14.4).

Table 14.4   Available preparations of pethidine (meperidine)

	Preparation	Strengths
Sy	meperidine hydrochloride (USNF)	50 mg/5 ml (standard strength)
T	pethidine hydrochloride	50, 100 mg
I	pethidine hydrochloride (sterile solution in water)	50 mg/ml in 0.5, 1, 1.5, 2 ml ampoules also 10 and 30 ml multidose vials (USA) 100 mg/ml in 1 ml ampoules and 20 ml multidose vials (USA)

Sy = syrup;   T = tablet;   I = injection

Overdosage
Because norpethidine (plasma half-life = 15 hours) differs from pethidine in having greater excitant and less depressant effect, overdosage with pethidine may present a mixed picture of depression and excitation. When toxic doses of pethidine are given parenterally, the rate of absorption exceeds the rate of norpethidine formation, and the result is primarily one of CNS depression. When toxic doses are given orally, the rate of absorption does not exceed the capacity of the liver to convert pethidine to norpethidine. Hence the ratio of norpethidine increases, producing a picture of mixed stupor and convulsions. Treat with naloxone (as for morphine overdosage). Naloxone does not, however, stop or prevent norpethidine induced seizures; thus if convulsions occur before or after the correction of the respiratory depression, intravenous diazepam should also be given.

Anileridine

This is related to pethidine and parenterally has a comparable duration of effect, namely, 2 to 4 hours. Orally it has a more prolonged action. It is more consistent in its effect than pethidine [4]. At one centre it is used with methotrimeprazine (levomepromazine) as the analgesic combination of choice in patients with severe pain in association with head and neck cancers [5]. It is our experience that pain from such cancers is generally no more difficult to relieve than other neoplastic pains using oral morphine, an anxiolytic if appropriate, together with a corticosteroid. If there is residual stabbing or shooting pain, valproate or carbamazepine is also prescribed (see Chapter 16).

Methadone

Drug portrait

Methadone is a synthetic narcotic analgesic (Figure 14.2). Despite substantial structural differences its effects are generally similar to those of morphine. Its central effects are mediated via CNS morphine receptors; peripherally it acts directly on smooth muscle. It is absorbed well from all routes of administration and orally is about one-half as potent as by SC or IM injection. The plasma half-life of a single oral dose is about 15 hours; though when given regularly the half-life increases considerably, up to 2 to 3 days in some patients. This implies that problems from cumulation are likely to occur especially in the debilitated and elderly. Given in a single dose, methadone is marginally more potent than morphine but, in repeated dosage, it is several times more potent. Its effective analgesic range is the same as that of morphine. Methadone is metabolized chiefly in the liver to a variety of metabolites. Most of the drug or its degradation products are excreted by the intestines, and only a small part by the kidneys. It is generally longer acting than morphine, useful analgesia lasting some 6 to 8 hours.

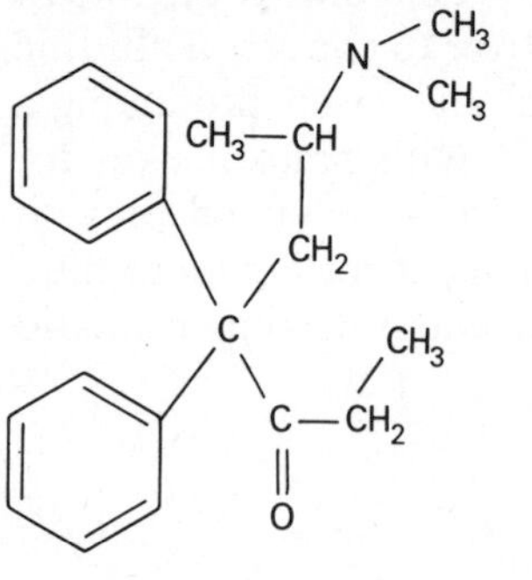

Figure 14.2 Chemical formula of methadone.

Methadone, like morphine, has no obvious ceiling effect. It is used by a number of centres as the strong analgesic of choice [6]. It differs from morphine in a number of ways (Table 14.5). The very long half-life seen in

Table 14.5 Methadone differs from morphine

Longer half-life
Cumulation when given regularly
No straightforward relationship between plasma level and degree of analgesia
Longer duration of action
Perhaps the strong narcotic of choice for children [11]

most patients taking methadone regularly is perhaps the most important difference to be borne in mind by prescribers. The relationship between plasma concentration and analgesia is not straightforward. Analgesia is maximal between 1 to 2 hours, whereas peak plasma levels occur after 4 to 6 hours. Moreover at 6 hours, when the plasma concentration is near maximal, pain relief has fallen to at least 25 per cent [7]. By contrast, the miotic effect of methadone correlates closely with plasma levels. It is not known whether the time course of unwanted effects bears a temporal relationship with methadone plasma levels.

Uses and Contraindications
Methadone may be used as an alternative to morphine for the relief of acute or persistent pain, or as an antitussive. It is also effective as an antidiarrhoeal, but is not normally used as such. Available preparations are listed in Table 14.6.

Table 14.6 *Available preparations of methadone hydrochloride*

	Preparation	Strengths
L	Methadone (BPC)	2 mg/5 ml
Sy	Methadone	1 mg/1 ml
T	Methadone (BP, USP)	2.5, 5, 10, 40 mg
I	Methadone (BP, USP) (sterile solution in water)	Strength variable: injection up to 50 mg/ml acceptable to licensing authorities

L = linctus; Sy = Syrup; T = tablet; I = injection

Because of the greater likelihood of cumulative toxicity, methadone should not be used:

1 in the elderly or demented;

2   in those with confusional symptoms;
3   in the presence of raised intracranial pressure;
4   in patients with 'organ failure', whether respiratory, hepatic or renal.

Case History. A 78-year-old female with carcinoma of the lung was given methadone, 3 mg orally every 6 hours for persistent chest pain. Instead of this, she took 12 mg orally every 6 hours. She was not receiving cytotoxic or radiation therapy. Twelve days later the patient was admitted to hospital with a history of increasing drowsiness. She was unresponsive with shallow slow respirations (3/min). Liver and kidney function studies were normal except for a mild elevation of the alkaline phosphatase level. She was treated with naloxone, 0.8 mg IV with an immediate response. She became alert and oriented with a respiratory rate of 16/minute. Over the next 24 hours she lapsed into a stuporous state several times. These episodes were readily reversed by giving 0.4 mg naloxone IV. She was discharged 3 days after admission. She and her family were given explicit instructions on the judicious use of methadone at the prescribed dose [8].

Case History. A 59-year-old female with carcinoma of the lung and chronic lung disease was seen in an outpatient oncology clinic 1 day prior to admission complaining of severe pain and a rash on the right buttock. The patient was found to have sacral herpes zoster. Because of the severe herpetic pain she was treated with methadone 10 mg orally every 4 to 6 hours. The patient began her methadone that evening at 5-hour intervals. After 3 doses she became weak and unable to move from her bed. On arrival at the clinic she was very drowsy and cyanosed. The patient had last received combination chemotherapy 5 weeks before and had been taking regular aminophylline. She was admitted to the hospital for evaluation of the altered mental status and respiratory insufficiency. Liver and kidney function studies were normal except for a slight elevation of transaminase. At the time of admission, naloxone 0.4 mg IV was administered. Respiratory rate and level of consciousness improved. Repeated doses of naloxone were required over the next 8 hours because of recurrence of respiratory depression. Further narcotics were withheld and the remainder of her hospital stay was uneventful. The patient was discharged 8 days after admission [8].

Precautions
Compared with morphine, greater care needs to be exercised when using methadone, certainly initially, and until a patient's response to it has been fully evaluated. The plasma concentration may not reach a steady state for 2 to 3 weeks in some patients. Particular care should be taken when psychotropic drugs are being administered concurrently.

Interactions

A number of important interactions between methadone and other drugs have been reported. Cimetidine inhibits the metabolism of methadone: this may lead to increasing drowsiness, or even coma [9]. Rifampicin, an antibiotic, speeds up methadone metabolism and may, on occasion, precipitate withdrawal symptoms [10].

Dose Regimen

It is not recommended for acute severe pain. In terminal cancer, the starting dose will depend on the patient's previous medication. As our own experience with methadone is limited, we record that of others, to demonstrate the variety of regimens that are currently being used.

Children. Methadone has been used successfully in a group of 23 children aged 1 to 17 (median 7) years with a variety of neoplastic conditions, for periods ranging from 4 days to more than 3 months. Most patients received the drug 6- or 8-hourly; three, 12-hourly. Doses ranged from 2.5 to 40 mg (median 10 mg). The majority (16 out of 23) also received hydroxyzine. No information is available as to the reasons for choice of timing. The children were well pain controlled and were not excessively drowsy [11].

Adults:
1   *4- to 6-hourly.* The more frequent dosage schedule tends to be used if patients have previously been taking analgesics 4-hourly, and have been changed to methadone because of inadequate relief. Six-hourly regimens tend to be the norm for patients previously on weak narcotics or who have been taking analgesics 'as required'.
2   *8- to 12-hourly.* At one centre methadone dosage is adjusted to achieve an 8- or 12-hourly regimen. Results are good and it has not been found necessary to give the drug more frequently.
3   *'Ad libitum'.* Patients with severe pain were advised to take a fixed dose (10 mg) when necessary. The need for flexibility was explained to them and fears about 'taking too much' allayed. After 5 to 7 days, the amount of methadone taken over the previous 2 to 3 days was noted. The patient was then advised how much to take every 8 or 12 hours.

In 14 patients, the total dose required during the first 24 hours varied between 30 and 100 mg (mean 44 mg). At the end of the first week, the average daily dose had fallen to 21.5 mg. Initial intervals between doses was short (3 to 7 hours) and increased to about 10 hours. Plasma concentrations of methadone increased 7-fold over 5 days. Eleven out of 14 had complete or virtually complete pain relief. Some patients experienced mild drowsiness. One patient discontinued medication because of vomiting [12]. In a series of 111 patients, treated over a 2-year period, the daily requirements ranged from 20 to 880 mg [13].

Other Diphenylpropylamines

Dipipanone
Dipipanone (Figure 14.3) is available, for oral use, in Britain as Diconal. This contains dipipanone 10 mg and cyclizine 30 mg. On a weight for

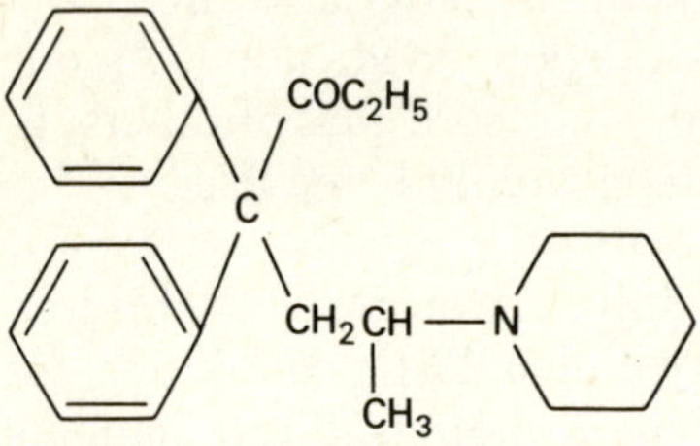

Figure 14.3 Chemical formula of dipipanone.

weight basis, it is approximately equipotent with papaveretum. There is no advantage in its use, unless an antihistamine antiemetic is also indicated. Even so, in patients requiring more than 2 tablets, the anticholinergic effects of the cyclizine tend to be troublesome, notably blurring of vision and dry mouth. Patients also complain of 'muzziness' and drowsiness.

Dextromoramide (Palfium)
Dextromoramide (Figure 14.4) is often prescribed as an alternative to morphine or diamorphine. For some patients, it seems to be a satisfactory

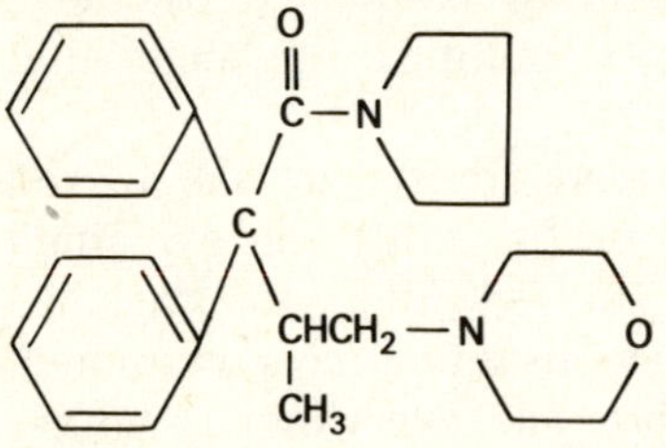

Figure 14.4 Chemical formula of dextromoramide.

substitute. By mouth it is more potent than morphine on a weight for weight basis. Pharmacokinetic data are scanty. Published data of a study involving one subject are available [14]. This study primarily concerned assay techniques for the analytical detection of drugs *in vivo* rather than pharmacokinetics in a clinical context. After a single 5 mg dose to 1 subject a biphasic plasma half-life was found for dextromoramide of

248

approximately 7 hours for the first phase and over 60 hours for the second phase. These results do not give sufficient information to draw general conclusions regarding plasma half-life in the therapeutic situation [15]. In any case, as with methadone, the plasma half-life of dextromoramide does not correlate closely with its duration of analgesic effect. Hospice doctors, including ourselves, have a strong clinical impression that the modal duration of action is some 2 to 3 hours [15–17]. A number of published uncontrolled studies quote 4 to 6 hours [18–20].

The phenomenon of the 'failed Palfium' patient is familiar to those looking after patients with advanced cancer. Typically, such a patient has severe or overwhelming pain and is taking 5 to 10 mg every hour, or 15 to 20 mg every 2 hours. Partial or even complete relief is obtained for up to 1.5 hours and for this reason the patient continues to take it. In short, dextromoramide appears to be a potent but relatively short-lasting analgesic. Not infrequently this results in a vicious 'switchback' effect which increases the likelihood of the pain becoming even more severe. As a general rule, dextromoramide should be used only as an 'as required' second strong analgesic. If used on its own regularly, its use must be closely monitored, particularly in relation to duration of effect.

Other Strong Narcotic Agonists

Semisynthetic
Oxymorphone (Numorphan)**
Oxymorphone is a semisynthetic opiate, obtained by a structural modification of the morphine molecule (Figure 14.5). A 1 mg dose of SC

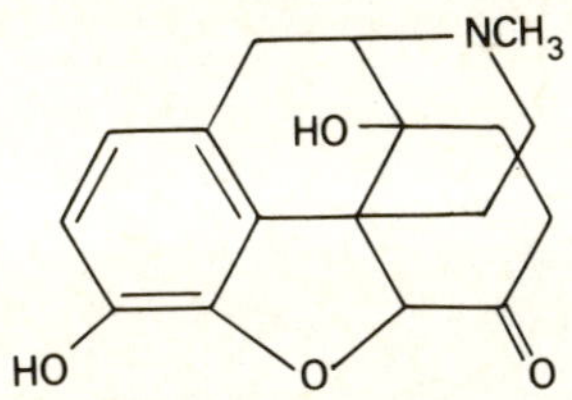

Figure 14.5 Chemical formula of oxymorphone.

oxymorphone is equi-analgesic with 10 mg of SC morphine [21]. It is at least as likely to produce unwanted effects, possibly more so. It is not available in an oral preparation. A 5 mg rectal suppository is, however, manufactured. Ten milligrams of oxymorphone per rectum is equivalent to 20 mg of oral morphine sulphate. If morphine suppositories are not readily available, oxymorphone is a useful alternative.

** not available in Britain

Hydromorphone (Dilaudid)

Hydromorphone is a semisynthetic opiate, a hydrogenated ketone of morphine (Figure 14.6). It is available as 1, 2, 3 and 4 mg tablets, in

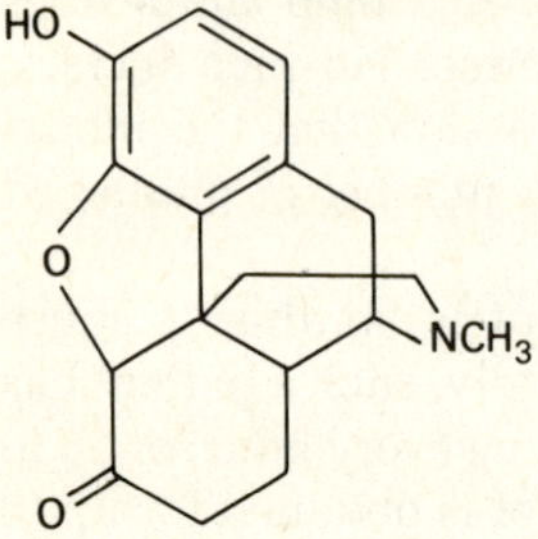

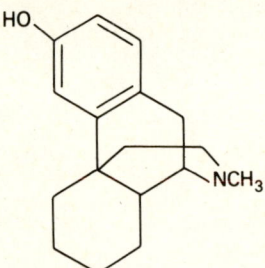

Figure 14.6 Chemical formula of hydromorphone.

ampoules containing 1, 2, 3 and 4 mg and as 3 mg rectal suppositories. The mean plasma half-life is about 4 hours. 1.5 mg IM is equivalent to 10 mg of IM morphine, both in analgesic potency and in propensity for unwanted effects. It is said to be less constipating than morphine. The analgesic effect lasts 3 to 5 hours, although it is generally slightly shorter acting than morphine. Its usefulness is hampered by lack of accurate information about relative potency on oral, parenteral and rectal administration.

Synthetic

Levorphanol (Figure 14.7)

This causes less nausea and vomiting than morphine and, after initial dose adjustment, will often provide relief for 6 hours. The longer duration

Figure 14.7 Chemical formula of levorphanol.

of action relates in part to lipid solubility and cumulation of the drug in body fat. Levorphanol has a plasma half-life of some 12 to 16 hours. As with methadone, this may result in excessive sedation in the elderly. We have used it successfully in a number of younger patients including one man who continued work as a construction site foreman for 9 months before he became too weak to continue.

Phenazocine (Figure 14.8)

This is as potent as levorphanol but, for oral use, is available only in 5 mg tablets; this is equivalent to 20 to 25 mg of oral morphine. The tablets are,

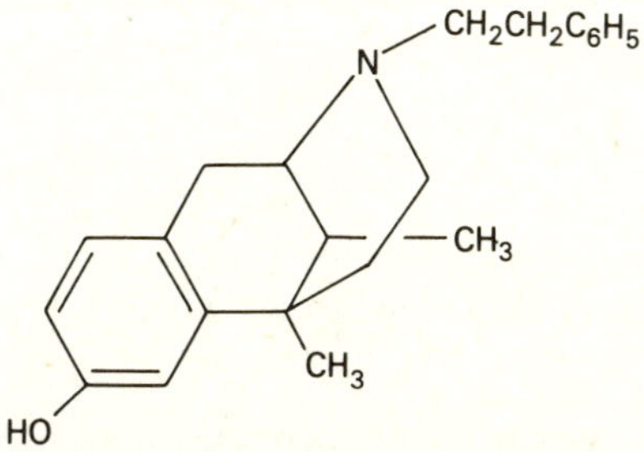

Figure 14.8 Chemical formula of phenazocine.

in fact, scored but it is not easy for a patient to break them. Although not stated on the data sheet, the standard tablets dissolve readily and are effective sublingually. Like all narcotics, phenazocine is bitter in taste. The incidence of vomiting with sublingual phenazocine is 5 per cent.

References

1 Szeto HH, Inturrisi CE, Houde RW, Saul S, Cheigh J and Reidenberg M. Accumulation of normeperidine, an active metabolite of meperidine in patients with renal failure or cancer. *Annals of Internal Medicine* 1977; **86:** 738–741.

2 Stambaugh JE, Wainer IW, Hemphill DM and Schwartz I. A potentially toxic drug interaction between pethidine (meperidine) and phenobarbitone. *Lancet* 1977; **1:** 398–399.

3 Stambaugh JE and Wainer IW. Drug interaction: meperidine and chlorpromazine, a toxic combination. *Journal of Clinical Pharmacology* 1981; **21:** 140–146.

4 Houde RW and Wallenstein SL. Minutes of 20th meeting committee on drug addictions and narcotics. Appendix B, 1959.

5 Evans RJ, Quoted in Mount BM. Narcotic analgesics in *The Continuing Care of Terminal Cancer Patients* edited by Twycross, RG and Ventafridda V. Pergamon Press, Oxford 1980, pp 97–116.

6 Bertler A, Eqelius N and Elwin CE. Coordinated activity at a university hospital of analgesic treatment in terminal care. Presented at *Symposium on Narcotic Analgesics*. Stockholm, November 1980.

7   Berkowitz BA. The relationship of pharmacokinetics to pharmacological activity; morphine, methadone and naloxone. *Clinical Pharmacokinetics* 1976; **1**: 219–230.

8   Ettinger DS, Vitale PJ and Trump DL. Important clinical pharmacological considerations in the use of methadone in cancer patients. *Cancer Treatment Reports* 1979; **63**: 457–459.

9   Foley KM. Personal Communication, 1982.

10 Kreek MJ, Garfield JW, Gutjahr CL and Giusti LM. Rifampin-induced methadone withdrawal. *New England Journal of Medicine* 1976; **294**: 1104–1106.

11 Martinson IM, Armstrong GD, Geis DP, Anglim MA, Gronseth EC, Macinnis H, Cersey JH and Nesbit ME. Home care for children dying of cancer. *Pediatrics* 1978; **62**: 106–113.

12 Jakobsson PA, Ginman C, Hanson J, *et al*. Clinical evaluation of methadone treatment in cancer pain. Presented at *Symposium on Narcotic Analgesics*. Stockholm, November 1980.

13 Breivik H and Rennemo F. Clinical evaluation of combined treatment with methadone and psychotropic drugs in cancer patients. *Acta Anaesthesiologica Scandinavica* 1982; **26** (Suppl. 74): 135–140.

14 Caddy B and Idowu R. Oxydative determination of dextromoramide (Palfium) in body fluids. *Analyst* 1979; **104**: 328–333.

15 Judd AT, Tempest SM and Clarke IMC. The anaesthetist and the pain clinic: dextromoramide analgesia. *British Medical Journal* 1981; **282**: 75–76.

16 Lamerton RC. Cancer patients dying at home. The last 24 hours. *Practitioner* 1979; **223**: 813–817.

17 Wilkes E. Some problems in cancer management. *Proceedings of the Royal Society of Medicine* 1974; **67**: 1001–1005.

18 Flavell-Matts SG. Dextromoramide analgesia in the acute general medical patient. *Practitioner* 1962; **188**: 524–526.

19 Kay B. A study of strong coral analgesics; the relief of postoperative pain using dextromoramide, pentazocine and bezitranide. *British Journal of Anaesthesia* 1973; **45**: 623–628.

20 Kolodny AL. Dextromoramide (Palfium) a new synthetic analgesic for relief of acute and chronic pain. *Antibiotic Medicine and Clinical Therapy* 1960; **7**: 695–701.

21 Swerdlow M. General Analgesics used in pain relief: pharmacology. *British Journal of Anaesthesia* 1967; **39**: 699–712.

Chapter Fifteen

Narcotic Agonist-Antagonists Narcotic Antagonists

Since the elucidation of the molecular structure of morphine in 1925, many attempts have been made to produce compounds which would share the analgesic efficacy of morphine but not the unwanted side

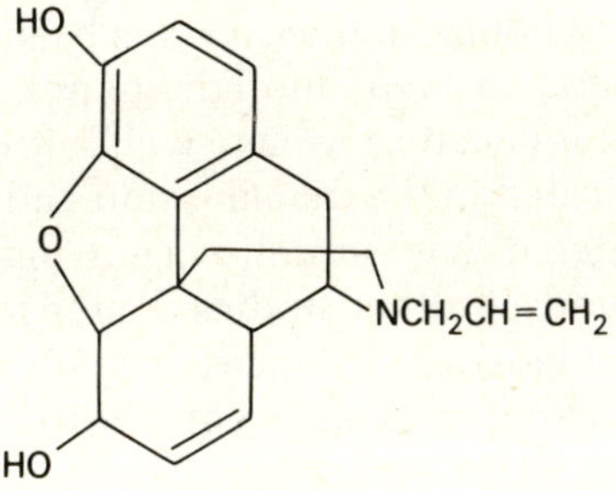

Figure 15.1 Chemical formula of nalorphine.

effects. In the 1950s, attention focused on nalorphine, the N-allyl derivative of morphine (Figure 15.1) Nalorphine was shown to have the following characteristics:

1 It is as potent an analgesic as morphine [1].
2 It causes disturbing psychotomimetic side effects in most patients.
3 When given after morphine, nalorphine reverses the effects of the previously administered drug.
4 Above a certain dose, nalorphine is *less* antagonistic to morphine [2].
5 Its capacity for producing physical dependence is much less than morphine.

6 In physically dependent animals and humans, the withdrawal syndrome associated with the use of nalorphine differs in certain respects from that seen with morphine.

The partial dissociation of analgesic and dependence-inducing properties seen in nalorphine acted as a spur to further research. The findings also suggested that two distinct receptors exist, one for morphine and the other for the agonist effects of nalorphine [3]. Nalorphine was seen as a competitive antagonist at the morphine receptor but an agonist at the second one, the so-called nalorphine receptor. Subsequent studies with a variety of compounds have extended this concept. A total of 5 opiate receptors have been postulated, of which perhaps 3 are noteworthy [3].

μ (mu)   —for morphine and responsible for supraspinal analgesia, feelings of wellbeing, morphine-type physical dependence, miosis and respiratory depression.

$\varkappa$ (kappa) —for ketocyclazocine and responsible for spinal analgesia, sedation, anaesthesia, and nalorphine-type physical dependence.

σ (sigma) —for SKF 10047 (N-allylnorphenazocine) and responsible for dysphoric and psychotomimetic effects, mydriasis and respiratory stimulation.

The distribution of density of the opiate receptors in the CNS has been mapped by means of *in vitro* binding [4] and *in vivo* autoradiographic techniques [5]. The sites of maximum receptor density correlate well with those areas of the CNS that have been implicated in the transmission and perception of pain. Moreover, it was considered that naturally occurring receptors must have naturally occurring ligands. Further studies demonstrated the presence of endogenous morphine-like substances, namely, β-endorphin and the enkephalins [6]. Naloxone acts as a competitive antagonist at all three receptors.

Agonist-Antagonists

The term 'agonist-antagonist' is used to describe narcotic drugs that have agonistic (morphine-like) effects when given alone but which are antagonistic when given with or after morphine (or another agonist). There are two main groups of agonist-antagonists:

1 of nalorphine type,
2 of morphine type.

Morphine type agonist-antagonists are *not* antagonist in low doses. It is for this reason that they are also called partial agonists. Nalorphine type agonist-antagonists are antagonistic at any dose. *They also antagonize*

Table 15.1   Extended classification of analgesics

1   NON-NARCOTICS
aspirin
paracetamol[1]
nefopam*

2   NARCOTIC AGONISTS

3   NARCOTIC AGONIST-ANTAGONISTS

	NARCOTIC AGONISTS	MORPHINE TYPE	NALORPHINE TYPE	OTHER
Weak	codeine dextropropoxyphene ethoheptazine oxycodone†	profadol propiram	pentazocine	
Strong	morphine diamorphine* methadone levorphanol hydromorphone**	buprenorphine	nalbuphine butorphanol	meptazinol

[1] acetaminophen (USA)
* not available in the USA
** not available in Britain
† see page 157 for comment

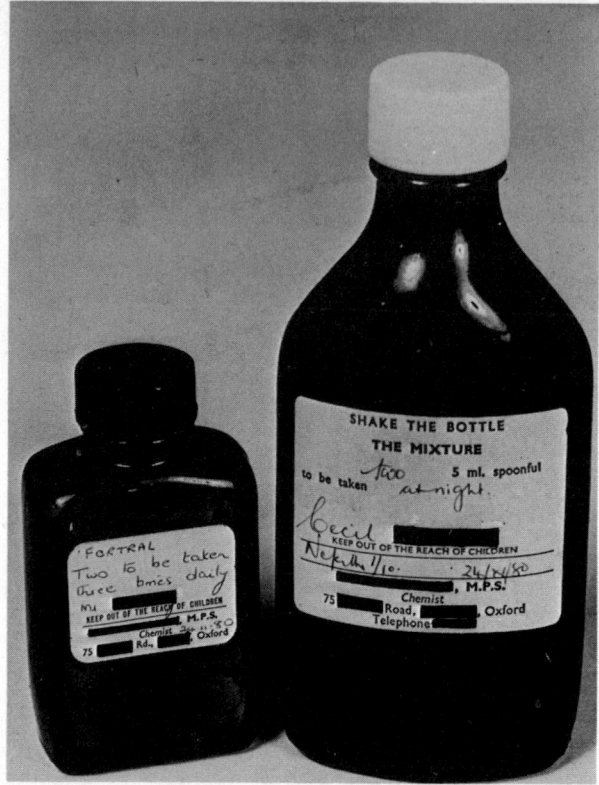

Figure 15.2 An example of concurrent prescription of a narcotic agonist (Nepenthe Oral Solution; a proprietary preparation of morphine hydrochloride) and an agonist-antagonist (Fortral/Talwin; pentazocine). If taken in conjunction, the latter will antagonize the former to a variable extent, depending on the relative doses. In this case, at least the Nepenthe was intended for night use and presumably to be taken several hours after the last dose of pentazocine.

partial agonists. It is important, therefore, to be aware which type of narcotic is being prescribed (Table 15.1). To administer narcotics of different types to the same patient could lead to *more* pain and, possibly, withdrawal symptoms (Figure 15.2).

Efficacy, Potency and Affinity
In order to understand the mode of interaction between morphine and the agonist-antagonists of morphine-type, it is necessary to bear in mind the distinction between *efficacy* and *potency*. A more potent drug is one that achieves the same effect with a smaller quantity. Some compounds which are very potent in low doses, have a relatively low intrinsic upper limit or 'ceiling' effect. Thus, a more potent drug with a low ceiling effect will, at higher doses, have less *efficacy* (that is, will be less effective) than a less

potent drug without a ceiling effect. In this situation, the less potent drug will be more efficacious when higher doses are used.

Affinity is a measure of potency and describes the strength of the attachment of a drug to its receptor. The greater the affinity, the more potent the drug. Drugs with a high affinity displace drugs with less affinity by competing for the receptors.

Morphine Type Agonist-Antagonists

Drug portrait
Morphine type agonist-antagonists (partial agonists) have subjective and physiological effects similar to morphine. They do *not* cause psychotomimetic reactions. Characteristically, they have a plateau or 'ceiling' effect. They also have a greater affinity for opiate receptors than morphine. They substitute effectively for low doses of morphine both for pain relief and in the prevention of withdrawal symptoms. Their effect is not additive as they act by competitive displacement at receptor sites. When used in conjunction with higher doses of morphine, pain relief may be reversed and withdrawal phenomena precipitated. This is because no more agonistic substitution is possible above their ceiling effect, but displacement of morphine continues. In view of the considerable receptor affinity of morphine type agonist-antagonist, the addition of a nalorphine type drug is likely *not* to have any noticeable effect. On the other hand, if a morphine type agonist-antagonist is given to a patient after a nalorphine type drug, perceptible antagonism may occur.

Three drugs currently come into this group: profadol, propiram and buprenorphine. Profadol is a congener of pethidine[1]. In single dose parenteral studies it is between one-half and one-fifth as potent as morphine [7]. Propiram is a congener of phenampromide. In two separate studies, one when it was given orally and the other by injection, it was estimated to have a potency ratio with parenteral morphine of 1:11 [7].

Buprenorphine

Buprenorphine is a derivative of the inactive opium alkaloid thebaine (Figure 15.3). It is a close analogue of etorphine (used in veterinary medicine) and diprenorphine. It is a strong narcotic with a relatively low ceiling effect. It is well absorbed sublingually and tablets are made for use by this route. The dose-response curve for subjective effects is bell-shaped; doses of 1.2 mg produce less effect than 0.6 mg [8]. Morphine-like

[1] meperidine (USA)

257

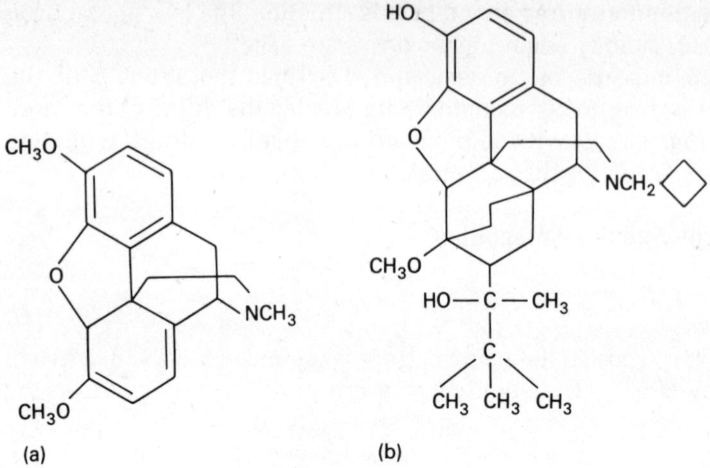

Figure 15.3 Chemical formula of (a) thebaine and (b) buprenorphine.

effects are maximal at a dose of about 1 mg subcutaneously. The plasma half-life is about 3 hours after IM injection. Onset of action is about 30 minutes, and peak effect after 3 hours (morphine = 1 hour). The duration of useful effect is some 6 to 9 hours (morphine = 3 to 5 hours). Most patients are satisfactorily controlled on an 8-hourly regimen. Subjective and physiological effects are generally similar to morphine, including drowsiness when used postoperatively or during the first few days of chronic use. There are, however, two important differences:

1 Vomiting is more common after sublingual than after IM administration.
2 Naloxone does not reverse the effects of buprenorphine when used in doses of 0.4 to 0.8 mg IV.

It is also said that buprenorphine does not constipate. We disagree: in our experience, when given regularly, patients usually require a laxative. Studies in animals have shown that buprenorphine slows intestinal transit in those species investigated [9].

One man who took 40 0.4 mg tablets sublingually had unimpaired respiratory function [8]. He recovered uneventfully after 24 hours and the only symptoms referable to buprenorphine were vomiting and drowsiness. Serious respiratory depression is unlikely to occur in clinical practice. If serious respiratory depression occurred as a result of self-poisoning, the use of massive doses of naloxone (up to 16 mg) would be necessary, and assisted ventilation considered. The manufacturers recommend the use of doxapram, a respiratory stimulant, by injection or infusion (*see* page 268).

In a study specifically aimed at assessing dependence liability, it was shown that tolerance can be induced by increasing the dose. When medication was stopped suddenly after receiving a total daily dose of 8 mg for two weeks, withdrawal symptoms typical of physical dependence occurred but not until the *fourteenth* day. It is generally considered to have a low abuse potential and is not a controlled drug in countries where it is available.

Sublingual administration allows absorption directly into the systemic circulation. The 'first-pass' effect (hepatic metabolism) seen after ingestion from the stomach or intestine is avoided. As a result buprenorphine is almost as potent sublingually as by injection; 0.4 mg is equipotent with 0.3 mg IM.

By injection, buprenorphine is 30 to 40 times more potent than morphine, and longer lasting. It would seem reasonable to assume that, compared with orally administered morphine, sublingual buprenorphine is some 60 to 80 times more potent. Thus, when changing from an unsatisfactory buprenorphine regimen to morphine sulphate, as a rule of thumb, the total daily dose of buprenorphine should be *multiplied by 100* and converted into a convenient 4-hourly regimen. Fortunately, although adding buprenorphine to morphine may lead to partial antagonism of the latter, changing from buprenorphine to high dose morphine does not result in a period of uncontrolled pain. The buprenorphine is already firmly attached to the opiate receptors and morphine substitutes for this as and when the buprenorphine becomes detached and is metabolized. As always, after a change from one narcotic to another, advice must be given to the patient and his family about what to do if the new medicine appears not to be as good as the old. In this circumstance, the patient should be advised to repeat the dose of morphine after 1 to 2 hours if necessary, and to increase subsequent regular doses by 50 per cent.

In one long-term open study, 70 patients with chronic pain (two-thirds with cancer) received sublingual buprenorphine [10]. The total daily dose ranged from 0.4 to 4 mg. While 10 per cent experienced little or no benefit, over half reported good or complete relief. Despite this, 'most patients' (number unspecified) withdrew from the study because of unwanted effects. Thus, in only an unpredictable minority did sublingual buprenorphine provide effective analgesia without unacceptable side effects. This suggests that the place of buprenorphine in the relief of cancer pain and chronic pain of non-malignant origin is limited. We have used it successfully on a few occasions. It should not be used in patients requiring more than 30 mg of morphine sulphate PO 4-hourly.

One mg is the maximum effective dose for subjective effects when given parenterally: higher doses are *less* effective. Although a comparable bell-shaped dose-response curve has not been demonstrated for analgesia, this remains a possibility and poses a number of practical questions:

1   What is the maximum effective *single* sublingual dose?
2   What is the maximum effective *daily* sublingual dose?
3   What is the optimum time interval between doses?
4   What do patients on maximum, or near maximum, doses do if they get breakthrough pain or a sudden severe new pain?

Although buprenorphine may well become the drug of choice for postoperative pain, it is clearly not ideal in a number of other situations. Its use in obstetrics is contraindicated in the absence of a specific, effective antagonist to treat neonatal respiratory depression. Similarly, in far advanced cancer, there are too many unanswered questions surrounding buprenorphine to recommend its general use.

Nalorphine Type Agonist-Antagonists

Drug Portrait
Nalorphine type agonist-antagonists are said to act as competitive antagonists at the mu receptor and as agonists at the kappa and sigma receptors. Analgesics of this type produce dysphoric and psychotomimetic effects (Table 15.2). Characteristically, they have a plateau or 'ceiling' effect. Individual drugs vary considerably in their relative agonist and antagonist properties. After a single dose, the dominant subjective and physiological effects are essentially morphine-like. On chronic administration they produce physical dependence and, if naloxone is administered, an abstinence syndrome is precipitated. They themselves are able to precipitate an abstinence syndrome in patients dependent on morphine or another agonist. They should not be used in conjunction with a narcotic agonist, nor with morphine type agonist-antagonists.

Table 15.2   Narcotic-induced psychotomimetic side-effects

Dysphoria
Feelings of unreality
Depersonalization
Vivid daydreams
Nightmares
Hallucinations
Delusions
Panic

Pentazocine

Pentazocine was the first drug of this class to be introduced for clinical use (Table 15.3). It is the N-allyl derivative of phenazocine (Figure 15.4).

Table 15.3   Pentazocine-containing preparations

Available preparations in Britain			
T	Fortral	pentazocine hydrochloride	25 mg
C	Fortral	pentazocine hydrochloride	50 mg
Supp	Fortral	pentazocine lactate	50 mg
T	Fortagesic	pentazocine hydrochloride	15 mg
		paracetamol[1]	500 mg
Available preparations in the USA			
T	Talwin 50	pentazocine hydrochloride	50 mg
T	Talwin Co.	pentazocine hydrochloride	12.5 mg
		aspirin	325 mg

[1] acetaminophen (USA)
T = tablet; C = capsule; Supp = suppository

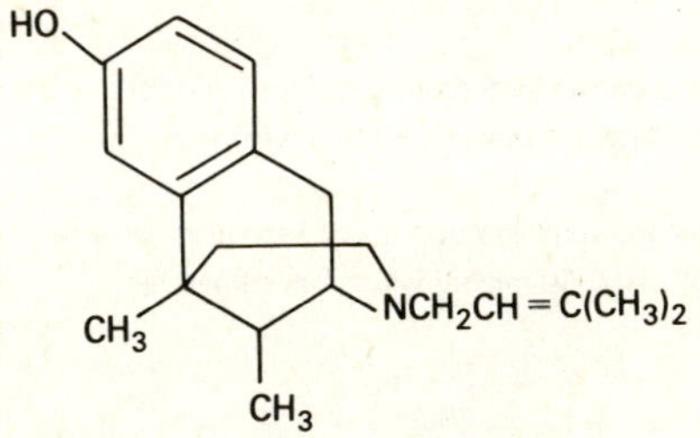

Figure 15.4 Chemical formula of pentazocine.

Pentazocine has been characterized as a weak competitive antagonist at the *mu* receptors, a strong *kappa*-agonist and a *sigma*-agonist [3]. Pentazocine is a strong analgesic by injection, some 50 to 60 mg is equivalent to 10 mg of IM morphine. By mouth, however, it should be regarded as a weak narcotic. In a single dose study in cancer patients, 50 mg of pentazocine was found to be less potent than two tablets of Codis (codeine phosphate + aspirin) or of Distalgesic[2] (dextropropoxyphene + paracetamol[1]) [11]. Further, considering there are safer alternatives, the proportion of patients experiencing nalorphine-like psychotomimetic effects is unacceptably high. In hospital patients who received pentazocine for acute pain including postoperatively, the incidence was between 7 and 10 per cent [12]. The incidence in patients with terminal cancer is almost

[1] acetaminophen (USA)
[2] 1 tablet Wygesic (USA) equivalent to 2 tablets Distalgesic (Britain)

Dr A J Herring
Dr J L Carter
Dr M Hilton

38 WALKER STREET
OXFORD
OX8 3NJ
Tel: 676584

22 March 1982

Dr C F McMichael
Sir Michael Sobell House
The Churchill Hospital
Headington
Oxford

Dear Dr McMichael

Mrs Hilda Jones
13 Rectory Road, Oxford

Very many thanks for accepting this lady who had a polya partial gastrectomy in July 1980 for Ca. stomach. Since then she has been quite well really, despite her anaemia, until 3 weeks ago.

When I saw her yesterday, she was complaining of nausea, melaena and back pain. I stopped her iron tablets and prescribed codeine phosphate 30 mg qid and fortral 50 mg qid which has helped her.

Unfortunately, her husband can no longer cope.

Yours sincerely

John Carter

JOHN L CARTER

Figure 15.5 A letter of referral from a family practitioner, showing that agonists and agonist-antagonists are still sometimes prescribed simultaneously. Letter heading and patient's name and address have been changed to preserve anonymity.

certainly higher because of other factors which are themselves potential causes of such symptoms. Although these side effects tend to be dose-related, they have occurred after even small doses by mouth. Psychotomimetic effects occur occasionally with *all* narcotic analgesics, including morphine and diamorphine. The incidence in relation to the more agonistic drugs is of the order of 1 to 2 per cent.

The potential value of pentazocine must be offset against its potential both for psychotomimetic effects and its ability to antagonize narcotic agonists. It is relatively common for patients to have 2 or 3 different weak narcotic-containing preparations in their possession at one time. Sometimes the patient is advised to alternate preparations, taking something every 2 hours; or the patient has a second preparation for 'as required' supplementary use. To avoid concurrent use of pentazocine and narcotic agonists (Figure 15.5), we would suggest that pentazocine should not be used at all in the management of cancer pain. Weak narcotic agonists, such as codeine and dextropropoxyphene, are the drugs of choice for pain of moderate intensity. Because of an increasing number of reports of abuse of pentazocine, this drug is now classified as a Schedule IV substance under the Controlled Substances Act in the USA. Some States have imposed stricter controls.

Nalbuphine

Nalbuphine is closely related to the pure antagonist naloxone and to the narcotic agonist oxymorphone** (Figure 15.6). Nalbuphine is slightly

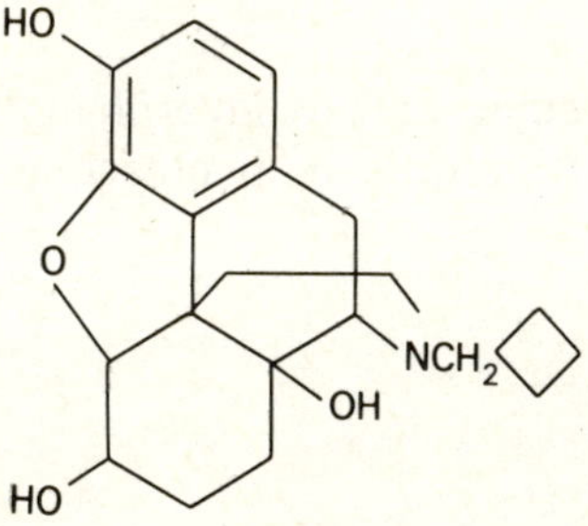

Figure 15.6 Chemical formula of nalbuphine.

more potent than morphine. Its pharmacological profile in man resembles pentazocine, although it has less propensity for psychotomimetic effects. The duration of effect is 3 to 6 hours [13]. Nalbuphine is given SC, IM and IV and it is available in ampoules containing 10 mg/ml.

The abrupt withdrawal of nalbuphine after prolonged administration causes opiate-like withdrawal symptoms. Nalbuphine is one-quarter as potent as nalorphine in precipitating withdrawal symptoms in morphine dependent subjects (Table 15.4), though it suppresses abstinence phenomena in subjects dependent on smaller doses of morphine. These apparently paradoxical actions are explained on the basis of differential affinity for the main opiate receptors. It is not presently classified under the Controlled Substances Act in the USA.

** not available in Britain

Table 15.4 Withdrawal phenomena in morphine dependent subjects

Mild		Moderate	
Yawning		Dilated pupils	develop
Lacrimation	develop	Gooseflesh	after
Rhinorrhoea	after	Tremor	24 to 36 hours
Perspiration	8 to 16 hours	Anorexia	
Irritability			
Severe		Prolonged	
Vomiting		Insomnia	
Diarrhoea		Restlessness	
Weight Loss		Hyperpnoea	
Twitching		Blood pressure ↑	
Cramps		Pyrexia	

Maximum after 2 to 3 days
Duration up to 2 weeks

Butorphanol

Butorphanol is structurally related to pentazocine and to levorphanol (Figure 15.7). It has a similar pharmacological profile to pentazocine

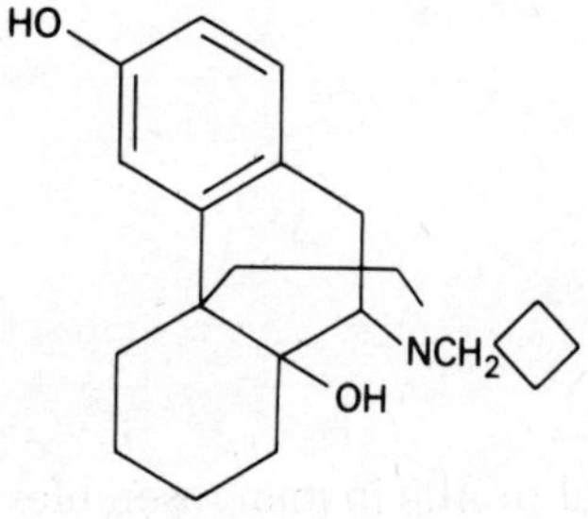

Figure 15.7 Chemical formula of butorphanol.

although it is considerably more potent. Butorphanol neither precipitates nor suppresses abstinence in morphine dependent subjects. Naloxone precipitates a moderately severe withdrawal syndrome.

Postoperatively butorphanol is 5 to 8 times more potent than morphine. In cancer, the potency ratio is about 4:1. This suggests that it is some 20 times more potent than pentazocine. Direct comparisons of the 2 agents support this, and give a range from 15 to 23 times [13]. The plasma half-life is 2.5 to 3.5 hours and the duration of effect after IM injection is 3 to 4 hours [14]. It is metabolized primarily to the inactive hydroxybutorphanol which is mostly excreted in the urine. Some is eliminated in the bile. It acts promptly and the only significant side effect is drowsiness. In cancer patients, there is a high incidence of psychotomimetic effects; 6 out of 18 after 4 mg and 6 out of 32 after 2 mg (by injection) [14]. It is available for parenteral use in solutions 1 mg/ml and 2 mg/ml. Butorphanol is not classified under the Controlled Substances Act in the USA.

Meptazinol*

Meptazinol is a synthetic analgesic derived from hexahydroazepine (Figure 15.8). Postoperatively, 100 mg IM meptazinol is as effective as

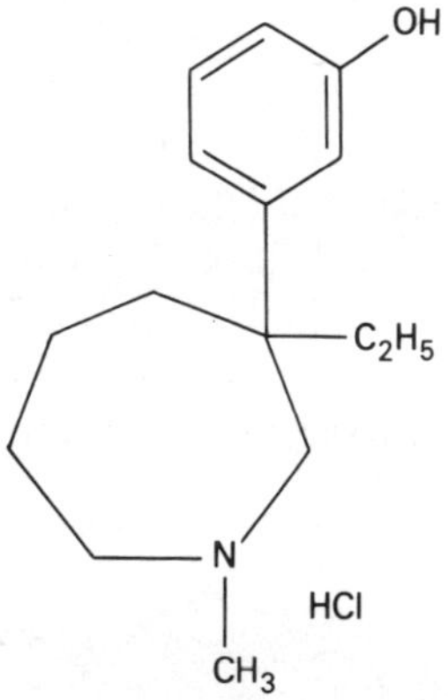

Figure 15.8 Chemical formula of meptazinol.

20 mg of IM papaveretum [15]. It is, however, shorter acting; the duration of useful effect being less than 3 hours in many patients. Like pethidine, meptazinol does not effect pupil diameter. It has remarkably little effect on respiration, nor does it cause constipation. Meptazinol precipitates withdrawal phenomena in animals, including primates, and reverses morphine-induced respiratory depression [16]. In complete contrast to morphine and pentazocine, meptazinol *potentiates* the electrically-induced twitch of an isolated guinea pig ileum [16]. Similarly, in other morphine sensitive tissues such as the mouse and the rat vas deferens, meptazinol has effects opposite to those of morphine and pentazocine. Meptazinol-induced analgesia is almost completely reversed by naloxone, although higher doses are required than are necessary to antagonize the effects of narcotic agonists. The analgesic effect of meptazinol in mice is also antagonized by low doses of centrally acting anticholinergic drugs such as hyoscine. This suggests that the analgesic properties of meptazinol may be mediated in part by central cholinergic mechanisms [17]. Work is currently under way to test this hypothesis.

Radioligand binding studies show that meptazinol has only low affinity

* not available in the USA

265

for opiate receptors. In contrast, in rodents, high affinity sites for meptazinol were identified in the cerebral cortex and the spinal cord [17]. This binding is not affected by morphine, buprenorphine or naloxone. In view of the fact that naloxone reverses meptazinol-induced analgesia, this is surprising. Unlike opiate receptors, meptazinol binding sites lack stereospecificity.

In summary, meptazinol is an exciting novel drug. It is both a narcotic antagonist and an analgesic, but the latter effect is not exclusively mediated via opiate receptors.

Antagonists

A pure antagonist is a substance which has a high degree of affinity for a receptor site but not intrinsic activity. Two compounds fit this description, naloxone and naltrexone. Naloxone is available commercially and is the standard narcotic antagonist in clinical use. Naltrexone is available in the USA. It is an oral narcotic antagonist used in post-detoxification programmes [18].

Naloxone

Drug portrait
Naloxone is a potent narcotic antagonist (Figure 15.9). It has a high affinity for morphine receptor sites and reverses the effect of narcotic analgesics by displacement. The degree of displacement is dose-related and partial antagonism may be obtained by using small doses. Activity after oral administration is low. It is only one-fifteenth as potent by mouth as by injection. Injected IV naloxone acts within 1 to 2 minutes, and has a plasma half-life of about 20 minutes. It is rapidly metabolized by the liver, primarily by conjugation with glucuronic acid. The conjugate is excreted by the kidneys. Naloxone is best given IV but, if not practical, may be given IM or SC. After IV injection, antagonism lasts for between 15 and 90 minutes.

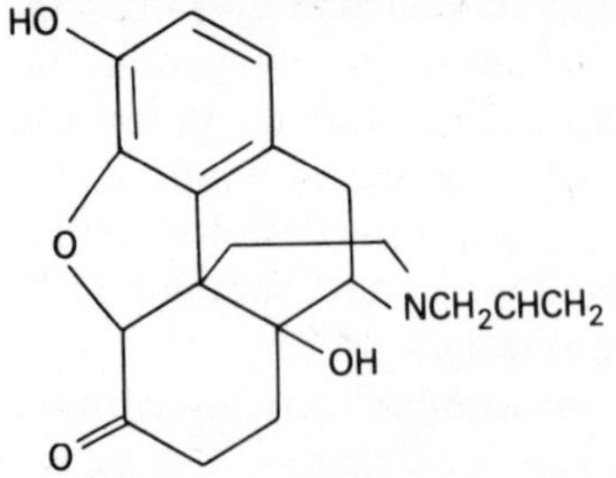

Figure 15.9 Chemical formula of naloxone.

Naloxone has no narcotic effect; it is a pure antagonist. Tolerance does not develop during clinical use and, if abruptly withdrawn after repeated administration, no abstinence phenomena occur. Overdosage has not been reported. A single dose of 24 mg IV causes only slight drowsiness [19]. The most important clinical property of naloxone is reversal of narcotic-induced respiratory depression. It also antagonizes the sedative, analgesic and miotic effects of systemically administered narcotic analgesics. Though, when used to reverse respiratory depression following *peridural* morphine, naloxone does not antagonize analgesia [20]. In contrast to the agonist-antagonists, it does not increase respiratory depression should the diagnosis of narcotic intoxication be wrong. It does not cause psychotomimetic effects. It is not effective against respiratory depression caused by non-narcotics such as barbiturates. Naloxone reverses the respiratory depression caused either by a large dose of a narcotic (including codeine and dextropropoxyphene) or by an exaggerated response to conventional doses. It also counteracts the narcotic effects of pentazocine and other nalorphine-type agonist-antagonists. Antagonism of buprenorphine is less complete.

The effect of intravenous naloxone lasts for 15 to 90 minutes and depends on the dose and the duration of action of the previously administered narcotic and the interval since administration. A dose in excess of that required to restore adequate respiration reverses sedation and analgesia. It also causes sweating and tachycardia. In narcotic dependent subjects, it precipitates withdrawal phenomena (Table 15.4). It is, therefore, important not to give too much when reversing narcotic-induced respiratory depression in someone who is taking narcotic analgesics regularly for medicinal purposes. The amount needed to improve respiratory function is unlikely to be more than 0.1 or 0.2 mg. A standard ampoule (0.4 mg) is usually too much, and causes the patient considerable distress. The patient becomes wide-eyed, twitchy, dysphoric and agitated. In addition the patient is hyperaesthetic to touch and pain, making further IV injections both very painful and difficult. In this situation, a Butterfly cannula or a heparin lock should be used and 0.1 mg IV of naloxone injected at not less than 2-minute intervals.

Narcotic Overdosage
Adults. In adult self-poisoning with narcotic analgesics, the overdose is considerably greater and the usual initial dose of naloxone is 0.4 mg. This should be repeated once or twice at 3-minute intervals if the patient's breathing does not improve sufficiently. If no response has been obtained after the third injection, the diagnosis of narcotic overdosage is probably wrong. As most narcotics act for longer than naloxone, respiratory depression may recur, especially with methadone and dextropropoxyphene. It can be prevented by a continuous intravenous infusion or

repeated IV or IM injections every 1 to 2 hours. Continued observation for up to 48 hours may be necessary, particularly when the amount or nature of the narcotic administered is unknown.

Buprenorphine overdose is reversed by naloxone, but relatively larger amounts of naloxone are required than for morphine overdose (Table 15.5). In the case of buprenorphine overdosage, the initial dose of

Table 15.5 Initial naloxone dose when treating narcotic overdosage

	IV dose
Iatrogenic respiratory depression	0.1 mg
Self-poisoning with narcotic agonist	0.4 mg
Overdosage with buprenorphine	4.0 mg

naloxone should be at least 4 mg (10 standard 0.4 mg ampoules). Subsequent doses of between 4 and 8 mg should be given, depending on the initial response. If necessary, doxapram, a respiratory stimulant, should also be administered. 100 mg IV should be given as an initial bolus, followed by an infusion of 200 mg/hour (3 mg/kg body weight). The rate may be increased up to 1 g/hour [21].

Children. The usual initial dose of naloxone for children is 5 to 10 μg (0.005 to 0.01 mg)/kg body weight. This dose may be repeated at 2- to 3-minute intervals in accordance with the adult administration guidelines.

References

1 Lasagna L and Beecher HK. The analgesic effectiveness of codeine and meperidine (Demerol). *Journal of Pharmacology and Experimental Therapeutics* 1954; **112**: 306–311.

2 Houde RW and Wallenstein SL. *Federation Proceedings* 1956; **15**: 440.

3 Martin WR. History and development of mixed opioid agonists, partial agonists and antagonists. *British Journal of Clinical Pharmacology* 1979; **7**: 2735–2795.

4 Kuhar MJ, Pert CB and Snyder SH. Regional distribution of opiate receptors binding in monkey or human brains. *Nature* 1973; **245**: 447–450.

5 Pert CB, Kuhar MJ and Snyder SH. Autoradiographic localisation of the opiate receptors in rat brains. *Life Sciences* 1975; **16**: 1849–1853.

6 Schachter M. Encephalins and endorphins. *British Journal of Hospital Medicine* 1981; **25**: 128–136.

7 Houde RW. Analgesic effectiveness of the narcotic agonist-antagonists. *British Journal of Clinical Pharmacology* 1979; **7:** 297S–308S.

8 Heel RC, Brogden TM, Speight TM and Avery GS. Buprenorphine: a review of its pharmacological properties and therapeutic efficiency. *Drugs* 1979; **17:** 81–110.

9 Anonymous. Buprenorphine injection (Temgesic). *Drug and Therapeutics Bulletin* 1979; **17:** 17–19.

10 Adriaensen H, Mattelaere B and Varmeenen H. A long-term open assessment of sublingual buprenorphine in patients suffering from chronic pain. *Pain* 1981; suppl. 1: 838.

11 Robbie DS and Samarasinghe J. Comparison of aspirin-codeine and paracetamol-dextropropoxyphene compound tablets with pentazocine in relief of cancer pain. *Journal of International Medical Research* 1973; **1:** 246–252.

12 Woods AJJ, Moir DC, Campbell C, Davidson JF, Gallon SC, Henney E and McAllison S. Medicines evaluation and monitoring group: central nervous system effects of pentazocine. *British Medical Journal* 1974; **1:** 305–307.

13 Lewis JR. Evaluation of new analgesics. Butorphanol and Nalbuphine. *Journal of the American Medical Association* 1980; **243:** 1465–1467.

14 Heel RC, Brogden RN, Speight TM and Avery GS. Butorphanol: a review of its pharmacological properties and therapeutic efficacy. *Drugs* 1978; **16:** 473–505.

15 Moyes DG, Miller MT and Aldridge NJ. A comparison between meptazinol and omnopon in the relief of postoperative pain. *SA Medical Journal* 1979; **55:** 865–866.

16 Stephens RJ, Waterfall JF and Franklin RA. A review of the biological properties and metabolic disposition of the new analgesic agent, meptazinol. *General Pharmacology* 1978; **9:** 73–78.

17 Green D. A pharmacology of meptazinol. A brief review of current concepts. (Unpublished Report 1981).

18 Kleber HD, Gold MS and Riodan CE. The use of clonidine in detoxification from opiates. *Bulletin on Narcotics* 1980; **32②:** 1–10.

19 Jasinski DR, Martin WR and Haertzen CA. The human pharmacology and abuse potential of N-allyl-noroxymorphone (naloxone). *Journal of Pharmacology and Experimental Therapeutics* 1967; **157:** 420–426.

20 Scott PV and Fischer HBJ. Intraspinal opiates and itching: a new reflex? *British Medical Journal* 1982; **284:** 1015–1016.

21 Dundee JW, Gray RC and Gupta PR. Doxapram in the treatment of acute drug poisoning. *Anaesthesia* 1974; **29:** 710–714.

Chapter Sixteen

Co-Analgesics

With certain pains, the prescription of 2 or more drugs together leads to better control and fewer unwanted effects than higher doses of morphine alone. Aspirin with morphine is perhaps the most important example of a 'co-analgesic' (Chapter 7). In this chapter, we examine a variety of other agents, particularly corticosteroids and psychotropic drugs (Table 16.1).

Corticosteroids

Glucocorticosteroids are widely used in far advanced cancer (Table 16.2). Inclusion in this list does not imply that they represent the sole or most important treatment for these indications. It simply means that a corticosteroid may be of benefit and should be considered as a treatment option, to be tried alone or in association with other recognized measures. Thus, in most patients with incipient paraplegia, superior vena caval obstruction or haemoptysis, a corticosteroid will be given in association with radiation therapy.

A corticosteroid should be considered as a co-analgesic wherever there is a large tumour mass within a relatively confined space. There is often an oedematous area around a tumour and pressure on neighbouring veins and lymphatics may lead to further local or regional swelling. In other words, total tumour mass = neoplasm + surrounding hyperaemic oedema. Corticosteroids reduce this oedema and thereby reduce the total tumour mass.

The classical situation is that of headache caused by raised intracranial pressure in association with cerebral neoplasm. There may be other central nervous symptoms or signs and patients often show improvement

Table 16.1   Co-analgesics in the relief of cancer pain

Types of pain	Co-analgesic
Bone pain	aspirin 600 mg 4 hourly *or* flurbiprofen 50–100 mg b.i.d. *or* naproxen 500 mg b.i.d.
Raised intracranial pressure	dexamethasone 2–4 mg t.i.d.–q.i.d. diuretic (?)
Nerve pressure pain	dexamethasone 2–4 mg daily– b.i.d. prednisolone 5–10 mg t.i.d.
Superficial dysaesthetic pain	amitriptyline 25–100 mg nocte
Intermittent stabbing pain	valproate 200 mg b.i.d.–t.i.d. *or* carbamazepine 200 mg t.i.d.–q.i.d.
Gastric distention pain	Asilone 10 ml p.c. and nocte; metoclopramide 10 mg 4-hourly
Rectal 'tenesmoid' pain	chlorpromazine 10–25 mg 8 to 4-hourly, or rectal belladonna alkaloids 0.2 mg†.
Muscle spasm pain	diazepam 5 mg b.i.d. *or* baclofen 10 mg t.i.d.
Lymphoedema	diuretic and corticosteroid (?)
Infected malignant ulcer	metronidazole 400 mg t.i.d. *or* alternative antibiotic

† can be pre-injected into standard morphine suppositories (Britain) or administered as B & O supprettes (USA)

lasting for weeks or months after starting treatment. Analgesics, a diuretic and elevating the head of the bed may help the pain when headache is the main symptom. Corticosteroids are also of benefit in relieving nerve compression pain (Figure 16.1). In our experience, 50 per cent of nerve compression pains respond to analgesics alone. Most of the rest respond to the combination of an analgesic and a corticosteroid. Only a minority of patients become candidates for neurolytic techniques because pharmacological measures have failed.

Metastatic arthralgia referred to in Table 16.2 is used to describe pain caused by metastatic involvement of the acetabulum (relatively common) or glenoid fossa (relatively uncommon). It occurs mostly in patients with cancer of the breast, bronchus or prostate (Figure 16.2). In addition to radiation therapy, sometimes maximum relief is obtained only by the combined use of a narcotic, a non-steroidal anti-inflammatory drug (NSAID) and a corticosteroid. Alternatively, injection into the joint space of a long-acting preparation of either methylprednisolone (Depo-Medrone) or a triamcinolone hexacetonide (Lederspan) may be considered.

Table 16.2 Corticosteroids in terminal cancer

Non-specific uses	*Other specific uses*
1 To improve appetite	1 Hypercalcaemia
2 To reduce fever	2 Carcinomatous neuromyopathy
3 To enhance sense of wellbeing	3 Incipient paraplegia
4 To improve strength	4 Superior vena caval obstruction
	5 Airway obstruction
Co-analgesic	6 Carcinomatous lymphangitis
1 Raised intracranial pressure†	7 Haemoptysis
2 Nerve compression	8 Leucoerythroblastic anaemia
3 Hepatomegaly	9 Discharge from rectal tumour‡
4 Head and neck tumour	10 To minimize radiation-induced
5 Intrapelvic tumour	reactive oedema
6 Abdominal tumour	11 To minimize the toxic effects of
7 Lymphoedema†	radiation or chemotherapy
8 Metastatic arthralgia	12 As an adjunct to chemotherapy

† may benefit by concurrent use of a diuretic
‡ given rectally

Which Corticosteroid?

Patients with cerebral oedema are initially given dexamethasone 4 mg q.i.d. This drug is 7 times more potent than prednisolone and has less mineralocorticoid activity. No controlled comparisons have been made. In other situations, prednisolone is usually given in a dose of 5 to 10 mg

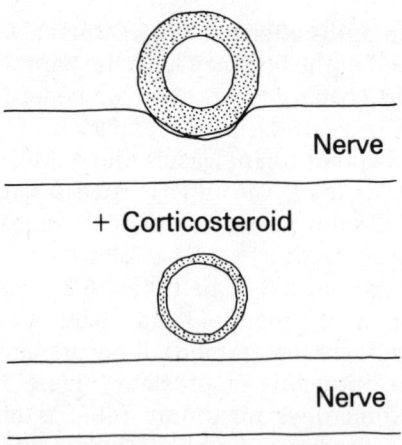

Figure 16.1 Presumed mechanism of action of corticosteroids in relief of nerve compression pain. Total tumour mass = neoplasm + surrounding hyperaemic oedematous tissue. General anti-inflammatory effect of corticosteroid reduces total tumour mass resulting in reduction of pain.

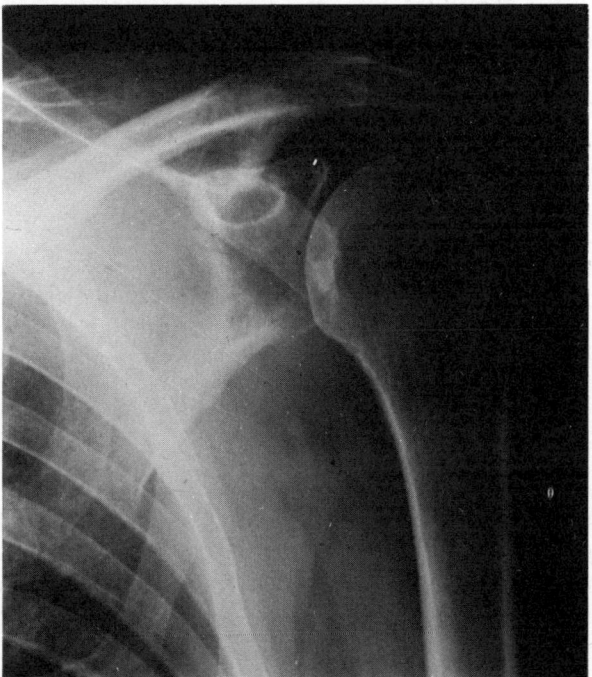

Figure 16.2 X-ray of the left shoulder of a man of 68 with carcinoma of the penis. He had excruciating pain if his arm was abducted more than a few mm. The glenoid fossa is totally replaced by a metastasis.

t.i.d. The dose needed to achieve maximum benefit varies from patient to patient. It is often advisable to commence with a higher dose to avoid missing a treatment effect. The dose can be adjusted downwards after 1 to 2 weeks, or sooner, if troublesome unwanted effects occur.

For 20 years, French physicians have used IV methylprednisolone as the corticosteroid of choice [1]. A dose of 125 mg IV is given daily for 30 days, followed by oral maintenance therapy with prednisolone 5 mg t.i.d. There is no evidence that the intravenous regimen is superior to the use of oral dexamethasone or prednisolone in terms of pain relief or general benefit. The IV regimen is, therefore, not recommended.

Unwanted Effects
Apart from oral candidosis and leg oedema, unwanted effects are not often troublesome in terminal patients receiving prednisolone. Weight gain and facial fattening may in fact be welcomed by the patient and family. Many patients receiving dexamethasone become more definitely Cushingoid. This may be a limiting factor. However, it is sometimes possible to reduce the dose without the original symptoms reappearing. Autopsies on over 500 patients with terminal cancer, of whom more than

half were treated with prednisone have shown that the only real risk from glucocorticoid therapy is an increase in complicated peptic ulcer. Death due to haemorrhage or perforation occurred in 5 per cent compared with 1 per cent in the patients not given a steroid [2]. In view of the patient's already poor prognosis, this is a small risk and one which most physicians are prepared to accept.

Steroid Withdrawal Pain

If the syndrome of pseudorheumatism (see Chapter 2) occurs with high dose corticosteroid therapy, the dose should be tapered slowly. If precipitated by too rapid a reduction, the dose should be increased and then reduced less rapidly.

Psychotropic Drugs

Various classifications have been proposed. In the interest of uniformity, we have opted for that of the World Health Organization (Table 16.3). The word neuroleptic replaces the term major tranquillizer. With the advent of more powerful benzodiazepines the division of anxiolytic drugs into

Table 16.3   WHO classification of psychotropic drugs [3]

Category	Representative members
Neuroleptics	phenothiazines
	butyrophenones
	thioxanthenes
	reserpine derivatives, benzoquinolines
Anxiolytic sedatives	meprobamate and derivatives
	barbiturates
	benzodiazepines
	hydroxyzine
Antidepressants	monoamine oxidase inhibitors (MAOI)
	tricyclics
	tetracyclics
	others
Psychostimulants	caffeine
	amphetamine, methylphenidate
	cocaine
Psychodysleptics	cannabis (marihuana, hashish, etc.)
(hallucinogens)	lysergic acid diethylamide (LSD)
	mescaline
	psilocybin
	dimethyltryptophan (DMT)

major and minor tranquillizers had become anachronistic. It is still helpful to retain the word tranquillizer as an umbrella term for both neuroleptic and anxiolytic sedative agents. Ataractic is also obsolete; it described the anxiolytic sedatives. The value of certain neuroleptic drugs and antidepressants in the relief of chronic pain states of non-malignant origin is well documented [4–6]. The conditions in which such drugs have been found beneficial are those which do not respond well to conventional analgesics. They include thalamic syndrome, postherpetic and trigeminal neuralgias, atypical facial pain, causalgia and phantom limb pain. These same drugs have a small but definite place in the treatment of a variety of pain syndromes in cancer (Tables 16.4, 16.5).

Table 16.4 Tranquillizers and the relief of pain in terminal cancer

	Chlorpromazine	Diazepam
Insomnia	+	++
Overwhelming pain	+	++
Anxiety	+	++
Tension headaches	+	++
Muscle spasm pain	+	++
Rectal 'tenesmoid' pain	++	+
Bladder 'tenesmoid' pain	++	+
Urethral spasm pain	++	+

++ Regarded as drug of first choice
+ Also used but less often than drug of choice, or if latter fails to relieve

Table 16.5 Need for antidepressants in terminal cancer

Depression
Insomnia
Nocturnal frequency
Nocturnal enuresis
Superficial dysaesthetic pain
Postherpetic neuralgia
Rectal 'tenesmoid' pain

The use of psychotropic drugs in the treatment of pain raises a number of questions:

1 Do these drugs have specific analgesic activity, acting centrally or on peripheral mechanisms?
2 Do they work by depressing the general level of arousal or by modifying sensory perception?
3 Is the apparent analgesic effect of antidepressants and tranquillizers a result of elevation of depressed mood or the alleviation of anxiety?

These questions remain largely unanswered. There is some information on the basic mode of action of antidepressants in pain [7, 8] but clinical evidence derives almost entirely from uncontrolled trials and from anecdotal reports.

Neuroleptics

This term refers to the phenothiazines and butyrophenones. The phenothiazines are commonly said to be analgesic potentiators. A careful review of published reports suggests that, in reality, the situation is not clear-cut. Early animal and volunteer studies indicated that in heat-induced pain (either hotplate or radiant heat) chlorpromazine, in particular, elevated the pain threshold [9, 10]. Surprisingly, the antihistamine antiemetic chlorcyclizine, 100 to 150 mg *by mouth*, was as effective as chlorpromazine 25 to 50 mg *by injection* [9]. In cancer patients, an *additive* effect with narcotic analgesics was noted [11].

Subsequently, the analgesic effect of 9 phenothiazines (as distinct from analgesic *potentiating* properties) was studied in women undergoing uterine curettage [12]. This study is of interest in that an experimental form of pain was used in an emotionally charged clinical setting. The results are more likely to reflect what happens in pathological pain than those from studies in healthy volunteers.

Intramuscular injections of the phenothiazines were given in the doses commonly employed in anaesthesia with atropine 0.6 mg as a premedication. Pain thresholds were measured between 60 and 90 minutes later by applying increasing pressure to the anterior surfaces of the tibia. The results indicated that the 9 compounds could be classified into 3 groups:

1 Those showing some analgesic activity:
    trimeprazine
    chlorpromazine
    promazine
2 Those mildly algesic:
    prochlorperazine
    perphenazine
    trifluoperazine
    triflupromazine
3 Those markedly algesic:
    promethazine
    pecazine

There was no clear relationship between analgesic action and chemical structure. Thus, while those with analgesic properties all have a dimethylaminopropyl side chain so does promethazine which is markedly algesic. There is, however, no definite evidence that promethazine is algesic in cancer patients with pathological pain when taken as a night sedative. Likewise, in many centres, prochlorperazine is used in patients with terminal cancer concurrently with morphine as the antiemetic of choice without any apparent loss of analgesic efficacy.

In the above study chlorpromazine 50 mg and promazine 100 mg were shown to be equally analgesic. Chlorpromazine, however, had neither analgesic nor analgesic potentiating effects in a double-blind randomized controlled trial in cancer patients (Figure 16.3). Subjects in this

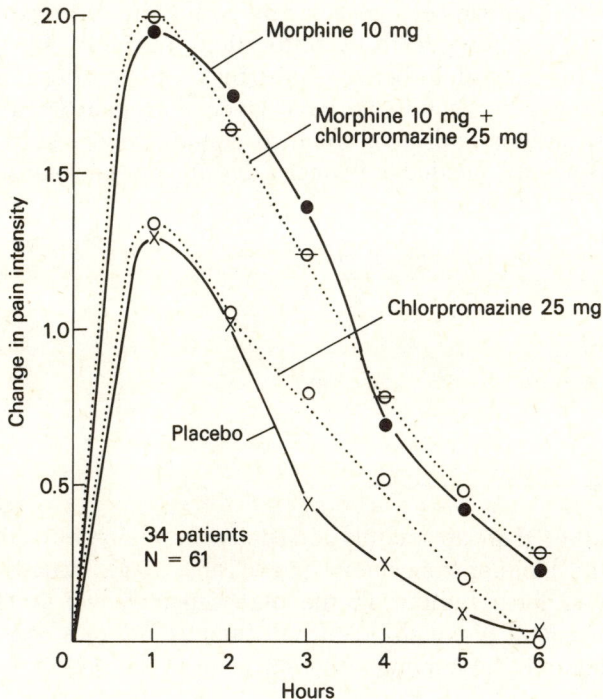

Figure 16.3 Time-effect curves for saline placebo, morphine sulphate 10 mg, chlorpromazine, 25 mg and a combination of morphine sulphate 10 mg and chlorpromazine 25 mg, all administered intramuscularly. Changes in pain intensity (ordinate) are plotted against time in hours (abscissa). Treatments were administered in a randomized order on a complete crossover basis to 34 patients with pain due to cancer. Twenty-seven patients repeated the crossover twice.
From Houde, 1966 [13]

study received, by IM injection in random succession, chlorpromazine 25 mg, morphine 10 mg, both agents and a saline placebo. The incidence of sedation as a side effect was several times greater for the combination than for morphine alone. One reviewer commented [14]:

'If a criterion of analgesia is that a patient is not bothering the staff by pushing the button and requesting more analgesic, a phenothiazine could be said to 'spare' analgesics. But if the patient is asked how bad the pain is, the reply will indicate that the phenothiazine seems not to be improving the situation, at least when administered on a single dose basis.'

Possibly there are differences when phenothiazines are given regularly. No controlled trial of the chronic use of phenothiazines in the relief of cancer pain has been carried out. We suggest that there is no place for the routine concurrent prescription of chlorpromazine with morphine. Some patients have an appreciable psychological component to their pain (for example, a patient with lung cancer experiencing both pain and dyspnoea, and who fears an agonizing death by suffocation). In these, chlorpromazine and morphine may yield better results than a higher dose of morphine alone. On the other hand, we have given diazepam ($\pm$ an antiemetic) in such situations and have obtained equally good results. Moreover, diazepam is usually needed only once a day and does not cause anticholinergic side effects (Table 16.6).

Table 16.6 Common anticholinergic side effects

Blurred vision
Dry mouth
Oesophageal reflux
Tachycardia
Urinary retention
Constipation

Chlorpromazine, rather than an anxiolytic sedative, remains our co-analgesic for rectal and bladder 'tenesmoid' pain (Table 16.4). Usually, such pain is related to local tumour in the unresected viscus, or to involvement of the presacral plexus by recurrent tumour. On rare occasions, it may be a phantom phenomenon after excision of the rectum or bladder.

Phantom bladder *pain* is an extremely rare phenomenon. It probably only occurs after cystectomy when, prior to surgery, the patient has experienced repeated painful perceptions originating in the bladder as a result of intractable urinary infection or bladder tumour [15, 16]. One such case responded well to a Comprehensive Pain Control Programme (Table 16.7) for chronic pain of non-malignant origin (*see* Chapter 3).

Phantom bladder *symptoms*—bladder distension and a desire to void—are described more frequently and occur after cystectomy, cord transection and in patients on haemodialysis [17]. These symptoms require explanation and reassurance to the patient but are not usually a source of ongoing painful distress.

Little interest has been shown in trimeprazine, despite its superior showing in the comparative study of 9 phenothiazines [12]. This is surprising in view of the marked analgesic properties of its congener,

Table 16.7 Comprehensive pain control programme for phantom bladder pain [15]

1 A series of six lumbar sympathetic blocks
2 A course of transcutaneous electrical nerve stimulation (TENS)
3 Relaxation training with Jacobson exercises supplemented by audiotaped instruction for home use
4 Assertiveness training through daily group meetings with an occupational therapist

methotrimeprazine (levomepromazine). By injection, methotrimeprazine 20 mg and morphine 10 mg are equally analgesic [18, 19], though the former tends to have a shorter duration of analgesic action, some 3 hours compared to morphine's 4 hours. The oral potency ratio has not been determined. When allowance is made for differences in the first-pass effect of the liver and in plasma half-life, methotrimeprazine by mouth is probably two-thirds as potent as morphine on a weight for weight basis.

Benefit in terminal pain is limited because it is too sedative for most patients, and causes unacceptable drowsiness. Methotrimeprazine commonly causes marked orthostatic hypotension and some believe it should be restricted to non-ambulant patients. This is unnecessary provided one is aware of this potential problem. Its use should be considered in the young, anxious patient requiring above average amounts of a narcotic, or in those who experience vestibular disturbance when given a morphine-like drug. In those aged under 40, it would be reasonable to prescribe 25 mg 4- to 6-hourly with 50 to 100 mg at night; in older patients a smaller dose should be given. Generally, it is wise to reduce the dose of morphine or other narcotic analgesic when first prescribing methotrimeprazine.

Haloperidol

This is a butyrophenone neuroleptic [20]. Compared with chlorpromazine, it is a more potent antiemetic but causes less sedation and less anticholinergic and cardiovascular effects. On the other hand, it has a greater propensity for causing extrapyramidal reactions. It is said that haloperidol is able to relieve chronic cancer pain, either alone or in combination with narcotics [21, 22]. The 6 case reports on which this claim is based indicated that the patients were all suffering from prolonged pain complicated by insomnia and physical and mental exhaustion. We would describe this situation as overwhelming pain (Chapter 3). Analgesics were generally modified and patients received between 10 and 30 mg of haloperidol at night, usually starting with 10 mg and increasing rapidly if sleep had been disturbed. Benzhexol 5 mg b.i.d. was also given to counter extrapyramidal side effects. The reports demonstrate that, in this situation, haloperidol is a useful alternative to diazepam or chlorpromazine. They do not support the contention that haloperidol is better or has specific analgesic properties. Our experience suggests that overwhelming pain will respond equally well to analgesic modification and a large bedtime dose of diazepam or chlorpromazine. The most important step in the treatment of overwhelming pain is to ensure a good night's sleep for the patient.

Anxiolytic Sedatives

Diazepam and hydroxyzine are perhaps the most important drugs of this type in relation to pain control. Diazepam is used as an anxiolytic and coincidental night sedative in patients who are very anxious or fearful and in those who have pain specifically related to muscle spasm or tension. In patients who find diazepam too sedative, even after adjustment of dose, clobazam* is an alternative. This has a comparable plasma half-life to diazepam (2 to 3 days) but is less sedative in comparable doses. Clobazam 10 mg is as effective as diazepam 5 mg.

It is fashionable to decry diazepam because of its depressing tendency. In our experience, it is not notably depressing, possibly because of the symptomatic relief which has a counteracting effect. As with chlorpromazine, and with narcotics themselves, it is important to be aware that depression may develop and an antidepressant may be needed.

Hydroxyzine is an anxiolytic sedative with antihistamine, antispasmodic, and antiemetic properties. In postoperative patients, hydroxyzine 100 mg IM has been shown to have analgesic activity approaching that of morphine 8 mg (Figure 16.4). Given together hydroxyzine and morphine have *additive* effects. This suggests that the two drugs produce analgesia by different mechanisms (cp. aspirin and codeine; Chapter 7). The sedative effect of the combination was only slightly greater than that of morphine alone. In a second postoperative study, morphine 5 mg and hydroxyzine 100 mg gave comparable relief to morphine 10 mg alone [24]. Several hospices in North America use hydroxyzine routinely with oral morphine, in a dose of 25 mg 4-hourly during the day and 100 mg at night. It would seem that this regimen has several advantages. It is narcotic sparing, and thereby reduces side effects. Separate antiemetic, anxiolytic and night sedative preparations are less commonly required.

Antidepressants

There is an association between the need for an antidepressant and the length of time a patient is maintained on a narcotic (Table 16.8). It is not clear whether the onset of depression is precipitated by the protracted terminal illness or whether this is a side effect of long-continued treatment with a narcotic and a phenothiazine. Physicians should be aware

* not available in the USA

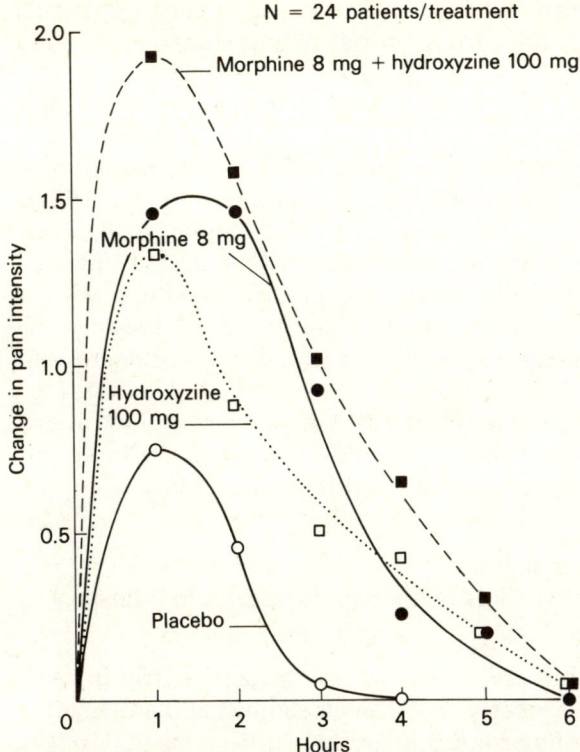

N = 24 patients/treatment

Figure 16.4 Time-effect curves for placebo, hydroxyzine 100 mg, morphine 8 mg, and a combination of hydroxyzine 100 mg and morphine 8 mg administered intramuscularly as single treatments to patients with postoperative pain. Mean change in pain intensity (ordinate), determined from subjective reports, is plotted against time in hours (abscissa).
From Beaver and Feise, 1976 [23]

Table 16.8 Incidence of antidepressant prescriptions in terminal cancer patients receiving diamorphine* for more than 12 weeks

Group	Number of patients	Length of treatment (weeks)	% prescribed antidepressant
I	23	12–13	17
II	22	14–17	32
III	32	18–25	41
IV	19	26–41	42
V	19	42+	68

From Twycross and Wald, 1976 [25]
* not available in the USA

that depression not only can, but frequently does, supervene in patients receiving so-called 'euphoriant' drugs. A trial of antidepressant therapy may then be indicated.

Our 2 most commonly used antidepressants are amitriptyline and mianserin. Nomifensine is reserved for those who are troubled by unwanted effects, such as dry mouth or sedation, or who might benefit by a stimulant rather than a sedative antidepressant. It is best to start with a small dose, amitriptyline 25 mg or mianserin 20 to 30 mg *at night*, or nomifensine 50 mg *in the morning*. The dose can be adjusted upwards once or twice fairly quickly; within a few days in hospital, after a week at home. Provided unwanted effects are not troublesome, the dose should be maintained for several weeks in order to evaluate the antidepressant effect.

Not all patients respond to an antidepressant. If no effect is noted after a reasonable trial of therapy, treatment should be stopped. In these circumstances, alternative measures to be considered include:

1   use of a corticosteroid;
2   prescription of dexamphetamine;
3   change of environment such as temporary admission to a hospice or similar unit.

Support and companionship are always necessary, particularly in cases where depression is more properly described as sadness at the thought of losing family, friends and hopes for the future.

Tricyclic antidepressants are also of benefit in terminal care in other ways (Table 16.5), particularly as the main analgesic agent in the management of superficial dysaesthesia and postherpetic neuralgia. Either amitriptyline or clomipramine may be used, beginning with a dose of 25 mg at night and increasing every few days until the pain is alleviated or unacceptable side effects occur (dry mouth, drowsiness, confusion) [23, 24].

Perphenazine (20 to 48 mg/day), chlorpromazine (300 mg/day) and haloperidol (12 to 20 mg/day) have been shown to decrease the rate of elimination of tricyclic antidepressants by between 25 and 50 per cent [28]. At the same time the plasma concentration in patients receiving perphenazine (the only ones examined) rose by 10 to 30 per cent. Most cancer patients receiving neuroleptic drugs take smaller doses than these, but possible potentiation must be borne in mind.

Psychostimulants
Cocaine (*see also* Chapter 11)
More than 80 years ago, Snow [29] began to prescribe cocaine with opium or morphine for patients with advanced cancer. He maintained that cocaine helped to 'sustain vitality', though he had to stop using it because

of the cost. Thirty years later it was reintroduced by Roberts, a surgeon at the Brompton Hospital, London, who used a morphine-cocaine elixir as a post thoracotomy analgesic. The mixture subsequently became known as the Brompton Cocktail (Chapter 11). Since 1973, the British Pharmaceutical Codex has included a standard formulation for both morphine-cocaine and diamorphine-cocaine elixirs.

Only recently has the effect of a standard 10 mg dose of cocaine hydrochloride been evaluated [30]. In this study patients were stabilized on morphine or diamorphine* with or without cocaine. After two weeks, patients receiving cocaine stopped it, and vice versa. Stopping cocaine had no effect at all, either in relation to pain, mood or other subjective states. On the other hand, starting cocaine resulted in a small but definite improvement in feelings of alertness and strength although it did not affect pain ratings. This order of treatment effect suggests that when cocaine is given in a small fixed dose tolerance develops after a few days. Cocaine would thus be of benefit during the initial period of treatment with morphine or diamorphine, but thereafter would be relatively ineffective. The results of a second trial comparing the traditional Brompton Cocktail with morphine sulphate alone also failed to demonstrate measurable differences in relation to pain, nausea, drowsiness or confusion [31].

Many physicians have experience of patients, usually elderly, who have become restless, agitated, confused and who hallucinate when prescribed a morphine-cocaine mixture. Symptoms have abated when the cocaine was withdrawn. In view of this, and the equivocal nature of the trial results, we no longer prescribe cocaine concomitantly. Instead, the patient is told that he may feel drowsy for 2 or 3 days following the start of treatment, but subsequently the drowsiness will become less. If troublesome drowsiness persists, dexamphetamine 2.5 to 5 mg may be prescribed once or twice daily.

Amphetamine

Dexamphetamine potentiated the action of narcotic analgesics in 450 young patients after abdominal or orthopaedic operations [32]. Pain relief scores were definitely improved when amphetamine was added even when smaller amounts of morphine were used (Figure 16.5). The effect on wakefulness was less apparent. Changes in pulse rate and blood pressure showed no uniform trends. Many of the patients experienced excessive sweating, and there was a tendency towards more dizziness and nausea. In addition, there were a number of other effects such as visual disturbance, body tremors and flushing. The authors do not state whether the subsequent requirement for morphine was diminished or if the characteristic responses to amphetamine might be cumulative. Important questions remain unanswered:

* not available in the USA

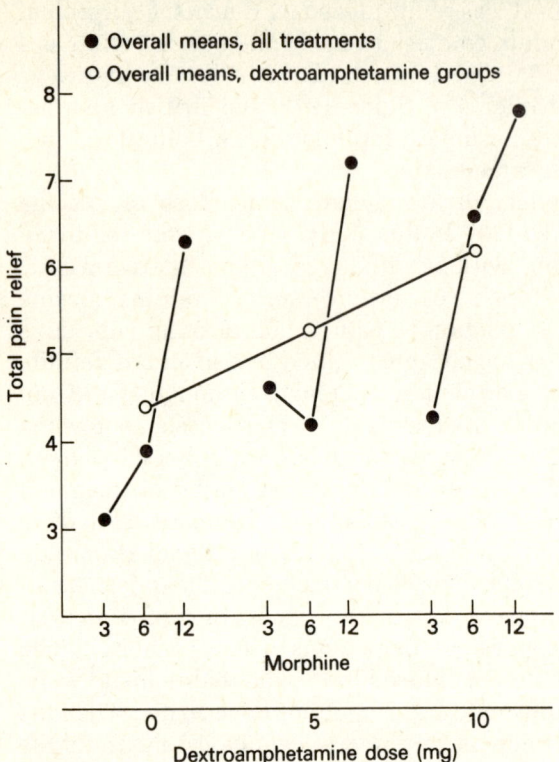

Figure 16.5 Dose-response curves for various combinations of morphine with dextroamphetamine administered intramuscularly on a single-treatment basis to patients with postoperative pain. Total pain relief scores (ordinate) are plotted against dose of morphine (on a log scale) and dextroamphetamine in each of 9 treatment groups, indicated by solid circles. Open circles represent mean effect of increasing doses of dextroamphetamine in the combination.
From Forrest *et al*, 1977 [32]

1   How would the combination work in the elderly, in whom the adverse psychological effects of drugs are more easily evoked, and in whom myocardial stimulation may more readily cause an arrhythmia?
2   Could the combined smooth muscle depressant properties of the two drugs result in a higher rate of urinary retention and ileus?

Its place in advanced cancer is probably limited as most patients appear to do better on a mildly sedative regimen. In those patients in whom there is continued troublesome drowsiness or lack of concentration, the addition of dexamphetamine 2.5 to 5 mg in the morning and at midday can be of considerable benefit. Tolerance may occur. If, after a number of weeks the patient complains 'it is no longer working', the dose should be increased.

Dexamphetamine antagonizes phenothiazine sedation and is itself antagonized by phenothiazines. Whether their analgesic potentiating properties are additive or not is not known. At the present time, the concurrent use of a neuroleptic and a psychostimulant as co-analgesics is not recommended.

Psychodysleptics

In recent years there has been renewed interest in psychodysleptic drugs such as lysergic acid diethylamide (LSD) and marihuana. LSD is the most potent member of the group. It has been successful in a small number of cancer patients, not as a co-analgesic but as an aid to psychotherapy. In one study [33], the following criteria were used in patient selection:

1 the patient must be suffering from some degree of physical pain, depression, anxiety or psychological isolation associated with his malignancy;
2 he must have a life expectancy of at least three months;
3 no evidence of brain metastases or organic brain disease must be apparent;
4 the patient must not manifest gross psychopathology or appear pre-psychotic.

The treatment procedure consisted of 3 phases:

1 a series of interviews over a period of 2 to 3 weeks in which rapport was established and the patient was prepared for the drug session. This preparation lasted from 6 to 12 hours;
2 the LSD session;
3 several subsequent drug-free interviews for the integration of the LSD session experiences.

Pain relief following LSD-assisted psychotherapy often lasted weeks or months. There was no clear dose-response relationship and the effect of LSD is not predictable. Almost certainly the relief resulted from a change in the patients' psychological outlook.

Marihuana is a much less potent psychodysleptic. Tetrahydrocannabinal (THC), the active principle in marihuana, possesses euphoriant, analgesic, appetite stimulant and antiemetic effects. Controlled trials have shown that in patients with prior marihuana exposure, THC has no advantage over codeine for analgesia. In patients without prior exposure THC carries with it a risk of unacceptable side effects, including sedation, thought impairment, and depersonalization [34, 35]. Nabilone is a new THC homologue with anxiolytic properties [36]. Studies of its use in terminal cancer are not available.

It is perhaps worth pointing out that the main thrust behind moves in the USA to legalize the medicinal use of THC relates to its potential role as an antiemetic in patients undergoing chemotherapy. There are a number of practical problems. Patients say THC in capsule form is not as effective as in a cigarette, even though the capsule contains 3 times as much THC. Moreover, the antiemetic effect appears to be closely related to the euphoriant effect, suggesting that the mechanism of action is mediated via the emotional or reactive component of nausea and vomiting.

It must be stressed that the casual use of either LSD or marihuana cannot be recommended. Rather, it must be condemned as likely to cause psychological harm. It must not be forgotten that patients can be greatly helped in their adjustment to advanced cancer by the more down-to-earth support and companionship offered by hospice and related programmes.

Anticonvulsants

The value of phenytoin and carbamazepine in the treatment of trigeminal neuralgia is well known. Less appreciated is the relief sodium valproate can provide for the stabbing pains of postherpetic neuralgia [26]. It may also relieve intermittent stabbing pain associated with neoplastic nerve compression. Treatment is initiated with a dose of 200 mg b.i.d., and is increased to t.i.d. after a few days if there is no or only partial response. In the majority of cases, this is sufficient. Occasionally, doses of up to 400 mg q.i.d. have been necessary.

The precise mode of action of valproate on the central nervous system is unclear, although it is known to increase the level of gamma-amino-butyric acid (GABA), a potent inhibitor of neurotransmission. Valproate is absorbed well after oral administration and has a serum half-life of 7 to 9 hours. The main initial side effect is gastric intolerance. Drowsiness or confusional symptoms occur occasionally, but these also tend to clear within 1 or 2 weeks. Valproate inhibits the secondary phase of platelet aggregation, but this is unlikely to be of clinical importance unless patients are on other medications which interfere significantly with haemostasis.

Carbamazepine up to 1 g a day in divided dosage can be used instead. In our experience valproate is easier to use. Patients usually obtain a response with the initial prescription of 200 mg b.i.d. and it is unusual to need more than 200 mg t.i.d. The range of effective doses of carba-mazepine is much greater and unwanted effects more troublesome. Carbamazepine and tricyclic antidepressants potentiate each other by a mutual reduction in the rate of metabolism [27]. The upper acceptable dose limit for carbamazepine in ill or elderly patients who are also receiving amitriptyline may be as little as 200 to 300 mg/day. When carbamazepine is commenced in someone already receiving a tricyclic, the dose of the latter should be reduced.

Gastric Distension

Epigastric pain in terminal cancer is sometimes related to gastric distension, either relative or absolute. The latter occurs after partial gastrectomy or with a large inoperable or recurrent intragastric neoplasm. Relative gastric distension occurs with or without gastric abnormality in patients with a grossly enlarged liver. It is important to recognize the postprandial discomfort for what it is because *explanation* to the patient is most important, even more so than with many other pains associated with cancer. Some patients, particularly those with a Celestin tube, also experience retrosternal pain due to acid-induced oesophagitis. The aim of treatment is to prevent overdistension; this requires a combination of dietary and pharmacological measures (Table 16.9).

Table 16.9 'Squashed stomach syndrome'

Definition: Dyspeptic symptoms associated with inability of stomach to distend normally because of hepatomegaly. Similar symptoms may be seen with carcinoma of stomach, linitis plastica, or post gastrectomy ('small stomach syndrome')

Symptoms:
Early satiation
Epigastric fullness
Epigastric discomfort/pain
Flatulence
Hiccough
Nausea
Vomiting (especially postprandial)
Heartburn

Treatment:
Explanation
Dietary advice
Defoaming agent
  (e.g. Asilone 10 ml after meals and bedtime)
Metoclopramide
  (4-hourly if also receiving morphine)
  (or after meals and bedtime)
Cyclizine 50 to 100 mg 4-hourly is occasionally also necessary

Case History. A 54-year-old woman gave a 6-month history of increasing lower oesophageal dysphagia. Investigation confirmed a carcinoma of the fundus of the stomach with extension into the oesophagus. A Celestin tube was inserted and the patient discharged a few days later.

She began to experience lower retrosternal and epigastric pain for which dihydrocodeine was prescribed. This helped a little but she then began to experience cramplike lower abdominal pain. Ten days after commencing dihydrocodeine, she was readmitted as an emergency because of increasing pain. The lower abdominal pain was caused by severe constipation with rectal impaction, and responded to enemas and oral laxatives. The reason for her epigastric and retrosternal pain was explained to her. Treatment was started with metoclopramide 10 mg before meals and 10 ml of postprandial Asilone, an antacid containing a defoaming agent. In addition, Gaviscon liquid, an antacid containing sodium alginate, was prescribed for use at bedtime in view of the history of nocturnal acid regurgitation and constant retrosternal discomfort. These measures relieved the pain. She learned to distinguish between gastric distension pain, for which she took an additional 10 ml of Asilone, and an intermittent epigastric pain apparently caused by the neoplasm itself and for which she took paracetamol[1] 1 g. She took this, on average, every other day.

This case history illustrates the fact that analgesics for neoplastic pain may also be necessary. It also highlights the point that some patients may need both Asilone (antacid + defoaming agent) and Gaviscon (antacid + inert gel). Gaviscon, however, requires both acid and foam to form a satisfactory 'flotation cushion' on the surface of the stomach contents. This was explained to the patient and she was instructed not to take Asilone, if at all possible, after 1900 hours. This arrangement proved satisfactory; she no longer experienced nocturnal regurgitation and the retrosternal discomfort gradually improved. Ultimately, it becomes necessary in almost all such patients to use analgesics regularly because of the local spread of the neoplasm or gross hepatomegaly. As always, close monitoring is essential.

Muscle Spasm

This may occur as a result of anxiety related increased muscle tension or it may be related to an underlying bone secondary. It is often possible to palpate a tender bone and to confirm metastatic involvement by X-ray or bone scan. Both diazepam and chlorpromazine have muscle relaxing properties and, if indicated for other reasons, may be the drugs of choice. At other times, a less sedative muscle relaxant such as baclofen will be indicated. This may be given in a range of doses from 10 mg t.i.d. to 20 mg q.i.d. The most common side effects are drowsiness and nausea. Occasionally, baclofen may precipitate confusional symptoms, particularly in ill patients receiving morphine and other psychoactive drugs.

---

[1] acetaminophen (USA)

When the spasm is associated with an underlying bone metastasis, treatment should be directed at the metastasis. If successful, a muscle relaxant may then prove unnecessary.

Lymphoedema

Many patients with advanced cancer develop a variable degree of oedema. Lack of exercise, hypoproteinaemia, sodium-retaining drugs, venous thromboses and concurrent heart failure account for most of the causes. In

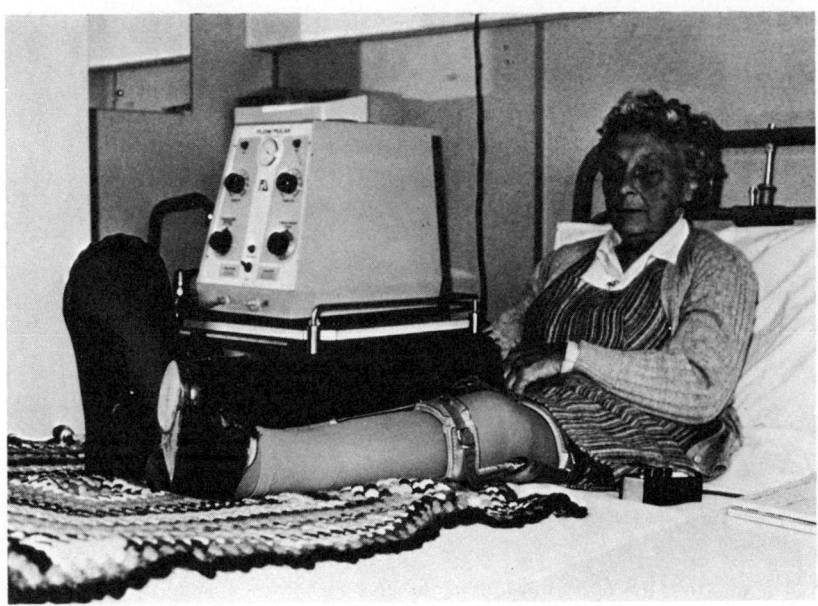

Figure 16.6 A patient using a Flow pulse compression sleeve to help reduce lymphoedema of the arm. The smaller Flowtron is more convenient for home use.

some patients malignant occlusion of the lymphatics either by infiltration or by external pressure is the main factor. Obstruction may also relate to post-radiation fibrosis. Thus, in patients with breast cancer, the ipsilateral arm becomes swollen, heavy and painful. In patients with intrapelvic disease, one or both legs may be affected in the same way. In the majority, the pain of the swollen limb is not the only pain and many are receiving morphine or an alternative strong narcotic. Occasionally, the lympho-edema is so painful that it is necessary to use a strong analgesic for this alone. This may, however, bring only partial relief.

The key to relief often lies in mechanical measures: the use of constricting bandages and compression sleeves (Figure 16.6). Tubigrip and Netelast are convenient forms of support. They are both available in several sizes and are readily accepted by most patients. The intermittent application of a compression sleeve without the continuous use of Tubigrip or Netelast reduces the likelihood of success. At Sir Michael Sobell House, Oxford, a standard treatment protocol is available for the Flowpulse and Flowtron compression sleeves (Table 16.10). In North

Table 16.10 Guidelines for treatment of lymphoedema†

---

1 All patients start diuretic therapy if not already prescribed.
  Initially: Dyazide 1 tablet daily
  Proceeding if necessary to:
  Moduretic 1 or 2 tablets daily,
  or
  Burinex K 1 or 2 tablets daily if delayed response or poor response to Moduretic.

2 Use the *Flowpulse* (the *large* one) rather than the *Flowtron* whenever possible.

3 All patients should adhere to the following sequence unless they are unable to tolerate it for any reason.

	Pressure	Duration	Frequency
Day 1:	40 mmHg	20 mins	daily
2:	40 mmHg	30 mins	b.i.d.
3:	40 mmHg	40 mins	b.i.d.
4:	50 mmHg	40 mins	b.i.d.
5:	60 mmHg	40 mins	b.i.d.
6: et seq.	60 mmHg	60 mins	b.i.d.

4 Tubigrip stocking should be worn between applications.

5 If lower limb involved the foot of the bed should be elevated 3 to 4″.

6 Dexamethasone 4 mg t.i.d. will be prescribed if there is a clear indication of possible benefit.

---

† Based on instructions in current use at Sir Michael Sobell House, Oxford

America, the Jobst compression pump is generally used. Success is measured principally in terms of comfort achieved; the limb does not always decrease in size but will feel more comfortable if the tissue turgor is reduced. Secondary success (reduction in limb circumference) occurs in most patients, and in some the arm returns to normal or near normal size within 3 to 4 weeks.

Infection

As a general rule systemic or local antibiotics are not clinically necessary for infected malignant ulcers. There are occasions, however, when the patient continues to experience much pain in association with extensive inflammation and induration. In these, a swab may or may not reveal a pathogen. It is sometimes worth a therapeutic trial of metronidazole as there may be an underlying anaerobic infection. In one or two patients, metronidazole has been necessary on a long-term basis, after a relapse within a week or so of completing a course of treatment.

References

1 Pierquin B, Baillet F and Maylin C in *La Corticotherapie en Cancerologie.* Malaine, Paris 1978.

2 Schell HW. The risk of adrenal corticosteroid therapy in far-advanced cancer. *American Journal of Medical Science* 1972; **252:** 641–649.

3 *Research in Psychopharmacology* Technical Report Series, 371. WHO Geneva 1967.

4 Merksey H and Hester RA. The treatment of chronic pain with psychotropic drugs. *Postgraduate Medical Journal* 1972; **48:** 594–598.

5 Kocher R. Use of psychotropic drugs for the treatment of chronic severe pain in *Advances in Pain Research and Therapy, Volume 1* edited by Bonica JJ and Albe-Fessard DG. Raven Press, New York 1976, *pp 579–582.*

6 Hanks GW. Antidepressants in patients with chronic pain in *Drugs in Pregnancy, Paediatrics and Geriatrics* edited by Edwards AM, Stevens EA and Burley DM. Trust for Education and Research in Therapeutics, London 1981, pp 123–132.

7 Spencer PSJ. Some aspects of the pharmacology of analgesia. *Journal of International Medical Research* 1976; **4** (suppl 2): 1–14.

8 Lee R and Spencer PSJ. Antidepressants and pain: a review of the pharmacological data supporting the use of certain tricyclics in chronic pain. *Journal of International Medical Research* 1977; **5** (suppl 1): 146–156.

9 Hougs W and Skouby AP. The analgesic actions of analgesics, antihistamines and chlorpromazine in volunteers. *Acta Pharmacologica et Toxicologica* 1957; **13:** 405–409.

10 Boreus LO and Sandberg F. The influence of three phenothiazine derivatives and of amiphenazole on the action of methadone. *Journal of Pharmacology, London* 1959; **11:** 449–455.

11 Sadove MS, Levin MJ, Rose RF, Schwartz L and Witt FW. Chlorpromazine and narcotics in the management of pain of malignant lesions. *Journal of the American Medical Association* 1954; **155:** 626–628.

12 Moore J and Dundee JW. Alterations in response to somatic pain associated with anaesthesia. VII: the effects of nine phenothiazine derivatives. *British Journal of Anaesthesia* 1961; **33**: 422–431.

13 Houde RW. On assaying analgesics in man in *Pain* edited by Knighton RS and Dumke PR. Little, Brown and Co., Boston 1966.

14 Beaver WT. Combination analgesics in *The Use of Analgesics*. Postgraduate Medicine Publications, Riker Laboratories, Inc., Northridge, California 1980, pp 27–37.

15 Brena SF and Sammons EE. Phantom urinary bladder pain—Case Report. *Pain* 1979; **7**: 197–201.

16 Arcacli JA. 'Phantom Bladder': Is this an unusual entity? *Journal of Urology* 1977; **118**: 354–355.

17 Dorpat TL. Phantom sensations of internal organs. *Comprehensive Psychiatry* 1971; **12**: 27–35.

18 Beaver WT, Wallenstein SL, Houde RW and Rogers A. A comparison of the analgesic effects of methotrimeprazine and morphine in patients with cancer. *Clinical Pharmacology and Therapeutics* 1966; **5**: 436–446.

19 Bonica JJ and Halpern LM. Analgesics in *Drugs of Choice 1972–73* edited by Modell W. Mosby, St Louis 1972, pp 185–217.

20 Ayd FJ. Haloperidol update: 1975. *Proceedings of the Royal Society of Medicine* 1976; **69**: 14–18.

21 Cavenar JO and Maltebie AA. Another indication for haloperidol. *Psychosomatics* 1976; **17**: 128–130.

22 Maltebie AA and Cavenar JO. Haloperidol and analgesia: case reports. *Military Medicine* 1977; **142**: 946–948.

23 Beaver WT and Feise G. Comparison of the analgesic effects of morphine, hydroxyzine and their combination in patients with postoperative pain in *Advances in Pain Research and Therapy, Volume 1* edited by Bonica JJ and Albe-Fessard DG. Raven Press, New York 1976, pp 553–557.

24 Hupert C, Yacoub M and Turgeon LR. Effect of hydroxyzine on morphine analgesia for the treatment of postoperative pain. *Anesthesia and Analgesia* 1980; **59**: 690–696.

25 Twycross RG and Wald S. Long-term use of diamorphine in advanced cancer in *Advances in Pain Research and Treatment, Volume 1* edited by Bonica JJ and Albe-Fessard DG. Raven Press, New York 1976, pp 652–661.

26 Raftery H. The management of postherpetic pain using sodium valproate and amitriptyline. *Irish Medical Journal* 1979; **72**: 399–401.

27 Gerson GR, Jone RB and Luscombe DK. Studies on the concomitant use of carbamazepine and clomipramine for the relief of postherpetic neuralgia. *Postgraduate Medical Journal* 1977; **53** (suppl 4): 104–109.

28 Gram LF and Fredricson Overø K. Drug interaction: inhibiting effect of neuroleptics on metabolism of tricyclic antidepressants in man. *British Medical Journal* 1972; **1**: 463–465.

29 Snow H. Opium and cocaine in the treatment of cancerous disease. *British Medical Journal* 1896; **2**: 718–719.

30 Twycross RG. The effect of cocaine in the Brompton Cocktail in *Pain Research and Therapy, Volume 3* edited by Bonica JJ, Lieberkind JC and Albe-Fessard DG. Raven Press, New York 1979, pp 927–932.

31 Melzac R, Mount BM and Gordan JM. The Brompton mixture versus morphine solution given orally: effects on pain. *Canadian Medical Association Journal* 1979; **120**: 435–439.

32 Forrest WH, Brown BW, Brown CR, Defalque R, Gold M, Gordon HE, James KE, Datz J, Mahler DL, Shroff P and Teutsch G. Dextroamphetamine with morphine for the treatment of postoperative pain. *New England Journal of Medicine* 1973; **296**: 712–715.

33 Richards W, Grof S, Goodman L and Kurland A. LSD-assisted psychotherapy and the human encounter with death. *Journal of Transpersonal Psychology* 1972; **4**: 121–150.

34 Noyes R, Brunk S and Avery D. The analgesic properties of delta-9-tetrahydrocannabinol and codeine. *Clinical Pharmacology and Therapeutics* 1975; **18**: 84–89.

35 Noyes R, Brunk S and Avery D. Psychologic effects of oral delta-9-tetrahydrocannabinol in advanced cancer patients. *Comparative Psychiatry* 1976; **17**: 641–646.

36 Lemberger L and Rowe H. Clinical pharmacology of nabilone, a cannabinol derivative. *Clinical Pharmacology and Therapeutics* 1975; **18**: 720–726.

Part Four

General

Chapter Seventeen

Home Care

Home care has been referred to repeatedly in this book. In this chapter we discuss selected aspects in more detail. Although home care is not for all, it is an alternative that has historic tradition and has proved a well received option in contemporary communities both in Britain and the USA. Moreover, in many areas, home care is the only vehicle by which hospice care is available for those patients who need such specialist support.

To deal adequately with the complex pain problems in advanced cancer it is necessary to provide extra help and support in the home. Hospice home care nurses complement the district nurses in Britain and the visiting nurses in the USA; they do not replace them. Hospice home care also requires close co-operation between general practitioner and consultant/attending physician. For details of organization, the reader is referred to several published accounts [1–5]. Existing services and hospice home care can together provide high quality care, and prompts tremendous verbal, volunteer and financial support from the community.

Pain at Home

'As regards pain, as long as my mother was taking drugs orally that was all right—I could cope. But when it got to the stage that she could not keep anything down and we had to have injections it was a terrifying situation. I could not phone my G.P. at all hours of the night. There was no 24-hour service as far as I knew. In fact, I was left alone in the middle of the night with my mother in absolute agony not knowing where to turn. I know now there were places that could have helped me, but I did not know at the time'.[6]

No advanced technology or new research was needed to relieve pain in the above situation. The issues were physician availability, information about community resources, 24-hour cover and instruction about how to give injections or, in some other way, administer analgesics to a vomiting patient. These are the problems that can be solved by a home care support team.

In an inpatient hospice it is relatively easy to assess the patient's changing condition; at home it is more difficult. If a patient very much wants to stay at home he can be remarkably uncomplaining. If the pain is bad he will attempt to conceal his distress or persuade himself that it is unavoidable. During the initial phase of pain control, and certainly when strong narcotics are first begun, *daily monitoring* of the patient's condition and reappraisal of his drugs is essential. Ideally this should be done by the same trained professional, whether nurse or doctor, in order to assess progress. If this is not possible, continuity must be preserved by visits from team members who meet regularly and gain experience of each other's methods and judgement [7]. On every visit adequate drug supplies should be ensured, with particular attention to weekends and holidays.

Drugs at Home

Analgesic regimens should be simple to understand and easy to administer. It is only necessary to adopt a 4-hourly regimen if morphine or a comparable analgesic is being used. With other patients, 'with meals and at bedtime' will cover all other drug requirements. Variations include:

1   'on waking, after lunch and tea, and bedtime',
2   'after breakfast and at bedtime'.

If some drugs are best given before meals and others after, it is usually advisable to forsake pharmacological purity and to opt for one or other time so as to avoid an impossibly complex schedule. It is necessary to look at boxes and other containers to check that the pharmacist has not given the patient contrary or complicating advice (Figure 17.1).

When a 4-hourly regimen is adopted, the first and last doses are linked to the patient's waking and bedtimes. The best additional times during the day are usually 1000 hours, 1400 hours and 1800 hours unless the patient wakes exceptionally late. When writing out the list of drugs and doses for the patient (and family) to work from, it is useful to add what the different preparations are for, even if this seems obvious to the doctor.

Capsules should be described as capsules and tablets as tablets, not vice versa. Doses should not be described simply as 'spoonfuls'. Patients have

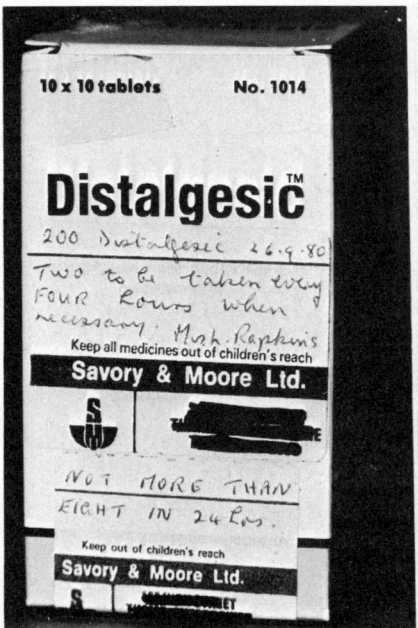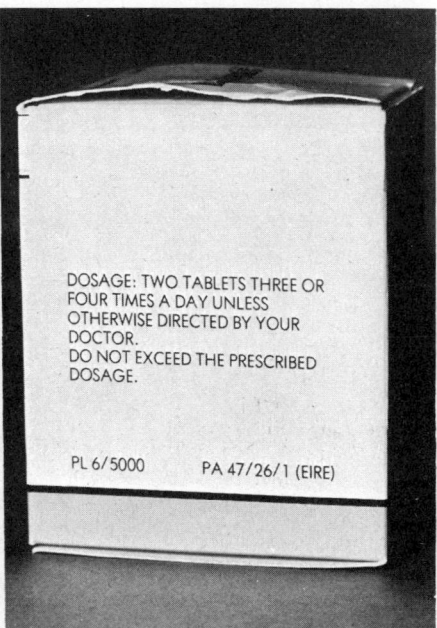

Figure 17.1 The front and side of a container of a commonly used non-narcotic-weak narcotic. The family practitioner prescribed '2 tablets every 4 hours'. The pharmacist added 'when necessary' and the conflicting 'not more than eight in 24 hours'. To be helpful, he should have covered the manufacturer's advice on the side of the box as the doctor had clearly prescribed more than this. The pharmacist's unwarranted additions caused the patient's family much concern and uncertainty.

been known to use a tablespoon (15 ml) instead of a teaspoon (3.5 to 5 ml). A plastic beaker/cup with each 5 ml clearly marked is generally the best way for the patient to self-administer liquid preparations (Figure 17.2). Sometimes, if the above recommendations are carried out, the patient can cope immediately with a new regimen. Not infrequently, however, the patient is found to be in confusion when visited the next day by a home care nurse.

Considerable ingenuity may need to be exercized to ensure patient compliance—as demonstrated by the example of Mrs D [8]. Poor vision and lack of co-ordination made it impossible for her to handle her medication in the normal way. Large colour-coded cards were marked with the medication times. Each day when visited by the nurse sufficient medication was put out in separate beakers for the ensuing 24 hours and arranged in a mini-dispensary on a small table next to the patient's favourite chair (Figure 17.3).

The relative giving medicine may also be elderly or infirm. On The Connecticut Hospice home care programme, one-third of 'primary care persons' (patient spouse or closest care giver) are over 65, 4 per cent are

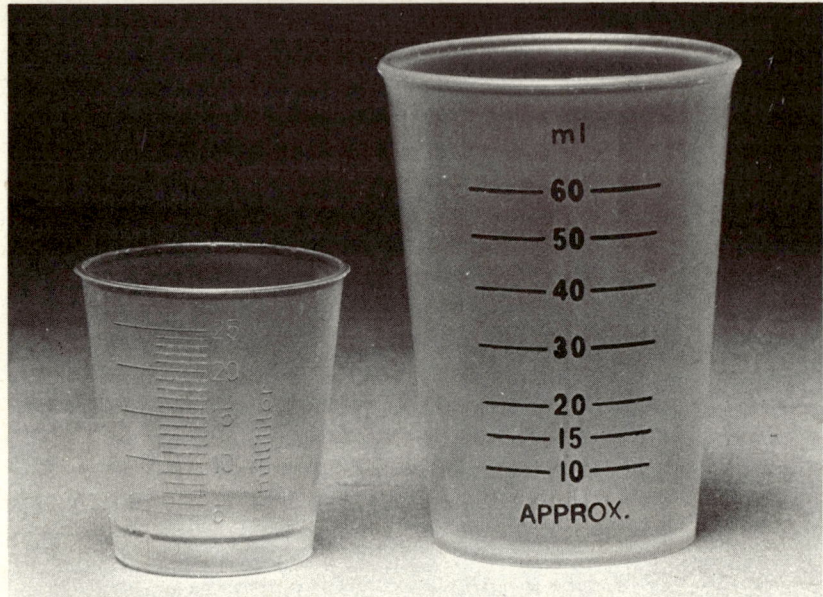

Figure 17.2 Visible or invisible? A clearly labelled plastic medicine cup (beaker) used at Sir Michael Sobell House, Oxford, in preference to the standard British National Health Service variety.

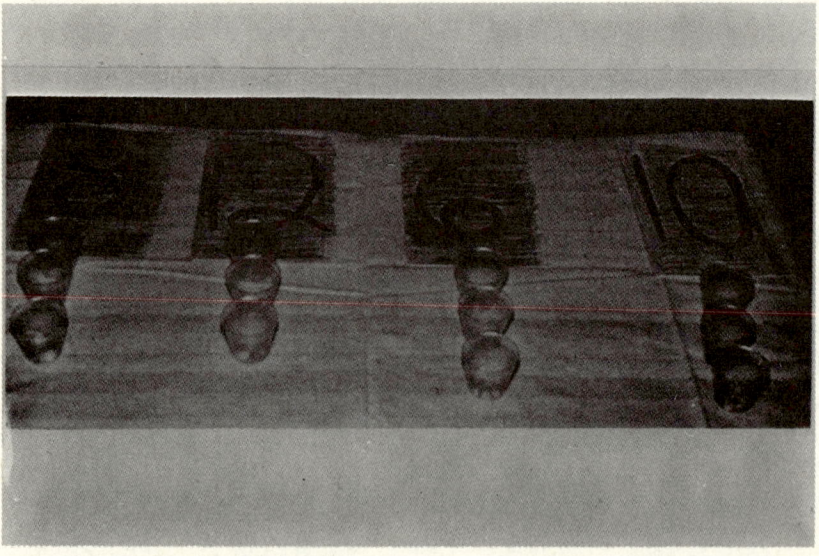

Figure 17.3 A minidispensary arranged by the home care nurse for a patient with poor vision and incoordination.
From Ajemian and Mount, 1980 [8]

over 80. One-third are not in good health themselves [2]. Medication must also be as simple as possible because exhaustion is commonplace among home caregivers. There are all kinds of attention which a patient requires at night; nourishment, adjusting position and pillows, company during restless hours. One wife who nursed her 46-year-old husband with lung cancer, did not sleep in a bed for over a month because her nights were broken by the frequent need for analgesics [9]. Thus short acting narcotics such as pethidine[1] are rarely satisfactory at home. A regular 'in between' tablet—in effect a 2-hourly regimen—is also impossible to maintain for long. Getting through the night needs careful planning. Suitable stratagems have been discussed elsewhere (*see* Chapter 9) and are summarized in Table 17.1.

Table 17.1 Stratagems for getting through the night at home without pain

Judicious use of a hypnotic
A double dose of morphine at bedtime
0200 hour dose pre-poured and the alarm set
Controlled release morphine sulphate tablets†
One or two oxycodone pectinate suppositories at bedtime‡

† used by authors only rarely
‡ not used by authors

Analgesic suppositories have a special place in the home, as an alternative to parenteral medication when the patient is unable to swallow (Table 17.2). The caregiver must be taught to place the suppository against the rectal mucosa. The drug is not absorbed if pushed into a mass of stool or if it is placed in the anal canal.

Instructions to the Family

Studies show that compliance is improved if time is taken to explain what each preparation is for [10]. We have also found that a list of medications serves as reinforcement when written with doses, times to be taken and purpose of prescription (Figure 17.4).

Anxiety is always present in the home even if not visible. Communication is blocked because the anxious person hears and assimilates only a percentage of what is said. All directions must be given several times [11]. A tape recorder is helpful if you know follow-up sessions are going to be limited. Constant repeated verbal and written instructions must be given to the patient and primary caregiver covering the following issues:

1 drugs, their names and what each is for;
2 which are to be taken regularly and which are to be taken when a problem arises;

[1] meperidine (USA)

Table 17.2   Analgesic suppositories

Analgesic	Available strengths
In Britain and the USA	
morphine†	10, 15, 20, 30, 60 mg
paracetamol[1]	650 mg
In Britain only	
oxycodone pectinate	30 mg
indomethacin	100 mg
In the USA only	
hydromorphone	3 mg
oxymorphone	5 mg
opium and belladonna (15 mg) (B & O supprettes No. 15A, 16A)	30, 60 mg
aspirin	650 mg

† can be made by a pharmacist in USA
[1] acetaminophen (USA)

TABLETS/MEDICINES	2 am	on waking	10 am	2 pm	6 pm	Bed-time	PURPOSE
							28 March, 1980
MORPHINE (20mg in 10ml)	(10)	10	10	10	10	10	for pain
FLURBIPROFEN (tab. 50mg)		1		1		1	for pain
PREDNISOLONE (tab. 5mg)			1	1	1		for appetite (DISSOLVE IN WATER)
DIOCTYL FORTÉ (tab. 100mg)			1				for bowels
DURBANEX (capsules)			2				for bowels
CHLORPROMAZINE (tab. 25mg)						3	for sleep
NYSTATIN (liquid)		2	2	2	2	2	for mouth

If pain returns, takes extra 10 ml dose of pain medicine

Figure 17.4 Medication chart for outpatients receiving 4-hourly morphine sulphate. Actual size = A4. A different chart is used for patients *not* receiving morphine or other 4-hourly analgesic. This has 4 unlabelled columns and the times of administration have to be added. These are linked to the patient's waking, meals and/or bedtime. The space at the bottom of the chart allows additional instructions to be recorded.
        (Modified from the chart used at St. Luke's Nursing Home, Sheffield.)

3 unwanted effects and what to do if they occur;
4 what to do if vomiting begins and medicines cannot be taken, or if the patient is unable to swallow;
5 where to go if supplies unexpectedly run out;
6 how liquid medicines should be measured;
7 how to keep track of whether a tablet has been taken;
8 keeping medicines away from children.

In short, the doctor has to educate the patient about his medication (Table 17.3). Education should include the family even when the patient handles his own medication, as this helps create an atmosphere of co-operation and support. Hospice home care nurses spend a lot of time with others who help at home, so that the private night nurse, the district nurse and the home help/home maker/health aide understand what is being done [5]. It is not unknown for a well meaning but misguided visitor

Table 17.3   Questions that must be answered for patients on analgesics at home

Which of my medicines are for pain?
How should I take them?
Do these drugs have side effects?
Isn't morphine very dangerous?
If I take morphine, will I get addicted?
How much is it safe for me to take?
What if the dose doesn't relieve my pain?
Can I take different pain medicines on the same day?
What about non-prescription pain relievers – shall I use them?
Will I need injections when my pain gets worse?
Is it true that really bad pain can only be relieved by heroin?
What can I do about drowsiness?
What can I do about constipation?
Should I eat fibre?
What can I do about nausea?
Will I get sick if I stop taking my morphine?
How do antidepressants help relieve my pain?
Can I take alcohol?
Will marihuana help?
What is the difference between aspirin and paracetamol?[1]
Which should I take, aspirin or paracetamol?
Can cancer patients take aspirin?
How should I take aspirin to cut down on side effects?
If I can't take aspirin – what other medicines contain aspirin?
What shall I do if I am still in pain and my doctor says there is nothing more that can be done?

[1] acetaminophen (USA)

to cast doubt on the whole regimen, thereby undermining the patient's and the family's confidence. The patient and family must, therefore, be able to contact a doctor or nurse *at any time* of the day or night should questions arise. If questions are not answered speedily and satisfactorily, the patient and family may stop following the doctor's advice and abandon completely a carefully constructed regimen.

Relatives should beware of the temptation to overprotect a patient, and of leaving him alone with nothing to do. They need to understand that drugs by themselves are not enough and that they can help with back rubs, moving the patient to a brighter room, television, radio and arranging for friends to visit. They need to know that such activities do more than just pass the time, they actually diminish the pain (*see* Table 5.1, page 80).

Planning for Crises

Change often comes quickly to the dying patient. With each visit one must expect the situation to have changed. The nurse must always try and anticipate the next stage in the illness and prepare the family and the home. A supply of essential drugs in parenteral form should be kept in the home. Family members should be taught early how to give suppositories and injections even though in most cases they will not be needed (vide infra). Common occurrences must be discussed fully with the relatives as they need to be prepared emotionally and practically. Likely crises in pain patients include:

1 refusal of medication,
2 disorientation,
3 inability to rouse the patient,
4 no bowel movement for a week,
5 severe breakthrough pain,
6 a new pain.

All these issues are manageable in the home, but poor planning and preparation can precipitate premature inpatient admission. Even the best laid plans can prove inadequate, but families can often manage to cope if they can talk at any time of the day or night with somebody who knows the patient. Families occasionally test out 24-hour availability and call for help at an unusual hour for some trivial reason. Once they discover that hospice personnel really are there, most stop testing and do not abuse the service.

'I Can't Stand Seeing Her Suffer'

Much can be done at home to relieve pain and in most cases all involved will feel satisfied. Sometimes, however, family and staff know pain control could be improved by inpatient admission, but the patient prefers to put up with the pain for the sake of staying at home. In this situation it is harder to watch than it is to suffer the pain. Family and staff may need much open discussion with and without the patient to prevent the admission of an unwilling patient. It may help to know that a willingness to be slightly more troubled and a desire to stay at home is normal amongst people at home with advanced cancer. In one study, mean anxiety and depression ratings were significantly higher amongst hospice outpatients than hospice inpatients, yet only 1 out of 20 desired inpatient care [12]. In some patients, however, the pain becomes so all-embracing that it is impossible to cope with it at home [13]. For these, inpatient admission is necessary (vide infra).

The experience of the family regarding available help must tally with what they are told. 'You're very difficult to get hold of,' insisted one daughter. She was trying in vain to tell her mother's physician that, prior to the present hospital admission, she had tried to reach him for 3 days because her mother had severe vaginal bleeding. Finally, a dash to the emergency room resulted in immediate admission. No amount of reassurance by the doctor, as he tried to persuade her to take her mother home again, could blot out the fear and anxiety of those three days.

Pain in the Last 24 Hours

Careful assessment is still necessary if the patient is, or seems to be, in pain. Temporary relief from a painful bedsore can be obtained by the application of a local anaesthetic gel. A distended bladder can be relieved by catheterization. Pain will not be troublesome at the very end if control has previously been good. There is no final crescendo of pain. On the contrary, analgesic requirements may decrease. Patients do, however, experience pain even when comatose. In addition, they may be physically dependent on narcotics and withdrawal restlessness may mar their peace if narcotics are suddenly stopped when they can no longer swallow. For these reasons we advise continuation of analgesia by suppository (Table 17.2) or injection. At The Connecticut Hospice, 60 per cent are able to swallow until a few hours before death and need no change in drug administration. Another 25 per cent require 1 or 2 doses of narcotic by suppository; only 15 per cent need an injection. There is no need to change to a long acting drug at this stage. It is possible that metabolism slows down as parenteral (dia)morphine every 6 to 8 hours will usually suffice. Only one-quarter of the original daily dose is needed to prevent withdrawal symptoms so rigid adherence to the previous schedule is not necessary for this reason either.

The doctor should tell both staff and relatives that, at this late stage, any injection may be the last and allay *in advance* any lingering fears about 'killing the patient':

> 'She might die just 5 minutes after you give her the 4 o'clock injection. How will you feel if that happens? You understand that it would be just a coincidence because she *is* going to die very soon anyway? We are using injections only to keep her out of pain.'

Physician Availability

Physician availability is a crucial element in pain management at home. It is vital to the psychological and physical well being of the terminally ill patient that the doctor remains a key figure throughout. The physician is needed to make routine and emergency home visits when on-the-spot pain assessment and management is required. In a survey of home-based terminal cancer care, physicians themselves rated medical (as distinct from nursing) needs as follows: heavy 12 per cent, moderate 59 per cent, and minimal 27 per cent [9]. Whereas 'minimal' needs may be met over the phone, it is difficult to justify not seeing a patient with heavy or even moderate medical needs. Yet if a patient elects to remain at home for his last weeks, this decision, in the USA, frequently cuts him off from effective medical care as many physicians do not make home visits. Many seriously ill bedfast patients, suffering from vomiting, pain and other potentially controllable symptoms do not see a doctor for many weeks. Others find that if they do struggle to the hospital clinic, they are seen by a registrar (resident) while the person they regard as their doctor is seeing patients who can be cured. Continuity of medical management also collapses if, when the family doctor is off duty, a substitute is in charge who knows little of the patient's history and the delicate nuances of the family situation. The development of the group practice has helped to avoid this.

A physician whose clinical experience has been in the protective security of the well-staffed medical centre may feel insecure and helpless when alone with a housebound patient who is experiencing the uncomfortable symptoms seen with advanced cancer. Physicians and nurses dealing with advanced cancer must become interested in pain control and skilled in the home management of distressing complaints. A problem oriented approach has been found useful at The Connecticut Hospice and other centres [3, 5]. Each pain is treated as a disease in itself, to be diagnosed and treated. Thus the patient does not become 'the terminal lung cancer' but 'Mr. Arnold, a man with severe pain for which a great deal can be done'. The doctor can then address the patient with a positive, optimistic, realistic attitude and the assurance that comfort is possible. The doctor's confidence will be transmitted to the patient. The benefits of such an approach for both patient and family can be dramatic.

Physician acceptance of the responsibility for the care of the patient with terminal disease does imply willingness to 'change gear' and make a commitment of time. Time to get to know the patient and family, and time to develop mutual trust. Skilful home care involves an almost unconscious preparation for each visit so that awkward questions can be anticipated, new situations or symptoms considered, gaps filled and comfort increased. Every family must have a sense of security in order to carry on. Most need professional reassurance and the hospice nurse is constantly sustaining the caregivers by encouragement and advice. For many families the doctor's approval is also essential for a sense of security, and the visits of a good family doctor give a great boost to morale.

In Britain, home visiting by the general practitioner is traditional and is a part of the National Health Service, though home visits have declined by 60 per cent over the last 20 years [14]. The added expertise of a hospice consultant can be of help and at Sir Michael Sobell House up to 4 home visits per week are made by the doctor. The focus of these visits is usually pain control. In many areas of the USA physician home visits have ceased altogether and the hospice doctor fills the gap. At The Connecticut Hospice, the attending physician is encouraged to make home visits, emergency visits and a pronouncement visit when the patient dies. If these essentials prove impossible, then permission is obtained for a hospice doctor to fulfil these duties.

The hard pressed family doctor and the busy community nurse are often not trained to deal with the details of pain control or they may not have the time to do it. In Britain, a general practitioner averages 10,000 consultations per year. In cities, a 5-minute appointment system is routine [15]. The hospice worker is given more time to deal more adequately with the patient and family than is often possible in the general hospital or in the community.

There is a time in a patient's illness when the physician begins to feel that there is nothing more that can be done. It is the loss of the doctor's interest that patients fear most. Patients and their families consistently report the pain of abandonment by medical personnel. A new hospice home care patient echoed the feelings of many when she said sadly, 'I feel as though I have lost Dr. Q somewhere along the way'. Conversely, following bereavement, relatives are profuse in their gratitude when good medical care has been given throughout:

'I'll never be able to thank him enough—he was more like a friend than a doctor.'
'She had great faith in him and felt better for whatever medicine he recommended.'[16]

Hospice care requires mature judgement by physicians, who must first deal with themselves to be sure they are comfortable with the patient dying. Only then will effective medical care be possible with support and counsel that will sustain the morale of the patient and family throughout the terminal illness and bereavement. People can put up with a great deal of inconvenience and discomfort if they are confident that their medical attendants respect them as individuals and have concern for their comfort. The 0200 hours home visit may do more in terms of reinforcing the reality of this concern than it does in pharmacological pain control.

Planning for Discharge

A proportion of patients admitted to hospital with terminal cancer improve as a result of the control of pain and other symptoms. They become physically independent again and no longer need to be in hospital. Many relatives have fears about what will happen should the patient be discharged. A trial day out or a weekend at home does much to allay these fears—or confirms that discharge is after all impractical. Clear advice should be given about whom to call in the event of a crisis. The physiotherapist can help considerably by instructing patients with gross skeletal abnormalities on X-ray, or even pathological fractures, on how to manage safely at home. The degree of bone damage that can be associated with mobility is impressive. The amount of pain on movement is a better guide to what can be attempted than the X-ray appearance [17]. (*See also* Figures 5.1 and 5.2, pages 96 and 97.)

If discharge does seem feasible, every effort must be made to ensure that the regimen constructed for pain control does not collapse when responsibility is transferred from inpatient staff to the patient and family. Home care may break down irretrievably if good foundations are not laid down [18]. At The Connecticut Hospice a half-time discharge planning nurse co-ordinates the exchange of information between inpatient staff and home care staff. The latter includes not only the hospice home care staff, but also other community agencies whom she may assist in becoming involved. Unfortunately, without such an individual, the services that are available are often not co-ordinated. There may be no one connected with the family who is aware of the available State, Federal and voluntary agencies. Many larger American hospitals now have a discharge planning department. Usually formal discharge planning is only done at the request of the attending physician, so it is incumbent upon the doctor to ensure that the patient benefits from this service. In British hospices the home care sisters assume this responsibility. Thus, at St. Christopher's Hospice, the sister-in-charge maintains continuity of care by linking up with the general practitioner and domiciliary services. She also runs an advisory service to family doctors and district nurses on all aspects of terminal illness [19].

Valuable continuity is provided if the home care nurse can visit the patient as an inpatient and learn first hand of the patient's capabilities and difficulties. Many are the times when a home care team wonders if the person they meet in the home can possibly be the same as the one described in the hospital transfer notes.

The family must be brought fully into the picture and made aware of the amount of extra work and worry that may be involved. Written and verbal information is given to the patient and the relative who will be the primary caregiver (Table 17.4, 17.5). It is helpful if other members and

Table 17.4 Instructions about morphine medication given to home care patients at The Connecticut Hospice

---

Starting to take morphine by mouth for pain control

1 You have just started taking morphine by mouth to help control your pain.
2 Your doctor has chosen an appropriate starting dose. This may not be sufficient to take all your pain away.
3 If this is the case, adjustments will be made to find the right dose for you.
4 If the medicine does not relieve the pain completely, it does not mean the medicine is not going to work. It means that the dose will need to be increased by the Hospice nurse or doctor.
5 If you find that you are groggy and cannot get out of bed, or are very dizzy, the dose is too high and it will be decreased by the hospice nurse or doctor.
6 If you get good pain relief but find that you feel a little light-headed, a little dizzy, or are sleeping more than usual, then the dose is probably about right.
7 Any unpleasant feeling in your head will go away in 2 to 3 days, so persevere and keep taking the medicine as ordered.
8 Do not let yourself get constipated. Take laxatives regularly like the pain medicine. (You will be given advice about this.)
9 If you feel nauseated, or if you vomit, this is the sign that you also need an antiemetic. (An antiemetic is a drug which stops nausea and vomiting.) If you were given a supply of antiemetic tablets, take as directed, otherwise call the hospice nurse or doctor immediately for a prescription.
10 Plan a few quiet days when you first start the medicine. Do not go straight back to work or plan a family dinner party.
11 Warn your friends and family that you may be a little lethargic at first. This effect will pass.

---

influential friends have a broad understanding of the aims of treatment. Addiction, tolerance and the fear of narcotic overdosage are issues particularly likely to surface in family discussions away from the protective hospital environment.

The Outpatient Pain Clinic

Besides the traditional function of a visit to the doctor, the hospice outpatient clinic provides another stimulus to everyday living. Many are arranged as a social occasion with provision made for families to talk to

Table 17.5 Instructions about morphine medication given to patients discharged from The Connecticut Hospice

---

Fact sheet about morphine by mouth

1 You are taking morphine by mouth for the control of pain.
2 The effects of morphine on the body used this way are quite different from its effects when injected by the street addict into a vein to get a 'high'.
3 Take the medication regularly, every 4 hours. Do not skip a dose or try to lengthen the time intervals to 5 or 6 hours, even if you have no pain.
4 Pour your middle-of-the-night dose before you go to sleep. Set your alarm. Then you can wake and swallow the medication and go back to sleep without too much disturbance.
5 Remember also to keep taking the other drugs. These are additional aids to your pain control. Don't get overtired, and make sure you don't get constipated.
6 If your pharmacist has trouble getting morphine, suggest he calls the Hospice pharmacist for assistance.
7 Carry a card stating that you are taking morphine for pain control so that if you are in a car accident, or some other disaster, the emergency doctor will be aware that you should continue taking this treatment.
8 If you find you are completely pain-free for several days, call the Hospice and we will advise you about whether to cut down on your medication. Do not stop it abruptly.
9 Your body will *not* become accustomed to the medication so that you lose pain control.
10 However, if you start moving around more and doing different activities, you may find that you need an adjustment in your medication.
11 Should your pain get worse there is plenty of room for increases in the medication. You should do this only after discussion with a doctor.
12 If at anytime your pain goes away entirely, you will be able gradually to come off the morphine without problems. You will *not* become an addict and unable to stop the drug.

---

each other informally. Numbers are kept small in order to foster a club-like atmosphere, and refreshments are served. Inpatient staff stop by to renew acquaintances and old friends are visited in the wards. Advice on pain relief is given along with medication renewal and letters to the family doctor. The cumulative effect is a boost to morale and elevation of the patient's pain threshold. Should inpatient admission later become necessary, the hospice is a place that the patient knows and trusts, with staff he has already met [20]. The potential benefits must, of course, be weighed against the possibility of exhaustion by the journey. The rigours of the journey can be minimized by using volunteer drivers if necessary. The journey can be therapeutic in itself especially if there is time to vary the route taken.

The Day Hospital

A day unit for those with advanced cancer provides an additional means of assessment without inpatient admission. One unit finds that 26 per cent of the cancer patients who attend come because their major problem is a need for more effective control of symptoms. Of the first 273 patients, 144 needed help with pain and other symptoms, although their major problem may lie elsewhere [15]. Eighty-five per cent of patients attend the unit once a week [21].

In addition to pain assessment the unit provides a therapeutic environment, occupational therapy and physiotherapy. All these are difficult to provide in the home yet can be vital in providing distraction and in modulating pain perception by improving morale (see Chapter 5). Distraction has been described as a kind of 'sensory shielding' [22]. By directing his attention to something else, the patient unconsciously shields himself from full awareness of incoming pain impulses and his pain threshold is raised (see Table 5.1, page 80). There are two settings where such distraction is hard to provide. One is in hospital where its absence has been termed the busy loneliness of the acute ward [9]. The other is at home where, with modern small families, lack of mobility can isolate the patient. A regular trip to the day hospital is a powerful counter to this lack of stimulus.

Inpatient Admission

A number of patients will need inpatient admission. This may be to die or temporarily for symptom control or family respite. The reassurance of quick admission is one of the essentials in maintaining a patient at home (Table 17.6). On a comprehensive home care programme 25 to 50 per cent of patients will need inpatient admission [2]. A figure greater than 50 per cent should prompt enquiry. Usually some essential service, such as physician visits or 24-hour cover, is not being provided.

Inpatient admission will depend on the patient's wishes, the degree of symptom control, family resources and strengths, and the availability of home care services. The more common reasons for admission in the pain patient are listed in Table 17.7. All these indications are relative and subject to the above variables. The person living alone will almost always have to die as an inpatient. Overwhelming pain (see Chapter 3) is usually better dealt with as an inpatient. This can be managed at home if there is a relative accustomed to serious illness, if the nurse can visit twice daily and if the pain responds quickly to treatment. If medications are not being given on time, intensive education may be the answer, though the situation may be more complex.

Table 17.6 Essentials for home care

1 Adequate trained staff who are familiar with the special needs of patients with terminal malignant disease.
2 Physician availability in the home when medical help is needed for optimal pain control.
3 Sufficient *time* for patients and families to be able to voice their fears, anxieties and difficulties to the staff.
4 Good communication between hospital, hospice, community and between all members of the team.
5 Full 24-hour cover, both medical and nursing, on an internal rota.
6 Frequent assessment of the changing needs.
7 Foresight and planning so that adequate drugs are available for emergencies.
8 A bank of nursing aids available for loan at a moment's notice.
9 Quick and easy access to beds should admission be needed suddenly, with the certainty of a continuity of attitude and care, and the possibility of discharge always in mind.
10 An outpatient clinic for those who are well enough, with volunteer car drivers to ensure quick and easy transport.
11 A follow-up service for the bereaved with help and support in starting life again.

After McNulty, 1978 [23]

Table 17.7 Some relative indications for inpatient admission of the pain patient

Overwhelming pain
Medication regimen has become too complex
Family fail to give medicines on time
Failure of simple pain control methods
Faecal impaction
Onset of extreme agitation or psychotomimetic side effects
Need for a change of environment

Case History. A 78-year-old woman with metastatic breast cancer was repeatedly admitted to The Connecticut Hospice with her pain out of control. Her pain was always alleviated in less than 24 hours on a simple 4-hourly oral morphine regimen. Her daughter, who appeared intelligent and in control was instructed in the importance of regular administration. Eventually the patient was sent in direct from her oncologist's office, again in pain. A visit to her daughter by the hospice social worker to inform her of the admission provoked an hysterical outburst. The daughter had hated her mother for many years, felt trapped by the illness and was systematically flushing the medications down the toilet. As more details emerged it became clear that this was a case of 'granny bashing' and home care was not a realistic possibility.

References

1 Schmale AH. Total community approach to psychosocial support in *The Continuing Care of Terminal Cancer Patients* edited by Twycross RG and Ventafridda V. Pergamon Press, Oxford 1980, pp 247–256.

2 Lack SA and Buckingham RW. *First American Hospice. Three Years of Home Care.* Van Dyck, New Haven, 1978.

3 Macauley CF and Ajemian I. Palliative care service home care program in *The Royal Victoria Hospital Manual on Palliative/Hospice Care* edited by Ajemian I and Mount BM. Arno Press, New York 1980, pp 323–360.

4 Martinson IM. Home care for children dying of cancer. *Pediatrics* 1978; **62:** 106-113.

5 Norton WS and Lack SA. Home care in *The Continuing Care of Terminal Cancer Patients* edited by Twycross RG and Ventafridda V. Pergamon Press, Oxford 1980, pp 239–246.

6 Hancock S. A death in the family: a lay view. *British Medical Journal* 1973; **1:** 29–30.

7 Lack SA. New Haven—Characteristics of a Hospice. Program of Care in *The Hospice Development* and *Administration* edited by Davidson GW. Hemisphere Publishing, Washington and London 1978, pp 41–52.

8 Ajemian I and Mount BM. Terminal care—essence. in *The Royal Victoria Hospital Manual on Palliative/Hospice Care* edited by Ajemian I and Mount BM. Arno Press, New York 1980, p 5.

9 Wilkes E. Terminal care at home. *Lancet* 1965; **ii:** 799–801.

10 MacDonald ET, MacDonald JB and Phoenix M. Improving drug compliance after hospital discharge. *British Medical Journal* 1977; **2:** 618–621.

11 Wilkes E. Terminal illness at home. *Modern Geriatrics* 1973; March: 133–136.

12 Hinton JM. Comparison of places and policies for terminal care. *Lancet* 1979; **1:** 29–32.

13 Saunders CM. A death in the family: a professional view. *British Medical Journal* 1973; **1:** 30–31.

14 Wilkes E. The role of the specialist of a hospice unit in *The Dying Patient* edited by Wilkes E. MTP Press, Lancaster 1982, pp 289–310.

15 Wilkes E. Preface in *The Dying Patient* edited by Wilkes E. MTP Press, Lancaster 1982, pp iv-vii.

16 Aitken-Swan J. Nursing the late cancer patient at home. *Practitioner* 1959; **183:** 64–69.

17 Wilkes E. Some problems in cancer management. *Proceedings of the Royal Society of Medicine* 1975; **67:** 23–27.

18 Gibson R. Supporting the patient in the home. *British Medical Journal* 1973; **1:** 35–36.

19 McNulty BJ. Continuity of care. *British Medical Journal* 1973; **1:** 38–39.

20 Lamerton R. Dying at home in *Care of the Dying*. Priory, London 1972, pp 25–34.

21 Wilkes E, Crowther AGO and Greaves CWKH. A different kind of day hospital. *British Medical Journal* 1978; **2:** 1053–1056.

22 McCaffery M. Relieving pain with noninvasive techniques. *Nursing* 1980; **10:** 55–57.

23 McNulty BJ. Outpatient and domiciliary management from a hospice in *The Management of Terminal Disease* edited by Saunders CM. Arnold, London 1978, pp 154–165.

Chapter Eighteen

More Fundamental Considerations

'We emerge deserving of little credit; we who are capable of ignoring the conditions which make muted people suffer. The dissatisfied dead cannot noise abroad the negligence they have experienced.' [1]

When seeking to relieve pain in cancer, it is axiomatic that science is not enough. The correct and appropriate use of drug and non-drug measures is only half the battle. In this final chapter, we turn our attention to some of the more general and fundamental issues that a doctor has to face when caring for a patient who is likely to die in the next few weeks or months.

There is no doubt the advent of the modern hospice has done much to raise expectations in both the public and the health-care professions. Often, however, it seems as if one caricature has been replaced by another. The old image of death, negative and despairing; the new, positive but 'rose-tinted'. Although care of the dying cancer patient should be approached positively, it does not help if the doctor, nurses and others involved underestimate the problems they are up against. Good terminal care is hard work, often very hard work, but perhaps all the more rewarding for being so.

The typical dying patient does not exist. Patients, like other people, are individuals. The aim is to help each patient do his best, given his illness, his symptoms, his fears, his frustrations, his family, his friends, his cultural background, his beliefs, and his ability or inability to accept what is happening. The aim is positive: to help the patient, despite increasing physical limitations, to go on living with cancer—until he dies. To see the time that is left as 'last days but not lost days'.

Bad Terminal Care Is Not The Prerogative Of The Bad Doctor

All humans fear death; it is part of the survival instinct. Unease is felt in life-threatening situations. Unease is also felt in the presence of death because it evokes fear about one's own future death. There is, therefore, a natural tendency to withdraw from the dying. In addition, there is a cultural factor: a collective fear of death. In every society, whether primitive or sophisticated, the corporate fear of death is focused on one or two particular diseases, or a group of diseases. In Europe and North America, cancer has taken over the role previously held by tuberculosis or, in generations past, by leprosy and plague. This has the effect of making cancer more feared than almost any other disease—despite the fact that up to 40 per cent of sufferers can now be cured [2]. The popular image of cancer is not just negative, it is doubly so. The doctor's instinctive reaction to cancer is equally exaggerated. More than with most other diseases, a feeling of helplessness creeps in:

'There's nothing that anybody can do.'

Some of the doctor's emotional discomfort relates not just to existential anxiety, but to spiritual unease. We are all, to some extent, children of our generation. That is, we absorb the fashionable ideas and aspirations. These become our *raison d'etre*. When confronted by death, our comfortable assumptions about life are often found wanting. The patient and his family ask:

'Why me?'
'What have I done to deserve this?'
'Where did I go wrong?'

A naive belief that man is born with a guarantee of 'three score years and ten', that death is never today but always in the future, is seen to be without foundation. These questions, present themselves also to the doctor, who is forced to reconsider:

'Why am *I* here?'
'What am *I* really doing?'
'What is life all about?'
'What is the purpose of life?'
'What is the meaning of my existence?'
'What am I going to do with the rest of my life?'

When faced squarely with the fact of death such questions inevitably intrude, and cause anxiety. If the doctor cannot face up to them, anxiety will increase still further. Some doctors find themselves unable to care for the patient at all. Others continue on only a very superficial level. This is a form of self-protection. Death is seen as the ultimate disaster, and terminal care a kind of macabre play in which the patient is 'jollied' along until the final curtain falls.

The Needs Of The Patient

These are many and varied (Table 18.1). It is common to talk of 'dying with dignity'. Another emphasis is to consider ways in which one can

Table 18.1 The needs of the dying patient

Physiological:	good symptom control
Safety:	a feeling of security
Belonging:	the need to be needed
	the need *not* to feel a burden
Love:	expressions of affection
	human contact (touch)
Understanding:	explanation about symptoms and the disease;
	opportunity to discuss the process of dying
Acceptance:	regardless of mood and sociability
Self-esteem:	involve in decision-making, particularly as physical
	dependency on others increases
	the opportunity to give as well as to receive

help to maintain a patient's self-respect or self-esteem. The patient should be involved in decision-making. This becomes increasingly important as the patient becomes more physically dependent on others. In short, the patient needs to be treated as a person; as a sane, sensible individual who has a right to be involved in discussions about what is happening to him, about what should be done, and about the immediate and future implications for the family. Yet, frequently, the patient is excluded from such discussions. If he is in hospital, he is removed to a remote corner of the ward or to a side room and visits by medical staff become infrequent and cursory. Nurses tend to avoid the patient except when duties demand or the call-bell is rung. An atmosphere of despair develops as helplessness is compounded by hopelessness. The patient feels he does not matter any more. Although it is his illness, he is not consulted, his co-operation is not sought. Resentment at everything and with everyone builds up. Symptoms tend to multiply and worsen. Yet this need not be. If the dying patient is treated as a person to be loved, not as someone to be feared and avoided, it is usually possible to maintain a patient's self-respect and morale.

Communication

The need for good communication between staff and patient cannot be overemphasized. Technical, scientific and clinical competence are not enough. Bad communication causes suffering. This is true not only with the dying but also with patients generally. Several studies have assessed the effect of encouragement and education on patients admitted for curative surgery. In one, 97 'special care' patients were told what to expect during the postoperative period. They were taught how to relax, how to take deep breaths and how to move so that they would remain more comfortable after the operation. Their postoperative analgesic requirement was half that of a control group and they were ready for discharge 3 days earlier [3].

The issue is good versus bad communication. Not, as sometimes suggested, a matter of to communicate or not. It is impossible not to communicate. Those who indulge in a conspiracy of silence often speak most eloquently by their every action and expression. The message conveyed is precisely the one they are most anxious to avoid. Children, also, are exquisitely sensitive to non-verbal communication [4].

The basic message a patient wants to hear at a time of increasing uncertainty is:

'No matter what happens to you I am going to do all I can to help you.'

Only part of this can be said in words:

'We will continue to take good care of you.'
'I will see you regularly.'
'One of us will always be available.'
'We will deal with any problems that arise.'
'We can relieve your pain.'

Essentially, this fundamental message of support and companionship is conveyed to the patient by means of non-verbal communication. This probably accounts for 80 per cent of all communication between doctor and patient. Touch, whether feeling the patient's pulse or holding his hand, is an important non-verbal form of reassurance.

When the patient's condition is initially diagnosed, he needs to be told what is wrong and what medical science has to offer in words that he can understand. The facts that are presented must be tailored to the intellectual, cultural and emotional background of the recipient, while at the same time expressing the truth. For most people cancer is an emotive word and to answer a direct question with, 'Yes, you have cancer', is unwise unless qualified. It is important to discover what the patient understands by cancer. If to him it means a painful and distressing death, he needs to be reassured that:

1 many patients are cured;
2 most of those who are not survive for several years, sometimes many;
3 many of those who are not cured never experience pain;

4   treatments are available to relieve pain should it develop;
5   treatments are also available to alleviate other symptoms.

Opinions have changed quickly over the past few years. In 1961 in the USA, 90 per cent of physicians responding to a survey did not tell cancer patients the diagnosis. In 1977, 97 per cent did so—a complete reversal of opinion [5]. The tendency in Britain seems to be in a similar direction. This trend towards truth telling is a welcome development, but must be tempered by improved communication skills (Table 18.2). Total candour

Table 18.2   Patients are people

Non-verbal communication:	Greet patient by name.
	Introduce self by name at first meeting.
	Shake patient by hand.
	Sit down if possible.
	Make eye-to-eye contact.
	Visit patient regularly.
Attention to detail:	Ask about known specific symptoms.
	Also ask about sleep, comfort, diet, mouth, bowels, micturition.
Verbal communication:	Generally, patients who want to know more about their condition will ask, if the way is opened to them.
	Do not compromise your relationship with the patient by making unwise (and unethical) promises to the relatives about non-disclosure of information to the patient.
	Truth has a broad spectrum with gentleness at one end and harshness at the other; patients always prefer gentle truth.
	The doctor-patient relationship is founded on trust. It is fostered by honesty but poisoned by deceit.
	The doctor's responsibility is to 'nudge' the patient in the direction of reality, but not to force him.

can be dangerous. Not infrequently, it damages the patient's and the family's psychological coping mechanisms. Unrelieved anxiety and unresolved anger mar the patient's remaining life. Total candidness reflects the doctor's inexperience and unease. A total catharsis of all that is negative, for the doctor's own emotional benefit, should be resisted. Evasion and deceit must not be replaced by total candour. The effect of both extremes is to isolate the patient.

When the cancer is advanced the situation is, in fact, easier because patients are already receiving clues from their bodies and from the behaviour of people around them. It is seldom a question of 'to tell or not to tell' but usually a matter of 'when and how to tell'. A patient's questions or statements often open the way:

'And what's the next step, doctor?'
'When will I be able to go home?'
'How long do you reckon this will go on, doctor?'
'I'm not getting any better, am I?'
'I want to stop chemotherapy, it's not doing me any good?'
'It's no use putting me back in hospital. In fact, I won't go.'
'I know I am going to die.'
'I know what I've got.'
'I've got cancer, haven't I, doctor?'

Such remarks often mean that the patient wants more information, that he is ready to accept more of the truth even if unpalatable. One study compared patient satisfaction with communication in two London settings. Communication policy at a hospice ensured that patients could readily discuss their condition and possible outcome, including dying. The policy of the other setting was for greater reticence about cancer and dying unless patients were clearly intent on knowing. The more open communication was firmly favoured by patients, and a significant preference for the hospice policy was shown. In addition, the setting with freer communication had less anxious and irritable patients ($p < 0.01$) and perhaps less depressed ones ($p < 0.1$) [6]. If, however, at a certain stage, a patient indicates by his manner and talk that he does not wish to regard his illness as fatal it is usually wrong to force the truth upon him [7]. Not many patients adopt such a stance permanently.

Pastoral Care

Few patients talk to a doctor about their fear of death. This may be due to lack of time or the fact that patients do not see this as something that falls within the doctor's province, or competence. Alternatively, it could be because, generally, doctors are unwilling to communicate at this level. The experience of some night nurses, social workers and clergy suggests that, given an unhurried atmosphere and a willingness to discuss such matters, many dying patients have a fear of death and appreciate being able to talk about it. The patient will, of course, decide for himself whether he feels 'safe' enough to express such a fear to the doctor or other member of staff. As always, regard for the patient does not allow the impositions of one's own faith or philosophy on him. But even unspoken confidence and conviction can help create a climate in which the patient can reach out trustfully to the One who is beyond.

If there is a link between the patient and a particular church, priest, minister or rabbi, this should be utilized. It is not generally possible to measure the contribution of the pastor. Yet it may be of obvious and paramount importance.

Avoid Inappropriate Treatment

In terminal illness the primary aim is no longer to preserve life but to make the life that remains as comfortable and as meaningful as possible. Thus, what may be appropriate treatment in an acutely ill patient may be inappropriate in the dying. Cardiac resuscitation, artificial respiration, intravenous infusion, nasogastric tubes, and antibiotics are all primarily supportive measures for use in acute or acute-on-chronic illnesses to assist a patient through the initial period towards recovery of health. Their use, without careful consideration of the intended purpose of that use, in the care of the terminally ill is poor medical care. It is not a question of 'to treat or not to treat?' but of deciding the most appropriate form(s) of treatment given the patient's 'biological potential' and bearing in mind his personal and social circumstances. Medical care is, in fact, a continuum ranging from cure at one end to terminal care at the other [8]. When cure is no longer possible, palliation should be considered; when palliation is no longer possible, the emphasis moves to symptom control as an end in itself.

Many types of treatment span the entire spectrum of care, notably radiotherapy and also, to a lesser extent, chemotherapy and surgery. It is important not to pigeonhole a particular type of treatment into a specific category, but to keep the therapeutic aim clearly in mind when employing treatment of any kind. Physical rehabilitation is part of medical care even in the dying. Sometimes, and eventually every time, it is inappropriate and the patient should be encouraged to remain in bed. However, many dying patients are unnecessarily restricted, sometimes by cautious relatives, even though they are capable of a greater degree of activity and independence. Provided, of course, that troublesome symptoms are controlled and gentle encouragement is given by an attentive doctor.

The Needs Of The Family

The care of the family is an integral part of the care of the dying. A contented family increases the likelihood of a contented patient. Relative-doctor communication generally needs to be initiated and maintained by the doctor. It is easy to neglect the relatives as they are reluctant to bother the doctor. There is much to be said, at the time of diagnosis, and later, for

321

joint interviews between the patient, the spouse and the doctor. The doctor should also make an opportunity to see both patient and the close relatives on their own. Further separate or joint interviews can then be arranged as necessary.

As with the patient, it is not generally necessary or wise to tell the family the whole truth (as you see it) at one time. If the family and patient are too far 'out of step' in relation to knowledge about the diagnosis and prognosis, it can create a barrier between the two. A common initial reaction is:

'You won't tell him, will you, doctor?'
'We'd prefer you not to tell him, doctor?'

This should be seen as the initial shock reaction and not as an excuse for saying nothing to the patient. If the family and patient are to be mutually supportive, it is necessary to help the relatives move forward from this initial reaction to a position of greater openness and trust. It is important to remember that the family cannot forbid the doctor from discussing diagnosis and prognosis with a patient. The doctor's therapeutic and professional contract is with the patient—not with the family, and the *patient's* wellbeing must be paramount. The family's desires are taken into account in so much as their attitudes impinge upon the patient's wellbeing, but the doctor must not avoid responsibilities to the patient by hiding behind the family.

Teamwork

Terminal care cannot be undertaken by individuals, only by individuals working together as a team. The approach to pain control advocated in this book exposes the physician to considerable physical demands and emotional suffering. There is a limit to the burdens that can be placed on one person. In an American survey, doctors with direct clinical responsibilities were found to have a higher rate of alcoholism, marital breakdown and suicide than non-clinicians of equivalent socioeconomic status [9]. Doctors do not have all the answers and are not exempt from human frailties. Working within the framework of a team is crucial for optimal care [10]. The composition of the team varies, but includes the patient himself, the immediate family, friends, doctor(s), nurses, volunteers, social worker, other ancillary staff, chaplain and, on occasion, lawyer. The team is collectively concerned for the total wellbeing of the patient and the family—physical, psychological, spiritual and social. In this situation, roles may become blurred, at least at the edges. Moreover, unless the nurses, and at home the family, actively participate in symptom control, the lead given by the doctor will be seriously undermined. Indeed for every step forward there may be a step backwards unless the nurses are encouraged to:

1 support the patient through the period of initial side effects commonly seen with morphine-like drugs;
2 advise the patient when to increase the dose of analgesic;
3 contact the doctor rather than wait for the next visit or round if the patient becomes less well when a new treatment is started;
4 contact the doctor if the patient fails to get a good night's sleep;
5 advise about diet and fluid intake;
6 monitor bowel function;
7 encourage the patient by quietly emphasizing that his symptom(s) will soon be better controlled;
8 give the patient opportunity to express anxieties and fears.

Without this degree of involvement, the doctor's task is made considerably more difficult and, occasionally, impossible.

The reverse is equally true. Much can be accomplished by the nurse in the management of pain [11, 12], but the continued interest and availability of the physician is crucial to optimal success.

Examples have been given in Chapter 3 of pain relieved by intervention of some team members. This is not the place for a detailed description of the individual role of each team member but this does not mean that the involvement of any is considered less important than others. The cook who prepares attractive food, the musician who fills the world with song, the financial manager who keeps the money flowing, the volunteer who drives many miles to bring a beloved pet are all equally important.

Our achievements frequently fall short of the goals we set ourselves. For information about their real needs and what truly constitutes quality of life, for realism, courage, generosity, and faith there are no better teachers than our patients, their families and their friends.

References

1 Hinton J. *Dying* (2nd edition). Penguin, Harmondsworth 1972, p 159.

2 De Vita V. Quoted in *International Herald Tribune*, September 22, 1980.

3 Egbert LD, Battit GE, Welch CE and Bartlett MD. Reduction of postoperative pain by encouragement and instruction of patients. *New England Journal of Medicine* 1964; **270**: 825–827.

4 Mott M. Caring for children with cancer in *The Dying Patient* edited by Wilkes E. MTP Press, Lancaster 1982, pp 45–55.

5 Novack DH, Plumer R, Smith RL, Ochitill H, Morrow GR and Bennett JM. Changes in physicians' attitudes toward telling the cancer patient. *Journal of American Medical Association* 1979; **241:** 897–900.

6 Hinton JM. Comparison of places and policies for terminal care. *Lancet* 1979; **i:** 29–32.

7 Maguire P. The personal impact of dying in *The Dying Patient* edited by Wilkes E. MTP Press, Lancaster 1982, pp 233–253.

8 Saunders CM. Appropriate treatment, appropriate death in *The Management of Terminal Malignant Disease* edited by Saunders CM. Arnold, London 1978, pp 1–9.

9 Rose KD and Rosow I. Physicians who kill themselves. *Archives of General Psychiatry* 1973; **29:** 800–805.

10 Lack SA. Philosophy and organisation of a hospice program in *Psychosocial Care of the Dying Patient* edited by Garfield C. University of California Press, San Francisco 1976, pp 2–8.

11 Charles-Edwards A. *The Nursing Care of the Dying Patient*. Beaconsfield Publishers, Beaconsfield 1983.

12 McCaffery M. *Nursing Management of the Patient with Pain*. Lippincott, Philadelphia, second edition, 1981.

Appendix

A series of figures are appended. These portray the more common muscle trigger points and their associated pattern of non-dermatomal referred pain. Reproduced by permission of Travell and the editor of *Postgraduate Medicine* [1].

A number of more recent articles are recommended for further reading [2–5], as is the monograph *Myofascial Pain and Dysfunction: the Trigger Point Manual* by Travell and Simons [6].

References

1 Travell J and Rinzler SH. The myofascial genesis of pain. *Postgraduate Medicine (Minneapolis)* 1952; 11 May: 425–434.

2 Sola AE and Williams RL. Myofascial pain syndromes. *Neurology* 1965; **6:** 91–95.

3 Melzack R, Stillwell DM and Fox EJ. Trigger points and acupuncture points for pain: correlations and implications. *Pain* 1977; **3:** 3–23.

4 Melzack R. Myofascial trigger points: relation to acupuncture and mechanisms of pain. *Archives of Physical Medicine and Rehabilitation 1981;* **62:** 114–117.

5 Sola AE. Myofascial trigger point therapy. *Resident and Staff Physician* 1981; **27:** 38–45.

6 Travell J and Simons DG. *Myofascial Pain and Dysfunction: the Trigger Point Manual.* Williams and Wilkins, Baltimore 1982.

Head and neck

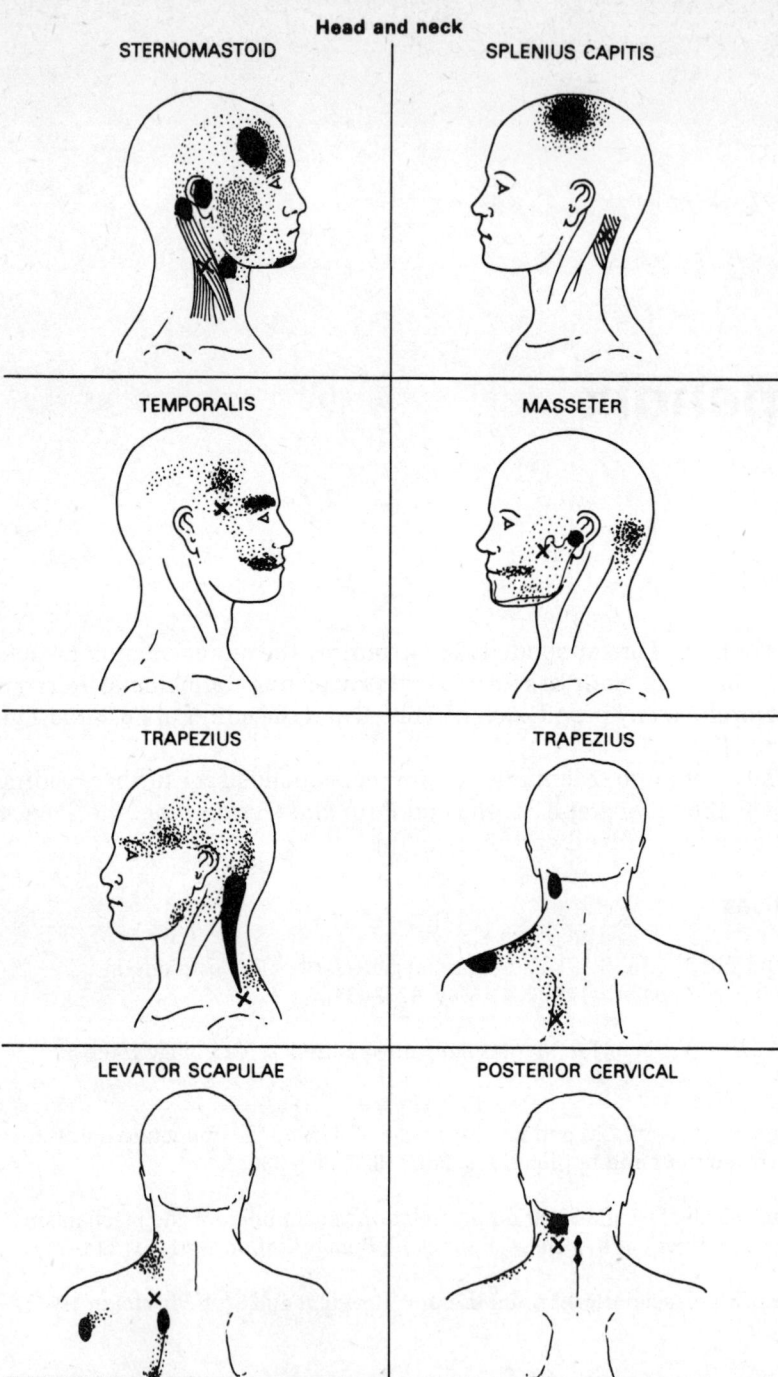

STERNOMASTOID   SPLENIUS CAPITIS

TEMPORALIS   MASSETER

TRAPEZIUS   TRAPEZIUS

LEVATOR SCAPULAE   POSTERIOR CERVICAL

Pain pattern ▬▨   Trigger area ✕

Figure A.1 Trigger points in the head and neck associated with local and referred myofascial pain. From Travell and Rinzler, 1952 [1]

326

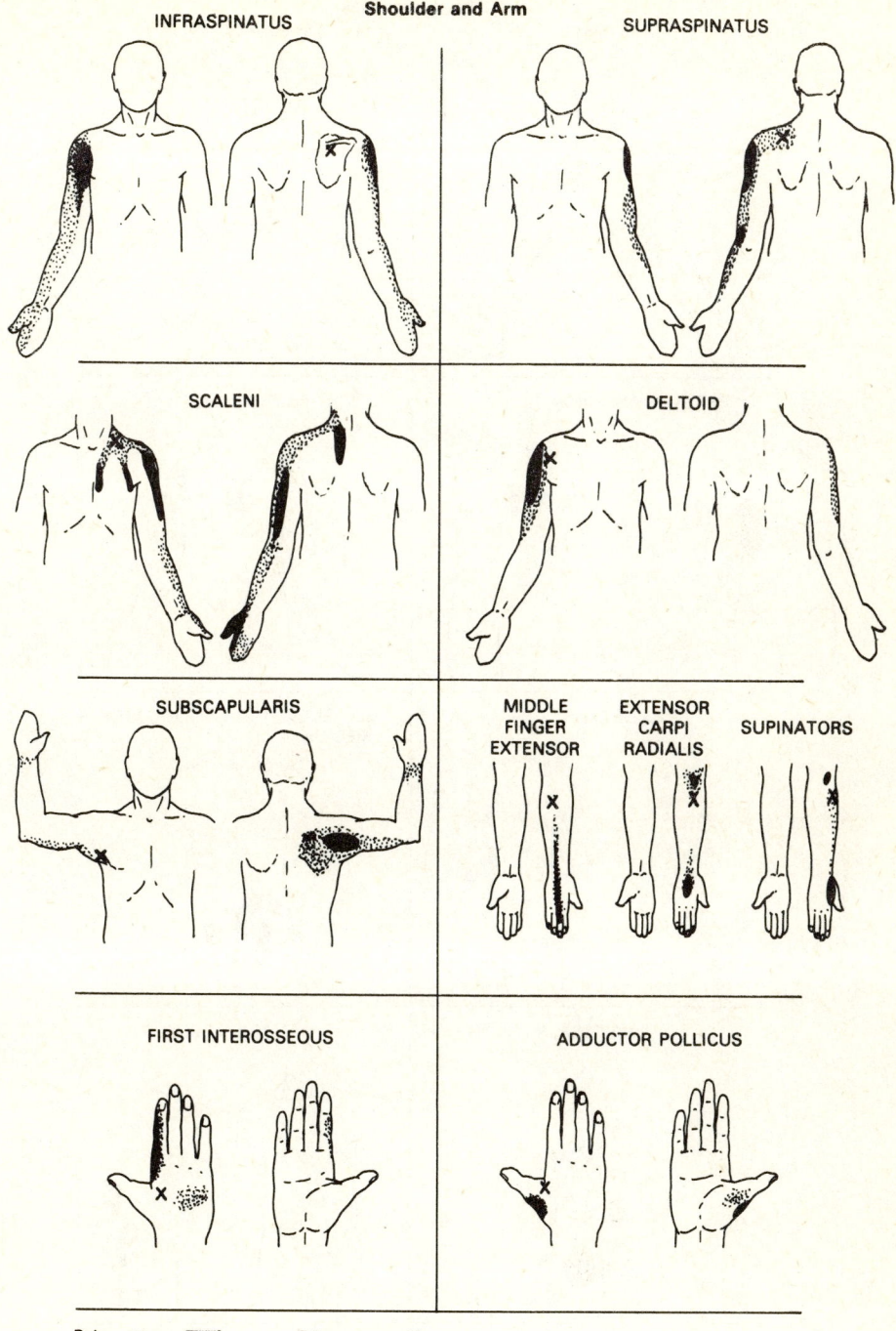

Shoulder and Arm

INFRASPINATUS   SUPRASPINATUS

SCALENI   DELTOID

SUBSCAPULARIS   MIDDLE FINGER EXTENSOR   EXTENSOR CARPI RADIALIS   SUPINATORS

FIRST INTEROSSEOUS   ADDUCTOR POLLICUS

Pain pattern ▬▓   Trigger area ✕

Figure A.2 Trigger points in the shoulder and arm associated with local and referred myofascial pain. From Travell and Rinzler, 1952 [1]

327

Chest and Back

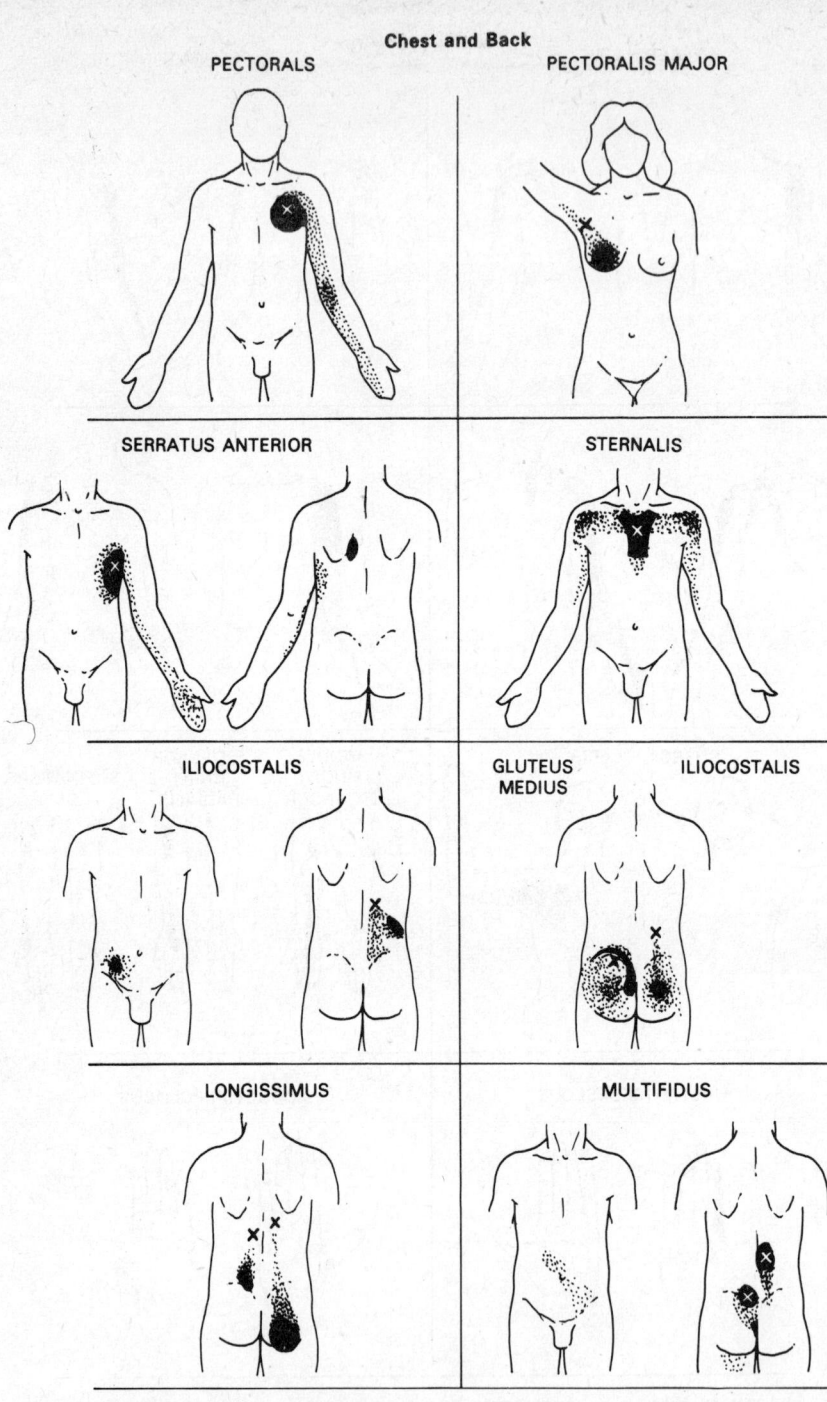

PECTORALS   PECTORALIS MAJOR

SERRATUS ANTERIOR   STERNALIS

ILIOCOSTALIS   GLUTEUS MEDIUS   ILIOCOSTALIS

LONGISSIMUS   MULTIFIDUS

Pain pattern ▓▒░   Trigger area ✕

Figure A.3 Trigger points in the chest and back associated with local and referred myofascial pain. From Travell and Rinzler, 1952 [1]

328

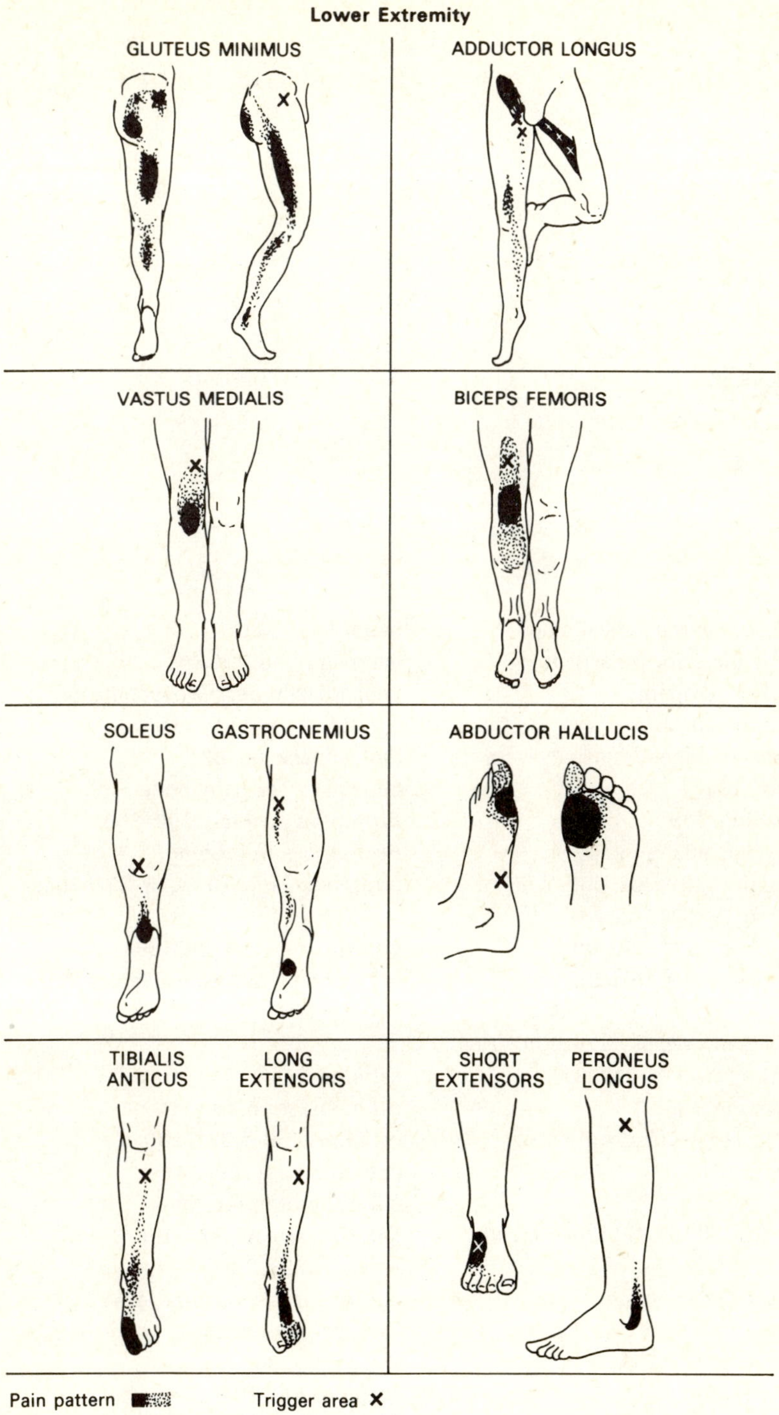

Lower Extremity

GLUTEUS MINIMUS

ADDUCTOR LONGUS

VASTUS MEDIALIS

BICEPS FEMORIS

SOLEUS   GASTROCNEMIUS

ABDUCTOR HALLUCIS

TIBIALIS ANTICUS   LONG EXTENSORS

SHORT EXTENSORS   PERONEUS LONGUS

Pain pattern ▪️▨   Trigger area ✖

Figure A.4 Trigger points in the lower limbs associated with local and referred myofascial pain. From Travell and Rinzler, 1952 [1]

Index

acetaminophen, *see* paracetamol
acetylsalicylic acid, *see* aspirin
Acupan, *see* nefopam
acupuncture, 80, 86
addiction, *see* dependence
alclofenac, 132
alphaprodine, 238
amitriptyline, 282
amphetamine, 183, 202, 282–285
anileridine, 238, 243–244
antibiotic, 100, 271, 290–291
anticoagulant, 119, 161–162
anticonvulsant, 100, 271, 286
antidepressant, *see* psychotropic drug
antiemetic, 176–177, 238, 271
antihistamine, 183
anxiolytic, *see* psychotropic drug
Arthropan, 121
ASA, *see* aspirin
aspirin, 101–102, 107, 117–129, 220–221
Atarax, *see* hydroxyzine

baclofen, 101, 271, 288
barbiturate, 274
barbotage, 94

benorylate, 121
benoxaprofen, 132
benzodiazepine, *see* psychotropic drug
biofeedback, 80–82
bone pain, *see* pain, bone
Brompton Cocktail, 200–206
Brufen, *see* ibuprofen
buprenorphine, 101, 255, 257–260, 268
butorphanol, 101, 255, 264–265
butyrophenone, *see* psychotropic drug

caffeine, 274
cannabis, *see* marihuana
carbamazepine, 271, 286
chemotherapy, 69, 271
chlorpheniramine, 183
chlorpromazine, 177, 198, 271, 275–278, 282, 288
chronic pain syndrome, 49–52
Clinoril, *see* sulindac
clobazam, 280
cocaine, 200–204, 282
codeine, 101, 149–152, 238, 285

Compazine, *see* prochlorperazine
compliance, 182, 184–186, 298–304
confusion, 176, 178, 203
constipation, 178–181
corticosteroid, 39–40, 119, 121–122,
    201, 203, 270–274, 282, 290
Cosalgesic, *see* Distalgesic
    counter-irritation, 84–85

Darvocet, 160
Darvon, 159, 160
day care, 311
Demerol, *see* meperidine
dependence, 226–230, 264
Depo-medrol, *see*
    methylprednisolone
Depo-medrone, *see*
    methylprednisolone
depression, 176, 226, 280–282
dexamethasone, *see* corticosteroid
dexamphetamine, *see* amphetamine
dextromoramide, 170, 238–239
dextropropoxyphene, 101, 107, 149–
    151, 158–162, 238
diacetylmorphine, *see* diamorphine
diamorphine, 101, 170, 190–199,
    200–204, 238–239
diazepam, 101, 183, 271, 275, 280,
    288
diclofenac, 132
Diconal, *see* dipipanone
diflunisal, 129–130
dihydrocodeine, 149–156, 238
Dilaudid, *see* hydromorphone
diphenylpropylamine, 238, 248–249
dipipanone, 170, 238–239
Distalgesic, 158–162
distraction, 80
dizziness, 176, 178
Dolasan, 159
Doloxene, 159
driving, 186–188
Dromoran, *see* levorphanol
drowsiness, 176–178, 203

dysaesthesia, 33–37

Elavil, *see* amitriptyline
Epilim, *see* valproate
Equagesic, 163–164
ethoheptazine, 101, 149–151, 162–
    164

Feldene, *see* piroxicam
fenamate, 132
fenclofenac, 132
fenoprofen, 132
Fenopron, *see* fenoprofen
fentanyl, 238
Flagyl, *see* metronidazole
Flenac, *see* fenclofenac
flufenamic acid, 132
flurbiprofen, 107, 121, 132, 134–136,
    141
Froben, *see* flurbiprofen

haloperidol, 177, 279–280, 282
heat, 80, 84
heroin, *see* diamorphine
hormone therapy, 67–69
hydromorphone, 107, 170, 197, 238–
    239, 250
hydroxyzine, 280–281
hypercalcaemia, 71–73
hypnosis, 80, 82–84
hypoglycaemia, 119

ibuprofen, 132
imagery, 80
immobilization, 95–97
Indocid, *see* indomethacin
indomethacin, 132, 134, 139–140
injections, narcotic, 194–196, 211–
    219

ketoprofen, 132

Largactil, *see* chlorpromazine
laxative, xi, 178–181

Lederspan, *see* triamcinolone
Levo-dromoran, *see* levorphanol
levomepromazine, *see*
    methotrimeprazine
levoprome, *see* methotrimeprazine
levorphanol, 170, 238–239, 250
Lioresal, *see* baclofen
local anaesthetic, 86–92
LSD, *see* lysergic acid
lysergic acid, 274, 285
lymphangitis, carcinomatous, 271
lymphoedema, 271, 289–290

marihuana, 274, 285–286
massage, 80, 84
Maxolon, *see* metoclopramide
Meclofen, *see* meclofenamate
meclofenamate, 132
mefenamic acid, 132, 134, 138
meperidine, *see* pethidine
meprobamate, 163–164, 274
Meprogesic, *see* Equagesic
meptazinol, 255, 265–266
Meralen, *see* flufenamic acid
methadone, 101, 170, 238–239, 244–
    248
methotrimeprazine, 183, 279
methylprednisolone, 89–91, 272
metoclopramide, 177, 183, 287
metronidazole, *see* antibiotic
mianserin, 282
mithramycin, 71–72
monoamine oxidase inhibitor, 274
morphinan, 238
morphine, 101, 167–189, 191–195,
    197, 200, 205, 207–219, 223–236,
    237–239, 264, 277, 281, 284
Motrin, *see* ibuprofen
myofascial pain, 90, 325–329

nalbuphine, 101, 255, 263
nalorphine, 253–255, 260
naloxone, 266–268
naltrexone, 266

Naprosyn, *see* naproxen
naproxen, 107, 121, 132, 134, 136
Napsalgesic, 159
Narcan, *see* naloxone
narcotic
  agonist, 237–252
  agonist-antagonist, 253–265
  antagonist, 266–268
  classification, 238, 255
  definition, 102
  strong, 237–252
  weak, 149–166
Narphen, *see* phenazocine
nausea, 176–177, 203
nefopam, 101, 144–145
Nepenthe, 219
nerve block, 86–93
neuroleptic, *see* psychotropic drug
neurolysis, 86, 92–94
neurosurgery, 66, 94–95
nomifensine, 282
non-steroidal anti-inflammatory drug,
    117, 120–123, 131–141, 272
NSAID, *see* non-steroidal anti-
    inflammatory drug
Nubain, *see* nalbuphine
Numorphan, *see* oxymorphone

Omnopon, *see* papaveretum
opium, 219–221
Opren, *see* benoxaprofen
Oraflex, *see* benoxaprofen
Orudis, *see* ketoprofen
osseous metastasis, *see* pain, bone
oxycodone, 101, 107, 149–151, 157–
    158, 170, 238–239
oxymorphone, 101, 107, 238, 249
oxyphenbutazone. 132

pain
  acute, 49–50
  bone, 23–25, 89–91, 119–123, 271,
    288–289
  chronic, 49–52

classification, 112
definition, 2–3, 34
dysaesthetic, 33–37, 271
financial, 48
modulation, 4–5
musculoskeletal, 80, 288–289
nerve, 28–39, 271
overwhelming, 52–54
psychological, 43–47
referred, 25–39
social, 47–48
spiritual, 48–49
threshold, 3–4, 43, 79–80
total, 46
treatment modalities, 61
Palfium, see dextromoramide
Panadol, see paracetamol
Pantopon, see papaveretum
papaveretum, 107, 170, 220–221
paracetamol, xi, 101–102, 142–143
paraplegia, 37–39, 65–66
Paynocil, 121
pentazocine, 101, 238, 255, 260–263
Percocet, 157
Percodan, 157–158
perphenazine, 276, 282
pethidine, xi, 170, 238–243
phenacetin, 142, 156
phenazocine, 107, 170, 238–239, 251
phenothiazine, see psychotropic drug
phenylbutazone, 132, 134, 140
phenylpiperidine, 238
Piriton, see chlorpheniramine
piroxicam, 132
pituitary ablation, 73–75
Ponstan, see mefenamic acid
Ponstel, see mefenamic acid
postherpetic neuralgia, 91–92
prednisolone, see corticosteroid
prednisone, xi, see corticosteroid
prescribing, 113
Primperan, see metoclopramide
Prinalgin, see alclofenac
prochlorperazine, 176, 198, 276

profadol, 255
Proladone, see oxycodone
promazine, 276–277
promethazine, 183, 276
propionic acid, 102, 132
propiram, 255
propoxyphene, see
    dextropropoxyphene
prostaglandin, 120–123, 133
pruritus, 183, 240
psychotropic drug
    antidepressant, 100, 271, 274–275,
        280–282
    anxiolytic, 100, 183, 271, 274–275,
        280
    benzodiazepine, 101, 183, 271,
        274–275, 280
    butyrophenone, 177, 183, 274, 279–
        280
    neuroleptic, 177, 183, 271, 274,
        276–280
    phenothiazine, 177, 187, 271, 274,
        276–279
    psychodysleptic, 274, 285–286
    psychostimulant, 183, 202, 274,
        282–285

radiation therapy, 63–65, 271
Reglan, see metoclopramide
relaxation therapy, 80–81
respiratory depression, 179, 182, 223–
    224

salicylamide, 129
salicylate, 127–130
salicylsalicylic acid, 127–129
saline, ice-cold, 94
salsalate, 127–129
Schlessinger's solution, 205
spinal cord compression, 37–39
squashed stomach syndrome, 287–
    288
Stadol, see butorphanol
Stemetil, see prochlorperazine

steroid, *see* corticosteroid
sulindac, 132
surgery, 66, 69–71
Synflex, *see* naproxen

Tandacote, *see* oxyphenbutazone
Tanderil, *see* oxyphenbutazone
Tegretol, *see* carbamazepine
Temgesic, *see* buprenorphine
TENS, *see* transcutaneous electrical
    nerve stimulation
Thorazine, *see* chlorpromazine
Tolectin, *see* tolmetin
tolerance, 227–233
tolfenamic acid, 132
tolmetin, 132
tranquillizer, *see* anxiolytic,
    neuroleptic
transcutaneous electrical nerve
    stimulation, 80, 85
triamcinolone, 89–91, 272

trifluoperazine, 276
triflupromazine, 276
trigger point, 90, 325–329
trimeprazine, 276, 278
Tylenol, *see* acetominophen
Tylox, 157

uricosuric, 118, 119

valproate, 271, 286
Vistaril, *see* hydroxyzine
Voltarol, *see* diclofenac
vomiting, 176–177

Wygesic, 159–161

Zactipar, 163
Zactirin, 163
Zomax, *see* zomepirac
zomepirac, 132, 134, 137–138